3 fat chicks
on a diet

Produced by The Philip Lief Group, Inc.

St. Martin's Press
New York

3 fat chicks on a diet

because we're all in it together

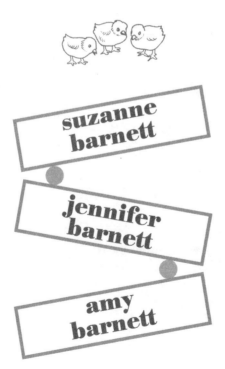

suzanne barnett

jennifer barnett

amy barnett

with bev west

Produced by The Philip Lief Group, Inc.

www.stmartins.com

Library of Congress Cataloging-in-Publication Data

Barnett, Suzanne.
3 fat chicks on a diet : because we're all in it together /
Suzanne Barnett, Jennifer Barnett, and Amy Barnett ; with
Bev West.
p. cm.
ISBN-10: 0-312-34807-X
ISBN-13: 978-0-312-34807-6
1. Reducing diets. 2. Weight loss. 3. Dieters—Biography.
I. Barnett, Jennifer. II. Barnett, Amy. III. Title.

RM222.2.B384 2006
613.2'5—dc22

2005033026

First Edition: May 2006

10   9   8   7   6   5   4   3   2   1

This book is dedicated to the wonderful, supportive members of the 3FC on-line community. Thanks to them, this book blossomed instead of our thighs.

acknowledgments

3 FAT CHICKS ON A DIET is the collective work of a lifetime of dieting. Many people gave us knowledge, inspiration, and support throughout our personal journeys and challenges of weight loss and the writing of this book.

Thank you, Mom and Dad, for always supporting us and encouraging us to stick with it. You've always loved us, fit or fat, and we are blessed to have you as our parents. We would also like to thank our brother, Doug Barnett, and his wife, Becky, for putting up with all the diet talk at the dinner table for all these years and for boldly trying any weird recipe that we showed up with. If anything, a few of them were a just return for the dirt and dog biscuits Doug tricked us into eating as little girls!

Suzanne would like to thank her son, Nicholas Barnett, for always encouraging her to be healthy and take care of herself, and for hiding the Little Debbie cakes from her while growing up. She'd also like to thank him for his love and support, and for taking care of things while she was holed away in the Batcave writing this book. No mother could be luckier than to have a son like you.

Jennifer would like to thank her husband, Rob Lesman, and son, Cody Honeycutt, for incredible patience and understanding while she was writing the book. Cody, you've been a sweetheart night after night while Mom worked, always being the funny guy just when it was needed. Rob, you've been Jennifer's rock through this process with your creative help and never-ending encouragement, and you've kept Jennifer's life in motion for the past year. There is no way she could have done this without you, and she is lucky to have you for a partner.

Amy would like to thank her husband, Jack Buchanan, for his support through the years, and for loving her regardless of her weight. The challenge of weight loss isn't always pretty, and you've been a great husband through it all.

We especially would like to thank Judy Linden for her help in the development of this book. Without her stumbling upon us, this book would not have been. Judy knew what the book could be, and she encouraged us to believe that we did have it in us. We also thank her for giving us Bev West and Judy Capodanno, to help us work together and make the best book we could.

Thank you to Mark Lockett, M.D., for his valuable help in providing a surgeon's insight into weight-loss surgery.

We would also like to thank the moderators of 3fatchicks.com and their constant help with 3FC and the many dieters who come our way looking for support and answers. These women are a fount of information, and without them, 3FC would not be what it is. All of these women work hard to make sure that all of us looking for answers get on the healthiest path that we possibly can. Thank you, Sherry Abernathy, Sandi Blair, Karen Canzoneri, Jane M. Catt, Eileen Cordes, Lauren B. Dale, Marti Dyche, Laurie A. Garner, Melanie Gumerman, Karen Kossowsky, Meg Heinz, Carol Lemon, Ellen McCorkle, Jane F. Perrotta, Amy M. Phillippe, Michelle Powell, Christina Preece, Ilene Robertson, Ruth Sheridan, Lianne Slaughter, and Geri Thueme.

Last but not least, we'd like to thank the members of 3fatchicks.com, for all you do in making 3FC a home for thousands of chicks across the globe.

contents

introduction
meet the fat chicks

Hi, WE'RE THE 3 FAT CHICKS, Suzanne, Jennifer, and Amy, three sisters of the South who have eaten enough empty calories among us in our lifetimes to drive old Dixie down. But not anymore. Because we're on a diet—again!

The truth is, we've been on a diet for most of our lives. We've tried them all, from Atkins to Weight Watchers, from the Ice Cream diet to Cabbage Soup, and everything in between. We've busted sugar, cut carbs, flushed fat, counted calories, and gorged on grapefruit. Secretly we dreamed of a diet that consisted exclusively of pecan pie, which we know was a little nutty, but hey, we're southerners and we believe in the miraculous potential of molasses and nutmeats.

Needless to say, we were somewhat less than successful in those early battles of the bulge, but now something has changed and that has made all the difference. That something is 3fatchicks.com.

We started 3fatchicks.com as a way for the three of us to track our own weight-loss progress. It introduced a little bit of accountability into our secret wars with our waistlines and gave us an opportunity to support and encourage one another, even when we were all alone in our own homes, with a bag of chips singing sweetly to us from the kitchen, daring us to eat just one!

The idea was that we would log our progress for better or worse, keep a written journal of our ups and downs, and post our favorite recipes and tips to help each other over the difficult moments, to help us just say no to the all-you-can-eat buffets of our former fat lives.

Imagine our surprise then, when our picture wound up in *USA Today* alongside the address to our Web site! Suddenly our secret support group wasn't such a secret anymore. We had been "outted" as fat chicks, coast to coast!

At first we were mortified. Well, in our picture we were standing in front of an all-you-can-eat buffet sign, which is not exactly a flattering backdrop for three women in muumuus and maternity shorts who weren't expecting anything but a third trip to the buffet table. But our embarrassment soon turned to enthusiasm as other fellow soldiers fighting the battle of the bulge began flooding our site. They offered their thoughts and feelings, successes and failures, hints and horror stories, all in the hopes of helping us win the war with our weight. And suddenly we began to feel a little bit better about, well, just about everything. We realized that we weren't alone. Our unexpected spirit squad cheered us on when we lost weight, and when we gained an inch or two, they cheered even louder! Suddenly we had more support than we ever dreamed of, and we began to lose weight and keep it off, with a little help from our on-line friends.

3 Fat Chicks on a Diet takes our Web site one step further. We have rounded up former and current fat chicks from across the nation—everyone from stay-at-home moms to biker chicks to sweet sixteens to high-powered executives—and asked them to share their ideas about the ups and downs of the total dieting experience, not only calorically but emotionally and psychologically.

The women represented in this real-women's guide to dieting are short, tall, young, old, single, married, separated, and divorced, but they all have one thing in common: they want to be thinner. We have organized their straight talk and ours into a no-holds-barred book about what it's really like to wage a war over our own impulses and lose weight.

In this book you'll find the information that other diet books and the celebrity gurus won't tell you. Here are helpful pointers about the little things that the big diet books forget to mention and honest assessments of the most popular diets on the planet from the women who have really tried to follow them. The questions and answers in this book are all based on our own 3fatchicks.com forum discussions as well as a survey that was conducted with thousands of our visitors and members.

Best of all, this isn't a book that requires that you go from the first page to the last page. You can weave in and out and flip around to the section you like, just as at an all-you-can-eat buffet, only you won't have to loosen your pants when you're through! Now that's something to cluck about! We hope you enjoy our book and the fun—yes, *fun*—of dieting together.

Love,
The 3 Fat Chicks, Suzanne, Jennifer, and Amy

3 fat chicks
on a diet

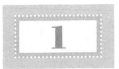

welcome to
the henhouse

WHEN YOU'RE CONTEMPLATING a climb up the slippery slope of weight loss toward your personal fitness peak, it's best not to spend too much time looking up at the steep trail ahead. When you look too far up the path in front of you, it's very easy to get winded just thinking about the climb, then turn around and go back to the lodge for a hot chocolate topped with a double scoop of "I'll start my diet tomorrow." But we did find it enormously helpful, when we started on our personal weight-loss journeys, to take in a quick view from the summit, through the eyes of somebody who has been there, to give ourselves the inspiration and the confidence to set out for the top.

The three of us have started more diets than Richard Petty has started races. We are sisters trying to drop over a hundred pounds apiece who don't have chefs, daily visits from our personal trainer, or elaborate home gyms. We understand what it's like to go it alone, without paid staff or even, in some cases, much support from our family and friends. And perhaps most important, we've learned that very few of us go on a diet and just lose weight. We also have to shed a lot of excess emotional baggage.

Most successful weight loss usually involves taking a long look at ourselves, making decisions to change the way we feel about ourselves and our eating habits, and discovering what success really means to us as individuals. This can be a very lonely experience at times, and for us, the help, support, and encouragement we got from each other and from our 3FC family made all the difference over the long haul. Hearing from women like us, who knew that learning how to just say no to a Big Mac can feel like nothing short of a religious conversion, made things easier. It really helped to know that we weren't alone, that there were women up on the trail ahead of us, who had found a way to climb beyond the world of pizza and popcorn and mac-and-cheese cravings and achieve their goal weight.

So for all of you chicks down there in the base camp getting ready for your final ascent, we'd like to share our three stories and the experiences of some very inspirational women, as well as the five most important steps we've identified that can prepare you for a successful climb. We hope our stories will fuel your motivation and your imagination, inspiring you to keep on going and never, never, never give up.

Jennifer 3FC

I've had weight issues almost all my life. I was probably a chubby fetus. My dieting experience started early. When I was eight years old, my doctor said I needed to lose weight, and he told my mother to water down my milk. Great idea! I went home and had a glass of watered-down milk with a Little Debbie cake!

Chubby girls aren't usually the most popular kids in school. I had only a few friends, but I made up for that with new friends, like Mr. Goodbar, Ronald McDonald, and Her Majesty the Dairy Queen. I was lonely, but that was okay, because it gave me plenty of time to snack.

Then hormones hit and I discovered boys, pimples, and PMS. My weight evened out. I sprouted boobs and a few curves. However, most of the other girls still had boyish figures, and I was fooled into thinking I was fat. As a gullible teenager, I tried every diet that was hot. I tried cabbage soup diets, grapefruit diets, fasting diets, negative calorie diets, and a tasty vinegar-water and kelp diet that I can still taste when I think about it.

When I moved out of my parents' house, I could no longer afford fancy luxury foods like fruits and vegetables. I lived on rice, noodles, bread, and whatever fatty meat I could find in the death row section of the meat department. I steadily gained up until pregnancy. Now I was knocked up, and so was my appetite, and I ballooned.

Finally, when my sisters and I started 3 Fat Chicks on a Diet, *I began to make some real changes in my lifestyle and my attitude toward food and health. I've spent years playing tag with my metabolism. Now I've caught up to myself, and most important, I've developed reasonable expectations. I don't want to be a skinny chick. I don't want to be a fat chick. I want to be a curvy chick. I just want to be me, and for the first time since I was eight years old, I finally feel like that's okay.*

Amy 3FC

There is something about me in a kitchen that just spells trouble. I could write the textbook for Cooking Disasters 101. *I almost caught my house on fire while broiling a steak. I didn't realize there was something called a broiler pan. Who knew? Then I was evicted from an apartment after forgetting about a pan of boiling eggs that exploded all over the ceiling. Experiences like these led me to develop a close relationship with my local pizza delivery boy. He was always punctual, he required nothing of me besides a tip, cleanup was a breeze, ordering out saved me a load of time, and most important, nothing ever ignited. Unfortunately, my cooking alternative was also addictive and extremely fattening.*

I did try to lose weight, and my choice of diets was as quick and easy as the dinners that got me there in the first place. I devised the "nothing but one Whopper a day" diet. I went on a laxative diet and a five-hundred-calorie a day diet. I mixed Slim-Fast with water instead of milk to save calories. My quick weight-loss schemes destroyed my metabolism quicker than one of those exploding eggs destroyed my ceiling. The more I dieted, the slower I lost weight. How's that for frustrating?

After I remarried, I found myself in the middle of a southern-fried Brady Bunch *episode. I was a newlywed and my husband delighted me daily with feasts big enough for a family of seven. Then suddenly that honeymoon was over, and that's when I developed a relationship with the Chi-*

nese buffet restaurant in town, and my weight blossomed faster than a magnolia grove in springtime. Finally, though, my quick fixes began to seriously impact my health.

I began to collect illnesses quicker than I did two-for-one pizza coupons, and I finally admitted that I'd lost control and I had to do something drastic. At nearly three hundred pounds I bit the bullet and had gastric bypass surgery. For the first time in more than twenty years, I am in control, I'm healthy, I'm confident. I've lost my delivery boys' phone numbers, and most miraculous of all, I've learned how to work a broiler pan!

Suzanne 3FC

My transition from a skinny kid to a fat chick was painless. I moved into my first apartment when I was eighteen years old, and for the first time I could eat anything I wanted to eat, whenever I felt like it. And I did! *Breakfast was frosting on a spoon, lunch was chips and dip, and dinners always concluded with an Oreo-thon that went on late into the night. Sure, I got pudgy, but I was enjoying every white, creamy middle and chocolate cookie outside along the way.*

As the years went on, my menus were dictated less by impulse than budget. When things were good, I experimented with recipes from Gourmet *magazine. When things were tough, I lived on mac and cheese. Rich or poor, I was always loaded with calories, which obviously resulted in weight gain. When I became a single parent, with a stressful job, my life was made easier by the help of a personal chef who always wore red and yellow and never forgot to ask if I wanted to super-size it. By the time I reached my early thirties, I was a full-fledged fat chick, but for some reason I did not consider dieting. I just ignored the situation. When the day finally came that I felt the urge to double-check the load capacity of an elevator before stepping in with my sisters, I realized that I needed to do something drastic—like go on a diet. Since then, I have fired my personal chef, learned to cook healthy and delicious meals, and taken back control of my health—all because I finally stopped ignoring my problems.*

┌─────────────────────────┐
│ **STRUTTING OUR STUFF** │
└─────────────────────────┘

The Chicks Sound Off on Their Personal Last Straws

We asked some of our chicks about their memories of the last straw that finally convinced them to change their lives forever. As you read through these snapshots, ask yourself what the first day of the rest of your life might be like. Maybe it's today!

I got really out of breath trying to tie my tennis shoes and realized that I wasn't even forty years old and if I can't breathe to tie my shoes now, what's it going to be like ten years from now? — CHAR

My mom came out for an extended visit from California a few years ago. It started off with me pretending, while my mom was visiting, that I don't usually eat like a pig. It ended with me realizing that I had dropped a few pounds while she was here and that the choice was mine whether to continue or not. It was a turning point, and at the time I didn't fully appreciate the magnitude of my power of choice. Now I can't help but wonder: what if I had chosen a different path? That thought alone is enough to make me put my fork down when I should, or go exercise when I really don't feel like it, and maintain my accomplishment. — BEVERLY

I had to go to a funeral. I had two pairs of black pants, a size 8 and a size 12. I didn't even consider the 8s. The 12s were the kind that button inside the pockets. I had already moved the buttons once, but that day they didn't even reach the holes anymore. I had to loop an elastic band through the buttonhole and around the last button and keep my coat on through the whole funeral. That day at the funeral buffet, I had a black

● *Continued on next page* ●

decaf. By the end of the month I was walking every day. The rest is history. —SUSAN

On the way back from a three-week trip to England, I couldn't zip my size 18 jeans for the return flight, and I felt dreadful for the entire time. Ten hours flying in coach in jeans two sizes too small changed my life forever. —MEL

The Five Essential Steps to Long-Term Weight Loss

1. Find a Support System

No chick is an island. You can't lose weight without a shoulder to lean on, so put a support system in place before taking the big leap. If you're not getting support from your family, find a new family. Seriously, there are options even if your family is less than enthusiastic about the bunless burgers that have begun to appear on the dinner table. Consider joining Weight Watchers, or look for a local support group at a hospital or church. Find walking buddies in the neighborhood, arrange your budget to accommodate gym fees, join an on-line support group, or visit 3fatchicks.com!

Howie and Kimberley are partners in diet and marriage. Between them, they've lost more than 250 pounds. Kimberley has lost 50 pounds, and Howie has lost 202 pounds, and they each have about 50 pounds to go. They have found that embarking on this journey together has helped them get through the tough times. The way they applaud and encourage each other is truly an inspiration to us all, and the perfect example of the kind of solid support system you'll want to try to develop. Not all of us are lucky enough to have a partner to succeed with, but having anybody in life who's there to pick you up when you stumble is a tremendous help. Here's what Kimberley and Howie had to say about the importance of their mutual support system.

Kimberley

Howie and I have dieted together off and on over the course of our marriage. The fact that he's my best friend helps a lot, and we can be either our own worst enemies or our own best coaches when it comes to weight loss. Having a partner, be it a spouse, friend, or another family member, really helps. Having 3FC and friends here helps us to stay accountable too. I have realized through this process that it isn't just my weight that's important, but my health. I love life, I love my husband, and I want to be healthy.

Howie

I have now lost over two hundred pounds from my heaviest. What a feeling! It is so much easier doing this with my best friend. She gives me strength to go on when I'm feeling weak. I am so proud of her for the weight she has lost and I know she will follow through with this to the end. I can't wait to see what we feel like when we lose "another person."

I really admire Kimberley for sticking to this even though the weight has been coming off really slowly for her. She is doing so well and is such a help to me. It makes it a lot easier when you have someone to make this trip with.

2. Load Up on Self-Esteem

A lack of self-esteem can wreck any chance you have at weight loss. Hating yourself really doesn't help the pounds come off. And remember, confidence doesn't have any calories. Before undertaking a serious weight-loss program, you need to heal yourself emotionally. Imagine if you were responsible for giving first aid to two people— one you hated and one you loved. Who would get the better care? Give that same care to yourself.

This means accepting yourself as you are, not as you wish you were. You're overweight: get over it. Everybody knows you're overweight, so there's no sense in trying to hide it. Accept who you are, and enjoy the fact that this will help you in your weight loss. Jessica, also known on our forum as Goddess Jessica, gives us some golden ways to learn how to love yourself.

Jessica

I had such a skewed idea of my body, so I took some examples from anorexic therapy books. See, anorexics think they are way bigger than they are. (Remind you of anybody?) Therapy includes a ton of very helpful exercises. Here are some things I do:

- *Get in front of the camera. A lot! Post pictures of yourself around areas of low self-esteem, such as the scale, the closet. I had this idea that I was so big that Geraldo was going to have to pry my walls off to get me out of the house. That is such a crock.*

- *Find some positive things to look at in the mirror. I had a huge problem getting out of the shower and feeling bad about myself. Now I wiggle and jiggle in front of the mirror, practicing my bedroom eyes and such. But also look at those areas you hate to look at. Quit imagining how bad they are and look. Yep, I'm fat, but I've got the nicest hourglass figure anyone could ask for.*

- *Finally, get out and do something you shouldn't do for a "woman of your size." I took belly dancing classes. Heck, I have a belly, shouldn't I use it? Gain some confidence for doing something you didn't think you'd enjoy doing. Then do it again!*

I'm lucky. I had a bad mental image of myself but lots of confidence. Now I'm reconciling the two.

3. Find a Less-Fattening Form of Comfort

We all have different reasons for needing an emotional rescue, but when we're on a diet, our answers can't be cream-filled or dipped in glaze anymore. Jane, one of the 3FC moderators, decided to get serious about her weight loss in January 2004. She is just fifteen pounds away from her goal weight and has maintained her diet because she learned how to reward herself without indulging in the comfort of empty calories. Here's what Jane had to say about combating her head hunger.

Jane

In order to finally lose the weight and keep it off, I had to find out what I personally got as a reward from staying overweight. For me, it was the comfort of eating. I used food to calm my nerves, soothe my bruised feelings, and also to celebrate. The way these foods made me feel was my payoff, so I had to find a different way to get the same satisfaction. My answer was limiting my portions, or finding a different kind of reward system, like an hour of junk TV instead of junk food, or going for long walks, or taking some time to tend to my garden when I needed a little comfort. The next thing I did was to enlist the support of my family. Also I got all the junk food out of my house. Yes, I can, and do, have treats, but a steady supply of them is just too tempting.

I have noticed in the past that when I lose for a specific event, such as a wedding, a reunion, or a vacation, I always gain the weight right back after the event is over. So this time I am losing for the rest of my life. Until the day I die, I will be doing Weight Watchers, because I want to!

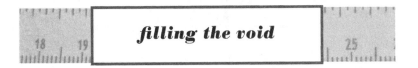

filling the void

Here are some tips from our chicks on how they overcame emotional eating:

Keep a journal and write down every bite that passes through your lips, and why you ate it. Even if you're pissed at the world, you're not likely to let that list get filled with unhealthy foods. — MARIA, VERMONT

I go to bed each night before I get too tired. I find that when I get sleepy, that is when I nibble, trying to stay alert to read or watch TV.

● Continued on next page ●

I'm less likely to eat bags of popcorn and frozen pizza at 7 A.M.!
—JULIA, TEXAS

I stay busy when my husband is away. I tend to nibble on bad things that I'd never dream of eating in front of him. I make sure when he is going to be away that I plan a project to keep my hands busy or go out with friends. —DONNA, VIRGINIA

---

4. Discover Something You Love and Stick with It

When you're feeling deprived on a diet, try thinking about the things that you are adding to your life, rather than the things that you are subtracting, like pecan pie and pizza. Change can be hard to get used to. By focusing on the positive, you'll find yourself feeling better about saying no to those empty calories, and success will come a lot easier. Rubia, one of our forum members, has taught us that success-ful weight loss is not about giving things up but about finding new and healthier ways to excite your passion for living.

Rubia

I'm five seven and since my teens I've always weighed around 160 pounds. When I went away to college I gained 35 pounds in nine months. I was a mess. My clothes didn't fit; I was depressed and looked like a whole different person. One day I watched a step aerobics class and decided to give it a shot. I absolutely loved it! I've been addicted to step ever since. I lost that 35-pound weight gain, then I went on vacation and somehow lost 10 more pounds! I realized I didn't always have to be 160 pounds. I was looking better, clothes were fitting me better, and I felt great! When people ask me for advice, I always say find something you love to do, and then do it as often as you can. There is something out there for all of us.

5. Try Gradual Change Instead of Going Cold Turkey

Weight loss isn't easy, but it can seem harder than it really is. We all know someone who has quit smoking cold turkey, but dieting is rarely that simple. If you are used to a certain kind of food, or lack of activity, it can seem daunting to change your habits and dive into a new diet and fitness program.

Change can be hard to get used to, so it's sometimes better to start off with small changes, rather than beating yourself up because you can't do it all at once. Focus on one meal a day and make that meal healthier. Wear a pedometer and try to add a few hundred more steps each day. By focusing on the small changes, you'll find yourself feeling better about yourself, and the rest will come a lot easier!

Jennifer, one of our forum members, has taught us that successful weight loss doesn't have to be instant, or an all-or-nothing venture. She decided it would be easier to concentrate on one small change at a time. Jennifer made little changes that would improve her health, such as adding a new vegetable to her diet or replacing white rice with brown. Jennifer even took her weight-loss goals slowly, making small goals of ten pounds at a time. These gradual changes helped make losing weight, and getting healthier, virtually painless. She soon realized there was nothing to stop her from reaching her goals.

Jennifer

I made "rules for myself" for weight loss. One of the top rules is that there will be no radical, unsustainable changes. When I first decided I wanted to change my eating habits to be stronger and healthier, I knew I needed something I could stick with forever. I couldn't radically change how I eat: there's no way to maintain that long term. With my boyfriend's support, we started changing foods one at a time to get used to our new, healthier eating habits. I am also making small changes toward exercise, which I do not like! I've taken the first baby steps by joining a gym.

Since I originally started, I got a tattoo to help me stay focused and committed. The tattoo is a Chinese proverb that means, "Dripping water can eat through stone," to help me remember it's every tiny step that leads to success. It is very meaningful to me: it represents all the hard work I've done this year. I have never given up, not for one second. I kept making changes, both big and little, to be the healthiest person I can be.

how not to diet

We totally understand the lure of easy weight loss. What chick isn't blinded by the sentence "Lose ten pounds in three days"? Amazing weight-loss claims are a sure sign that a diet isn't healthy or that it doesn't promote fat loss. If you really want to know if a product works, ask your doctor—not the savvy marketers who wrote the testimonials and product claims. Remember, if diet pills, gadgets, and miracle diets worked like they claimed, our doctors and insurance companies would be pushing them on us. We'd hear about them on CNN, not infomercials and e-mail spam. And America wouldn't be the most obese country on the planet.

- **Over-the-counter diet pills.** If you need a diet pill, get it from your doctor, not from a truck stop or flea market stall. Some contain properties that could be harmful to your body—particularly your heart. The fine print always tells you to go on a reduced-calorie diet and exercise program. That's how you lose the weight.
- **Weight-loss jewelry, clothing, and shoes.** We don't care how many women in the ads claim to have kept slim with these products. Believe us, a pinky ring will not make your butt smaller.
- **Diet patches.** These usually contain various herbs that won't help you lose weight and may not even be absorbed through your skin anyway. The only way a diet patch can help you lose weight is if you use it to tape your mouth shut.
- **Extreme diet schemes.** Cabbage soup, grapefruit, water, and juice diets might sound good in theory, but after three days of eating nothing but citrus fruit, it starts to get a little difficult to unpucker, and cabbage, well, let's just say cabbage can

be a little windy when eaten in mass quantities. Also, unbalanced meals like these do nothing for you nutritionally. Limiting your foods to only one type can be harmful, not to mention boring, and so can extremely low-calorie diets. Our bodies need protein, carbohydrates, and fat to thrive. The only thing you really wind up losing on these crash diets is your sense of humor.

* **"Detox" plans.** That's just a fancy version of Ex-Lax and a jug of water. There is no scientific evidence that "detoxing" will help you lose weight, but it has been proven in extreme cases to cause coma or even death. Besides, if you were truly toxic, you'd need a trip to the ER, not the health food store. Make water and fiber a part of your healthy diet to keep your system clean. If you are concerned, please ask your doctor for advice.

* **Diets that claim you'll lose weight effortlessly.** That's just not how it works. If it did, we'd all be running around in size 2 bikinis. Weight loss takes a change in lifestyle, through diet and exercise.

Picking the diet that works for you is one of the most important first steps in successful weight loss, but how do you pick from the wide array of plans available today? Before you put all your eggs into one diet basket, take some time to listen to what our chicks have to say about the most popular programs around. In the pages to come, you'll hear from real chicks who have been eating on the beach, dining with Dr. Atkins, or counting their points on Weight Watchers. Their candid thoughts about what worked for them and what didn't, along with answers to their most frequently asked questions, troubleshooting suggestions, helpful hints, and personal stories about the agony and the ecstasy of weight loss, will help you figure out which program is right for you. The questions addressed in these chapters are based on our own forum discussions as well as a survey that was conducted with thousands of our visitors and members. The answers are designed to give you the real-world information, support, and insight that you will need to ride the crest of those crave waves all the way to the shores of better health. Make the diet you choose this time your last.

Words to Live By

I have gained and lost the same ten pounds so many times over and over again, my cellulite must have déjà vu. —JANE WAGNER

To eat is a necessity, but to eat intelligently is an art.
—LA ROCHEFOUCAULD

fat chicks on the beach
the south beach diet

THE SOUTH BEACH DIET is one of the most misunderstood diets in the coop because everybody thinks it's a variation on the low-carb philosophy of the Atkins diet. Well, we fat chicks on the beach are here to tell you that the South Beach diet is not *at all* like the Atkins plan. This diet limits the types of carbs, not the amount, and also limits the types of fats you eat, which makes for a very different dieting experience.

Unlike Atkins, the South Beach diet does allow a few glorious carbs. But don't get too excited. South Beach–friendly carbs aren't exactly the carbs we dieting-down-in-Dixie chicks know and love. There will be no French fries, or fritters, no pound cake or pralines, and definitely no Moon Pies.

Basically, on the South Beach plan, you're not going to eat anything white or greasy (including anything named Bubba). No white potatoes, white bread, white rice, sugar (white *or* brown), or white flour. But here's the kicker. Unlike the Atkins plan, the South Beach diet limits your fat in addition to your carbohydrates. This means no full-fat dairy, no bacon or standard oils with a lot of saturated fats either. Ready to turn to the next chapter?

Well, hang on a minute, there is some good news . . .

You *are* allowed to eat a whole lot of earth tones on the beach. You can eat some bread and even rice, as long as they're brown and wholegrain. And you can eat some potatoes too, so long as they're sweet potatoes (which make delicious french fries, by the way, simmered in a little monounsaturated fat). You can also eat olive oil, nuts, avocados, lean meats, veggies, and most fruits. Is your mouth watering yet? Ours isn't either, but remember, this is a diet that was originally devised to maintain heart health, so it's very good for more than maintaining your waistline: it improves your overall health and can even increase your longevity. And because it is a more balanced diet than Atkins, it's an easier and healthier plan to maintain long-term. Are those sweet potatoes starting to sound a little better now? Well, read on.

Dr. Arthur Agatston, a cardiologist, who could be called the accidental millionaire, developed the South Beach diet (SBD) to help improve his patients' cardiac health. Coincidentally, the diet was also very effective for weight loss. His patients lost weight, felt great, and shared their secret with friends. This plan was probably passed around Southern Florida on folded-up photocopies, just like the "Mayo" diet from the eighties, which wasn't really from the Mayo Clinic at all. But who cares about pedigree if it works?

On the South Beach diet you can eat three meals plus snacks each day, and you don't have to count calories, which is good, because who can do math when they're woozy with carb and fat depletion? The South Beach diet does have one very important rule: *stop eating when you aren't hungry anymore*. While moderation might seem like an obvious boundary, for most of us fat chicks on the beach, overeating is what made us fat in the first place, so learning when to say no to seconds and thirds is a little tricky. Once you master this simple rule of thumb, though, the South Beach diet is very effective long-term, and remarkably easy to follow.

The South Beach diet is divided into three phases. Phase 1, which lasts for two weeks, restricts most carbs and most fat. As we carb- and fat-aholics can attest, when you first hit the South Beach surf, it can feel like a real diet tidal wave, and the level of restriction has knocked more than a few of us off our boards. One bad case of the Krispy Kreme blues, and you can find yourself caught in the undertow and wind up miles from the beach before you even realize it. And then sometimes you have to start all over again. After an experience like this, a lot of chicks decide to go in search of friendlier diet waters. In fact, in a recent poll we conducted on 3fatchicks.com, 75 percent of us who wound up quitting the diet quit during Phase 1. So hold on through this early phase as long as you can, and try your best not to get frustrated. And more important, be realistic. The Fat Fairy didn't zap the pounds on overnight, so shedding them might take some time. If you stick with the program during Phase 1 boot camp though, you can lose up to thirteen pounds in just two weeks! Now that's what we call a hang ten!

If you make it through these two weeks, you will be rewarded with Phase 2, when the diet becomes much easier. Phase 2 allows additional complex carbohydrates and monounsaturated fats. So you *can* have your cake and eat it too, but only if that cake is made with whole-wheat flour and olive oil.

Phase 3 of the South Beach diet is designed for long-term maintenance. During this phase, you add more foods so that you stop losing weight but don't gain any pounds back either. Basically, Phase 3 is like Phase 2, only with larger portions. Phase 3 of the South Beach diet is no longer a weight-loss diet but a new way of eating that you will continue with for as long as you wish to remain at your goal weight—which is probably forever!

As with any weight-loss plan, there are issues with the South Beach diet that make it, well, a diet. Some of the issues cause dieters to give up too easily or, like some of us do, stick with it but bitch all the way. So it's not surprising that our community of South Beach beauties had very strong emotional responses to this diet. Those of us who thrive on a sense of control would reassure ourselves, at the end of a hectic and otherwise helpless day, that if nothing else, we managed to stay on program. Some of us recognized that we would sooner stick needles in our eyes than say good-bye to spuds and abandoned the beach for a diet that understood that sometimes french fries are two dozen of the best reasons to get out of bed in the morning.

In our responses we grappled with being so close, yet so far away from that real piece of cake. We struggled with food charts and meal planning, carb cravings, headaches, and feelings of inadequacy when we didn't lose as much weight as quickly as we had hoped. We really would have preferred the pounds to come off as enjoyably and deliciously as we packed them on!

So for all of you chicks who have just hit the beach, or for those who are thinking about rolling up your blanket and calling it a day, below is the collective wisdom of our fat chicks on the beach, who have made it through Phase 1, broken through the boredom of Phase 2, and reached their weight-loss goals.

meet the fat chicks on the beach

Laurie from New York

I once weighed 326 pounds (or more!). My ankles were swollen, I was out of breath, and I structured my life at home around avoiding the stairs because climbing them was too painful. I had terrible pain in my back, hips, shoulders, and ribs, and it took about five minutes of excruciating pain for my back to straighten out when I lay down at night. I had increasingly bad cholesterol, blood pressure, and heart rate, and I had a terrible self-image. On top of it all, my husband and I wanted to get pregnant, and I knew there was no way I was ever going to be able to healthily become pregnant at that weight. I picked up a copy of The South Beach Diet *at Wal-Mart one night after my doctor recommended it. I was thinking I would look it over, just to see, but my husband was very excited that I had bought it, so I figured I might as well try it. Now I'm healthier than I've been in more than a decade. I work out and all of the problems mentioned above are either much improved or completely gone.*

Jane from Arizona

I had been low-carbing on and off for a few years but I found that I gained immediately after even the tiniest "cheats" and I never figured out a way around them. I decided South Beach might work better for me, and it did! I'm so thrilled! I love it!

Amy from Michigan

When I first started the South Beach diet, I did everything exactly like it's written in the book. And you definitely need the book to do this diet successfully. I never ate any more or less for the first two weeks and I dropped 16.5 pounds and I was thrilled. This diet taught me that not only what you eat matters but also how much of what you eat. Portion control has made this a very successful plan for me.

Q: I'm a week into Phase 1 of the South Beach diet, I'm tired all the time, I don't feel any skinnier, and my cravings are so intense that I'd trade my first-born for a cheeseburger deluxe. Help!

3FC: The good news is that you aren't the first South Beach beauty who wanted a warm, soft bun so much she'd seduce Ronald himself to get it. We have all seen our families freeze like deer in the headlights when we walk through the door at suppertime with that look in our eye. We've all found ourselves growling at our pooch when he gets near his dog biscuits. And we've all looked up and actually seen the word *surrender* forming in the clouds above our aching heads. But don't worry, Dorothy, you're not in Oz, you're in Phase 1, and unfortunately the only answer is, *Do not give up.*

What you're going through is called carb detox, and we know it's not pretty. Carb detox is difficult, but the upshot of going through it is that once you cleanse your system, you won't feel those cravings anymore. You'll be free from carb addiction and actually crave healthier foods, the same way that you're craving that Big Mac right now.

Think of Phase 1 as hazing session at a frat party, minus the part where you have to wear underwear on your head. It might be difficult at the moment, but enduring this brief humiliation pays you back with a lifetime of membership privileges. Once your blood sugar stabilizes, your cravings will go away. For most people, the side effects only last a week or two. Would Scarlett have given up on Tara in two weeks? We don't think so. So when the going gets tough, remember: Phase 1, like everything in life except death, taxes, and dryer lint, shall pass.

In the meantime, if it gets too bad, just lock yourself in a room and have your family slide omelets and turkey rollups under the door while you watch *Super Size Me* over and over from the safety of your bedroom. And when you feel like you just can't hold out another moment, try our bacon cheeseburger salad on page 38 or a few of the detox remedies our fellow beach beauties have found to help you get through those long, hard, carbless nights when you're afraid you're going to rush out and mug the pizza delivery boy.

detox remedies for recovering carbo-holics in crisis
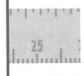

- One sure way to kill a carb craving is sugar-free Jell-O. We're not talking about the little sundae dish of Jell-O cubes with a dainty dollop of fat-free whipped cream. We want you to make a few boxes of the stuff, just litter the fridge with big bowls of multihued Jell-O. Then, when you can't go a moment longer without a carb or sugar fix, raid the fridge. And we mean *really* dig in, like a liposuction machine in reverse. Jell-O is sweet and it's filling, and if you eat it without moaning, you'll probably hear the choir of angels singing in the background.

- Take a nap. You're still allowed to eat carbs in your dreams.
- Drink a lot of water. You need to flush your system, and water will give you the illusion of being full.
- Play Scrabble. Spell words like *coronary, plaque, muumuu,* or *obese.*
- Get the most bang for your buck with sugar-free Fudgsicles, hot cocoa, and hazelnut syrup for your coffee. These are long-lasting treats; by the time you have finished them, the cravings will be gone.
- We suggest snacks, snacks, and more snacks! You need a few extra munchies when you are kicking the cravings in the beginning. Try almonds, low-fat cheese sticks, sugar-free Jell-O, or fresh veggies and lean lunchmeats. Salad veggies and a good dressing low in saturated fat are very important! And since you are living with people you care for, until those early cravings pass, we'd suggest sedatives and a padded room!
- Here's a good dip for your turkey rollups: Find a jar of tapenade. It's a thick spread made of olives, olive oil, and spices. Mix a heaping tablespoon of tapenade with one ounce of light cream cheese that's been softened a bit. This is a *wonderful* dip or spread for your turkey rollups!

Q: Breakfast is boring me to death. Every morning is eggs, eggs, eggs, and more eggs. I have been doing the first phase of SBD and am very happy with the program. But I have eaten so many eggs in one week that I feel like I really will turn into a chicken. I am in grad school and have class every morning at 8 A.M. and I have a forty-five-minute commute, so cooking a big breakfast every morning just isn't cutting it anymore. Help!

3FC: Breakfast is a killer. And when you're cutting carbs, you can find yourself eating so many eggs that you'll make them scrambled just for the pure pleasure of beating them with a blunt object. Eggs get old *real* fast. Fortunately, eggs are very versatile and forgiving, and with the right combination of ingredients, you can totally fool your rebellious taste buds into believing that they are sensing something fabulous! So before you move on to explore a beach without eggs, try a few of our recipes for eggs with a twist on pages 35–36.

Of course, you don't even have to eat traditional breakfast foods. Sticking to traditional foods shows a worker-bee attitude. You can be a rebel and try something totally different! Make up a batch of chicken salad, tuna salad, shrimp salad, or (if you really have a hard time breaking tradition) egg salad made with low-fat mayonnaise. Fill a romaine lettuce leaf or two, and you have a quick and tasty breakfast.

If you'd like something warm and rich for breakfast, try reheating a vegetable casserole, or even the crab cake recipe from the official South Beach cookbook. It doesn't have to be limited to dinner. Try a crab cake for breakfast, and start your day in the lap of luxury! You can also have a spicy chicken breast or even a bowl of warm black bean soup with salsa and fat-free sour cream on top. We also like veggie burgers for breakfast, with a smear of mustard and tomato on top. Diets are a lot like life. The key to happiness is to think outside the box. Think of what you *can* have and don't focus on what you can*not* have. With that perspective, the possibilities are endless!

STRUTTING OUR STUFF

I often eat last night's leftovers if they appeal to me, or sometimes I'll have cottage cheese, low-fat cheese, or lunchmeat rollups and V-8 juice. Once you are on Phase 2, you can have things like a fat-free yogurt blended with berries, Splenda, and vanilla. —MARTHA IN OHIO

Sometimes I just grab a couple of slices of low-fat cheese and a handful of nuts when I can't face cooking. Mostly I have eggs and cheese or low-fat sausages with mushrooms or tomatoes, or I'll make quiche cups ahead of time, for a quick and easy breakfast. —FRANK IN WASHINGTON

If I'm running late, I usually have a V-8 and cheese sticks, or what I call an Egg McNuthin. (Buy an Egg McMuffin, and throw out the muffin!)—BONNIE IN IDAHO

Q: Is it healthy to cut out a food group in Phase 1? My mother always told me I should eat my fruit and bread!

3FC: Now, we know that Mother always knows best, and most of our mothers taught us from an early age to eat a well-balanced diet that included all four major food groups. If we didn't, they told us, our eating habits would lead to a lot of unladylike symptoms, such as bad breath, poor complexion, and slow bowels. Of course, in our family, one of those food groups was pecan pie, so we've learned to take Mom's menu suggestions with a grain of salt. Let's not forget that many of our moms also taught us that a balanced lunch included a PB&J on fluffy white Wonder bread, an apple, and a glass of whole milk. So it's no wonder, then, that Phase 1 of the South Beach diet, which eliminates fruit and bread and severely limits dairy, can cause us to feel fundamentally uneasy, as if we're breaking the Ten Commandments of food. This has caused a lot of chicks to flee before finishing Phase 1. Apparently they never heard of Phase 2.

You need to remember that the unbalanced diet of Phase 1 only lasts two weeks. You're eating not to build strong bodies twelve ways but to cleanse your system from carbs and sugars. Once you get into Phase 2, you'll be able to gradually add fruits and whole grains back into your diet, along with more dairy products. The only thing you'll eliminate will be high-glycemic carbs and trans fats. Until you get to the end of Phase 1, you can improve your vitamin consumption with alternative foods that are on the Phase 1 program. Add vitamin C with broccoli, cauliflower, or bell peppers. You can increase your fiber with carbs such as black beans and fibrous vegetables from the Phase 1 list. Hang in there until Phase 1 has passed. Then you can safely invite your mother over for a nice sandwich on whole-wheat bread, washed down with a glass of nonfat milk, and we're sure she'll approve!

alternachick tips: vegetarians on the beach

The menu on the average reduced-carb diet is a vegetarian's nightmare. It's much easier on South Beach. Vegetarians follow the same plan as everyone else on South Beach, except in the choice of protein, and some of which may be limited due to fat or carb content.

Read the labels! You can have soy-based meat substitutes, but they can have no more than six grams of fat per two- or three-ounce serving. Others may contain rice or other ingredients not allowed during Phase 1.

My husband loves Mexican food, but my choices are obviously limited now. When we eat out, I choose the vegetable fajitas, without the tortilla. The filling is full of flavor, and they don't mind filling up my plate. Just double-check that the fajitas are not fried in lard! —JILL

I couldn't wait to reach Phase 2 so I could eat oatmeal with walnuts sprinkled on top. It has a bit of protein, some good omega-3 fats, and a powerhouse of heart-disease-fighting oats. —RUBY

I hate to cook and loved the convenience of tofu marinated in teriyaki or other sauces. Most contain sugar, so I had to learn how to season my own tofu, without sugary sauces, and avoid the premarinated kinds. —JEN

Q: I'm at the end of Phase 1, and I didn't lose eight to thirteen pounds like the book said I would! I feel like such a failure and I'm ready to give up!

3FC: Okay, so Phase 1 didn't move the earth and the sky for you. The book jacket said you could lose up to thirteen pounds, but you weren't even close. Welcome to Marketing 101. We read the same book jacket as you did, and it gave us the same funny feeling in our stomachs that we had when Publishers Clearing House told us we might *already* be millionaires! While there are certainly a couple of fortunate folks out there who did open their front door to find Ed McMahon standing there with a big fat check in his hand, most of us eventually have to face the fact that we are going to have to earn our luck the hard way. While it is true that dieters *might* lose eight to thirteen pounds in Phase 1, many of our South Beach beauties lost much less. But just because you weren't a big loser in Phase 1 doesn't make you a loser. Dieters who haven't been on a diet recently or haven't been watching their carb intake or those who are very overweight are the ones who drop the most weight in Phase 1.

In other words, the fatter you are, the more weight you lose up front. So if you didn't lose very much weight in Phase 1, it could just mean that you didn't have that much to lose! Keep in mind too that this early weight loss is mostly due to water lost because of your body's sudden drop in excess carbs. If you were already watching carbs, or if you had less excess water to spare, then you won't have as much water weight to shed. After all, there is only so much weight a fat chick can whiz away.

And of course, it's important to level with yourself. Are you sure that you ate everything on the plan to the letter? Are you sure there weren't any Mallomars moments that you've conveniently forgotten about? Did you really exercise, or was your activity confined to remote control curls and the occasional jog to the refrigerator? Did you drink enough fluids? Were you poaching chicken or makin' bacon?

Other common Phase 1 beach beauty blunders include eating too many nuts, eating cheese that was not low-fat, having too much dairy, or indulging in too many two-for-one cocktails at happy hour. Some of our beach beauties have discovered that journaling daily food intake makes a big difference. Try writing down every bite that you eat. You might be able to pinpoint where things went wrong, and correct those problems before they slow you down where it really counts—in Phase 2, and over the long haul.

 deep thoughts from our heavy hens

The main thing I have learned through my weight-loss journey is that there are two major components: consistent exercise and the support of people who are in the same boat as you. —JENNIFER MOORE

The scariest thing about embarking on this journey is that I have no idea where it will end. In my entire life I have never been thin or even at a healthy weight. I was overweight as a child and have been that way all through my teenage years. Even when I lost weight in the past, I still remained in the "obese" category. So I don't even know how it's going to feel! I'm scared that once I start feeling good, I'll stop because I won't know how much better I could still feel. —RISHE

For the first time in my personal history, I'm hoping that my weight loss will be a by-product of changing my relationship with food, rather than

of dieting to lose the weight. I've had a dysfunctional relationship with food for most of my life. Breaking up with that has been liberating, and even if no weight loss occurs, I've already made the biggest change to help myself live a longer, healthier life. —AMY STEVENS

Q: Phase 1 just isn't working for me when it comes to lunch, because I am a sandwich freak. If I don't get my sandwich, somebody's gonna get hurt. Should I trash this diet?

3FC: Many dieters would chew off their left arm for a mere crumb of bread by the end of Phase 1. On the other side of the coin are those dieters who have the mutant ability to *not* crave carbs and who aren't quite ready to give up the rapid weight-loss regimen of Phase 1. For both ends of the carb cravings spectrum, we recommend that beach chicks consider what we call Phase 1.5. Phase 1.5 is completely unofficial. Phase 1.5 is basically Phase 1, with only one or two servings of Phase 2 carbs per day. It isn't full force, so you get the best of both worlds.

Q: I'm really reluctant to graduate from Phase 1! I am having a very hard time with that issue. I feel very good, my body is really trimming down (my husband is thrilled, as am I), and I am still enjoying the diet on Phase 1. I never really was a fruit eater, and I don't miss it. I suppose it might be nice to have an apple, but I don't really care. Also, I don't get all excited about whole grains. To me, what I can add in Phase 2 just sounds kind of boring, and I don't want to stall my weight loss. I know this sounds crazy, but can I just stay in Phase 1?

3FC: Dieting may not always be fun, but actually losing weight really is like one long, glorious day at the beach, and potentially one of the greatest experiences in your life. Knowing that you can make hard decisions and carry them out because it's the right thing to do for yourself is one of the best self-esteem builders around, but the only thing better than taking the weight off is keeping it off long-term. Phase 1 usually results in quick weight loss, and we lose more per week during this period than in Phase 2. So why would we want to give that up?

Well, because Phase 1 simply wasn't intended to be the whole diet, and it isn't nutritionally sound for long-term use. Phase 1 was intended to flush out water and get you past your carb cravings. If you are still having cravings, stay on it for another week or two, but no more. The name of the game here is better health. Besides, Phase 1 is primarily water loss, and there is only so much water you can shed! Staying on Phase 1 will not help you lose weight quicker, it will only burn you out.

Phase 2 is designed for healthy weight loss. You wouldn't want to continue to lose weight at the rate of Phase 1 anyway. That would be too hard on your body. Slowing down on the weight loss will give your skin a chance to catch up with your body and will keep your metabolism in balance. You wouldn't want to fool your body into thinking you were starving. If you eat too few calories, your body begins to believe it's going to be deprived long-term, and it begins to act like a squirrel gathering nuts for the winter. It will store your fat and save it for later. Unfortunately, later never comes, and we can wind up with a very full basement! So keeping your body nourished is as important on this diet as restricting your intake. If you do start to gain weight again on Phase 2, just cut back a little and you'll be fine. Be aware that a small gain may just be water, as your body replenishes part of what it lost in Phase 1.

To Market, to Market

Our Favorite Phase 2–Friendly Items

Let's face it, supermarkets can seem like a Shangri-La of forbidden fruits when you are starting out on a diet. And passing up the potato chip pleasure dome for the produce aisle can be a real exercise in self-control. So here's an easy rule of thumb: Do not walk where even South Beach angels fear to tread. Most South Beach–friendly food will come from the outer sections of the grocery store. "Good carb" produce, lean meats and sea-food, low-fat yogurts, cheeses, eggs, and quality deli meats are usually arranged on the margins of the supermarket, which will keep you out of the midsection, where they keep the Lay's and the Chips Ahoy. Only dip into the tempting middle for grains, condiments, and miscellaneous frozen foods. And while prepar-ing food from scratch is the best way to ensure you don't have hidden fats and carbs, we all know that there are times when we just can't or don't want to cook. For times like these, here is a list of our Chick Picks for the best South Beach–friendly prepared foods easily found in your local grocery store.

- Uncle Sam's Cereal
  www.usmillsinc.com
- Smucker's Reduced Fat Natural Peanut Butter
  www.smuckers.com
- Pepperidge Farm 100% Whole Wheat Bread
  www.pepperidgefarm.com
- Bob's Red Mill Steel Cut Oats and Stone Ground Flour
  www.bobsredmill.com
- DaVinci Sugar Free Syrups
  www.davincigourmet.com
- Blue Bunny Health Smart Bars
  www.bluebunny.com
- Progresso Lentil Soup
  www.progressosoup.com
- Diet Rite with Splenda
  www.dietritecola.com
- Mission Whole Wheat Tortillas
  www.missionfoods.com

Q: Okay, I admit it. I'm a week into Phase 2, and I don't know what came over me, but last night I snuck into my kitchen when everyone was asleep and devoured three Boston cream doughnuts in the blink of an eye. I woke up with chocolate in my hair and Krispy Kreme remorse in my heart. Can I just forget about the whole thing and move on with Phase 2, or do I have to start over again from the very beginning and go back to Phase 1?

3FC: You can cheat on your husband, you can cheat on a test, and you can cheat on a diet. If you cheat on your diet, though, you have only to answer to yourself. The truth is you're going to feel inclined to cheat when you hear the word no. You've been saying yes to food for quite a while. Plus, it's a lot easier to cheat when you don't have to worry about divorce or detention hall. On the bright side, you're not alone. A whopping 50 percent of our beach beauties cheat occasionally. Only about 30 percent of them never cheat, while a naughty 20 percent cheat often. None of this should give you an excuse to cheat, but you can relax and know that you are not a failure (and you're not alone!) if you do.

Realistically, you're going to have to suck it up and deal with it. You can stick with this plan. You can also plan to have a little something every once in a while. When we feel the need to go off plan, we plan it. We're still on plan! Get it? We'll never have to beat ourselves up afterward. We planned on that piece of birthday cake; now we're going to eat it and enjoy it, and tomorrow we're back on sugar-free Jell-O. If you do succumb to an unplanned, perhaps naughty cheat, don't fret. You don't have to start over; you didn't undo the progress you made. Just learn from your Krispy Kreme moment, and move forward.

Q: My husband and I eat out frequently and I am trying to get some new ideas. I usually play it safe and stick to salads, but I would like suggestions for eating in regular or chain restaurants. I know that a lot of restaurants have Atkins-friendly meals, which might work, but many are still high in fats and are not suitable for the South Beach diet. I am serious about my weight this time, and I vow to get down to my goal and not give up or slip!

3FC: Many restaurants are now advertising low-carb selections on their menus. Many of these meals may not be wise for South Beachers for two reasons. First, the portions served by most restaurants are sinfully large. Always plan to bring home enough for lunch the next day. You can wipe out most of a day's calorie allowance with one restaurant meal. Second, the ingredients in many low-carb selections are high in saturated fat, because restaurants follow the Atkins approach instead of the South Beach method. Before you dive in, be sure to ask if the meat is a lean cut. Is the skin removed before cooking? Is the dish fried, or cooked in butter?

For smart selections, you can usually find something at a steakhouse. Order grilled chicken with a sweet potato without the butter or sugar, and a salad with light dressing. Shish kebabs are also usually acceptable. If rice is served, make sure it is brown rice. Steer away from pilafs that might have ingredients that aren't allowed, like pasta or high GI vegetables. The vegetable of the day can be good, but check to see if it comes in a vat of butter before ordering. Lastly, there is always the trusty salad. Question the server about the ingredients in the dressing. Most restaurants offer a grilled chicken salad or have a salad bar to enjoy. Okay, salad isn't imaginative, but it works in a pinch.

You can also check out our list of food dos and don'ts that our South Beach beauties have compiled during their stay on the beach.

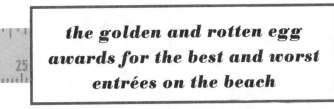

the golden and rotten egg awards for the best and worst entrées on the beach

Tony Roma's Ribs

Rotten Egg: Ribs! The sauce is too high in sugar.
Golden Egg: Grilled chicken and grilled vegetables.

● *Continued on next page* ●

Boston Market

Rotten Egg: Anything in gravy, which is most of the menu.
Golden Egg: Southwest Grilled Chicken Salad, hold the tortillas.

Ruby Tuesday

Rotten Egg: Most of it. Atkins-approved doesn't mean South Beach–approved.
Golden Egg: White Chicken Chili for a low-carb, low-fat meal.

Chicks' Tip: Kudos to Ruby Tuesday for including their nutrition information right on the menu. It's horrifying, but good education (or entertainment, depending on how you look at it) while you wait for your meal.

Red Lobster

Rotten Egg: Anything fried or broiled, and also the biscuits.
Golden Egg: Crab legs, grilled fish. Veggies, hold the butter.

Lonestar Steakhouse

Rotten Egg: The Cajun Ribeye, with over 1,000 calories and 100g of fat!
Golden Egg: Sweet Bourbon Salmon, steamed veggies, and black bean soup.

Golden Corral

Rotten Egg: Everything but the green beans and lettuce.
Golden Egg: Green beans and lettuce.

Wendy's

Rotten Egg: The sandwiches.
Golden Egg: Chili, Spring Mix Salad, and a reduced-fat dressing.

Outback

Rotten Egg: BBQ'd anything, potatoes, and rice.

Golden Egg: Chicken on the Barbie, hold the sauce, and veggies, no butter.

Chicks' Tip: While the Web site www.outback.com doesn't provide nutritional data, it is full of tips on how to order your meals for special needs. Three cheers for their cooperation!

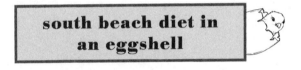

south beach diet in an eggshell

Professional Counseling No. However, if you subscribe to the official South Beach diet Web site, you can post nutrition questions for their dietitians to answer.

Support System No meetings, but there are a lot of South Beach support forums on the Internet, including our own Fat Chicks on the Beach group at www.3fatchicks.com.

Fitness Factor Barely there. Dr. Agatston suggests exercise but doesn't require it. Other than the two pages in the book of reasons why exercise is good for you, you're on your own.

Family-Friendly Very! Once you hit Phase 2, you can feed your family on the same healthy foods you will enjoy.

Pros It's very heart healthy, provides energy, and is easy to follow.

● *Continued on next page* ●

Cons Forbidden food list can make it harder to stick to. You need more time to plan meals.

$$ Can be initially more expensive, because you are restocking your pantry with new foods, but it evens out over time.

The Person This Diet Is Best For Someone who likes a very structured diet, doesn't mind eating from a limited list of foods, and may be interested in improving her heart health.

recipes from the front lines

Eggs don't have to be just scrambled or sunny-side up. Here are a couple of recipes that practically let you forget about those white oval things in the ingredients list!

When you really need a dose of good ol' breakfast food, try this "French toast." It might not be made with thick slices of bread, but it's extra tasty with turkey bacon and coffee!

mock french toast

4 egg whites
1 egg
1 teaspoon vanilla
¼ cup ricotta cheese
Dash cinnamon
1 packet of granular sugar substitute
Butter spray
Sugar-free maple syrup

Mix everything but the butter spray and the syrup in a bowl. Pour into pan on medium heat just like you are making pancakes. Top with butter spray and syrup and *enjoy!*

This is a standard recipe in the South Beach book, but many of our members were not pleased with the flavor. We created our own version, which is a variation of a family recipe we've eaten for many years. These mini quiches are perfect for breakfast, snacks, or even as a side dish. They freeze well, so you can prepare them in advance. Just thaw them and zap them in the microwave for a few seconds to serve.

anytime spinach quiche cups to go

Two 10-ounce packages of frozen chopped spinach, thawed
  and squeezed dry
1½ cups egg substitute, equal to 6 eggs
1½ cups nonfat cottage cheese
¼ teaspoon salt
Freshly cracked black pepper to taste
4 tablespoons freshly grated Parmesan cheese

Preheat oven to 375°F. Spray a 12-cup muffin pan with nonstick cooking spray. Combine all ingredients except Parmesan cheese. Divide among muffin cups and bake for 20 minutes. Sprinkle each cup with 1 teaspoon of Parmesan cheese and return to oven. Continue to bake 10 minutes more, or until firm and lightly browned. Loosen cups with a narrow spatula and remove to plate to serve. If preparing in advance, remove to wire rack to cool, then refrigerate or freeze as desired.

This is a sweeter variety of chili, suitable for all phases of the South Beach diet. If dried chipotle pepper is unavailable, you may substitute your favorite chili powder. If you are in Phase 2 or 3, you may serve the chili with low-fat sour cream and shredded reduced-fat cheddar cheese. Are you drooling yet?

vegetarian chili

Serves 4 generously

2 tablespoons olive oil
1 large sweet onion, chopped
2 red bell peppers, seeded and chopped
4 cloves garlic, minced
1 cup canned vegetable broth
32-ounce can crushed tomatoes
14-ounce can black beans, drained
14-ounce can kidney beans, drained
Freshly cracked black pepper to taste
1 to 2 teaspoons dried chipotle pepper powder, or to taste

Over moderate heat, add olive oil to a stockpot or Dutch oven. Add onion, peppers, and garlic and sauté for 3 to 5 minutes, or until soft. Stir in ½ cup of the vegetable broth, and the crushed tomatoes. Add beans to mixture and combine well. If too thick, add additional vegetable broth, up to ½ cup more. Gradually season with chipotle pepper, to taste. Reduce heat and simmer 10 to 20 minutes, stirring occasionally.

When you're about to pull into your local diner's parking lot for a bacon cheeseburger deluxe, try driving home instead to make this delicious salad. It has everything your body is craving—except the bun and extra calories!

bacon cheeseburger salad

Serves 1

FOR THE SALAD:
6 ounces 95% lean ground beef, cooked and crumbled
2 slices turkey bacon, cooked and crumbled
4 cups salad greens
1 cup diced tomato
½ cup chopped dill pickle
6 tablespoons chopped red onion
½ cup reduced-fat cheddar cheese

FOR THE TOMATO VINAIGRETTE:
½ cup chopped tomatoes
2 tablespoons white wine vinegar
½ teaspoon dried basil
½ teaspoon dried thyme
¼ teaspoon ground mustard
Pinch coarse black pepper
½ packet Splenda or other sweetener

Combine Tomato Vinaigrette ingredients in a blender and pulse for a few seconds until combined; set aside.

Combine salad ingredients in a bowl. Add vinaigrette and toss well.

Per serving: 282 calories, 12 grams fat, 16 grams carbs, 5 grams fiber, 29 grams protein

Words to Live By

My weakness has always been food and men—in that order.
— DOLLY PARTON

Never eat more than you can lift. — MISS PIGGY

low-carb chicks
the atkins diet

ONE OF THE BIGGEST dieting trends to take American waistlines by storm in recent history is the carb cutting approach to weight loss. For all of you who are still eating your burgers on a bun, carb-limiting diets are radical programs that let you eat all the bacon and eggs you can fry up in a pan, but won't let you get anywhere near a biscuit. Carb-cutting plans have always been a challenge for us Dixie chicks because they eliminate most of the staples of southern cooking, like cornbread, sweet potato pie, hush puppies, and yes, much to our horror, even pecan pie!

Now, we aren't nutritionists, but we understand enough about food to know that any diet that doesn't let you eat biscuits and gravy with your bacon and eggs can't be too balanced. The mere thought of starting on a low-carb diet is enough to make the Colonel himself roll over in his Kentucky grave.

The low-carb approach does have some definite advantages, however. Like bacon, for example—and chicken wings. The Atkins plan, which is king of the low-carb diets, lets you eat juicy steaks dripping in herb butter, roasted chicken complete with crispy skin, and omelets stuffed with cheddar cheese, which is probably one of the reasons why so many of us put this plan on our personal weight-loss throne. Who could get hungry or be tempted to cheat when your diet buffet includes all that delicious fat? But hang on to your tenderloins, because there's a catch. While it's true that you can have unlimited protein and fat, you should only eat them in moderation, and you can never eat a burger on a bun.

Wait a minute, did we say moderation? Yes, we did. We realize that's a word that many people don't realize is associated with the Atkins diet, but we're here to tell you moderation matters, even when you're dining with Dr. Atkins.

Sadly for all of us fat chicks in search of the diet rainbow, the Atkins plan isn't the steak and cheese free-for-all that it appears to be. There are portion restrictions. And while there are now lots of your favorite trigger foods at your local grocery store marked with the scarlet A, meaning Atkins-approved, those low-carb treats, although exciting and satisfying in theory, can go over like a lead balloon when what you're really craving is a double chocolate brownie or a super-sized order of fries. In fact, the first time we tasted a rich, chocolaty low-carb brownie, we had childhood flashbacks to the time our big brother talked us into eating dirt by telling us it tasted like chocolate. So just be prepared; there are going to be moments of temptation, even on Atkins, when no approved substitutes will do, and your willpower will have to prevail over your sweet tooth.

The Atkins plan is divided into four phases. The beginning phase, Induction, covers the first two weeks of the plan. This, as any chick who has ever cut carbs will tell you, is when you come face-to-face with the beast—the dreaded carb cravings!

Induction is a lot like diet boot camp and you can bet dollars to doughnuts that it will *not* be a cakewalk! But the good news is that many chicks see drastic weight loss during this initial phase. Dropping a few pounds sure does make it easier to just say no, even when you want a french fry so bad you would eat a birthday candle if it was dipped in ketchup. In fact, many low-carb chicks are so happy with the rapid results during Induction that they are reluctant to move on to the second phase, which is called Ongoing Weight Loss (OWL), hoping to become supermodel slim in record time.

Ready for the next fly in the ointment? Because you know there is one. While it is true that there is usually a hefty weight loss in this early phase, what you're losing is mostly water, and you can only lose so much water weight before you have to level out and move on to the more measured OWL phase of the diet, where results are less rapid and romantic but more sensible and sustainable. If you have a lot of weight to lose, Atkins says you can stay on Induction for up to six months. Lighter low-carb chicks, however, are encouraged to move on to the next phase after the first two weeks.

During Induction you are only allowed twenty carbs per day. For nondieting chicks, twenty carbs is equal to half of a Moon Pie or a six-ounce Coke. Kind of depressing to think about that, isn't it? I mean, who can eat *half* of a Moon Pie? And how many ounces of Coke are in a Big Gulp anyway? But there is some good news. While you can't polish off that Moon Pie and chase it with a Yoo-Hoo, you can eat four cups of vegetables, a few ounces of select cheese, and virtually unlimited amounts of meat and butter—all for twenty carbs. Starting to feel a little better about a low-carb future now? We neither. So let's sweeten the pot a little, because there are a few irresistible elements of a carb-cutting plan that have led fat chicks to just say no to white bread for nearly three decades and counting.

The goal during Induction is to achieve a physical state called *ketosis*. Ketosis is a condition in which you are burning your fat stores, using them as fuel rather than holding on to them in your hips for that rainy day that never comes. This gives a whole new meaning to the phrase "running on empty," doesn't it? When you restrict your carbs, you trick your body into using your stored fat as energy. This triggers a release of those magical *ketones* (substances released when the body breaks down fat for energy), which are then released as waste products into your urine. We know, this doesn't sound too ladylike, but if you think about the fact that in ketosis you are literally whizzing away your fat stores, you can really start to appreciate this brand of bio-chemistry. And if you think this sounds like a dream come true, just wait!

On Atkins, you can have almost any kind of meat you want, even a double cheeseburger with the works (except, of course, the bun and the fries), with very few limits on quantity. You also can eat lots of veg-gies. Of course, you can't just eat any old thing that grows in the garden. Corn is a definite no-no, as are potatoes and other starchy vegetables. There is, however, a long list of other vegetables to choose from. You can get the full list in the Atkins book, or visit www.3fatchicks.com/atkins for recent updates.

We don't want to kid you, though. Carb-cutting plans are not easy, quick-fix diets. No matter which way you slice the white bread, Induc-tion is difficult. Even though carb-cutting diets let you eat a lot of foods that are taboo on most other plans, you can only eat so many buttered steak and salad dinners before you start to miss the bread and baked potatoes. And a cheeseburger can never really become deluxe without fries and a sesame seed bun. As enticing as the selec-tions are on Atkins, the approved food list is short, and we low-carb chicks with a taste for culinary adventure do tend to get a little bored. If you can stick it out through Induction though, the next phase will allow the addition of more choices, so hang on to your lamb chops and put down those dinner rolls!

In the Ongoing Weight Loss phase of the Atkins plan, you will be-gin to gradually add carbs back into your life, so you'll have more fun creating your menus. Don't get too excited; by gradually, we mean you'll be adding carbs at a snail's pace of five per day, raised on a weekly basis. This may seem painfully slow, but then again, in the world of weight loss, good things come to those who are willing to wait.

On the Atkins plan, you are almost guaranteed to lose weight if you stick to the food list. Why? Because, frankly, there isn't anything on the food list that we love to pig out on. We know we're not going to gorge on boiled eggs and pork chops for a midnight snack. And a hunk of cream cheese on a spoon just isn't the same as a nice big slice of cheesecake.

As long as you stay in ketosis, you can keep adding more carbs each week. You are able to measure whether you are in ketosis with special ketone test strips that you can find at your local pharmacy. Due to some unfortunate side effects of ketosis—bad breath, for example—not all chicks choose the ketosis route, even though this is how the plan is written. If you are unsure about ketosis, a quick trip to your doctor should help you make the decision. In any case, as long as you are losing weight, you can add nuts, berries, and of course, *more vegetables* to your diet.

As you near your goal weight, you need to put the brakes on and get ready for lifetime maintenance. The name for this phase is Pre-Maintenance. In this phase, you can add a little more variety while you add more carbs to your diet. The idea is to slow down your weight loss and begin to massage the program from a crash diet into a lifestyle.

The final phase of the Atkins plan is called Maintenance. In this phase, now that you have discovered a goal weight that you can maintain comfortably and consistently, you learn to eat so that you can stay just the way you are. If you start to gain or slip back into old eating habits, it is suggested that you start Induction again. Now there's some incentive to stay on plan!

The most common problem that chicks encountered on this plan was, obviously, the carb cravings. A huge chunk of some of the world's most delicious foods are forbidden to us on this plan, and you never get to dip anything in syrup, so how could we not start to experience a few cravings? And it can be very depressing to contemplate living the rest of your life without eating at least a hush puppy or two. Our chicks tell us that the carb cravings were the most severe during Induction, where the Atkins camp refers to a single bite of illegal food as "the taste of failure."

The rigid structure and food restrictions, however, also helped a lot of our low-carb chicks. If they managed to do without those periodic nibbles of forbidden fruit, many were able to get past their carb cravings entirely. Atkins also encourages portion control, because let's face it, it's just easier to say no to a third meatball than another helping of peach cobbler.

Among the low-carb chicks who quit the Atkins plan, most said the lack of choices made them want carbs even more, and they feared bingeing. And as we are three chicks who have been known to eat a four-course meal off a dessert cart, we certainly understand. The Pre-Maintenance and Maintenance phases allow more carbs, but many chicks never make it that far.

But what about the low-carb chicks who reach their goal weight? One very common mistake we chicks make is to think that we can go back to our old way of eating once the diet is over, so we make a bee-line for the nearest bakery once we're finally free. Low-carb chicks have it especially hard because they didn't lose weight by just cutting back portions of their standard fare. Having eliminated entire groups of food from their diet, they often end up feeling like they deserve a reward for all the deprivation—a reward that often involves a carb-athon filled with cake, fritters, and fluffy biscuits.

Can you stick with the Atkins plan for the rest of your life? Studies show that low-carb diets promote rapid weight loss initially, more than low-fat diets offer. These same studies also show, however, that low-carb dieters regain their weight faster than low-fat dieters. A study based on records kept by the National Weight Control Registry showed that not many low-carb dieters were able to maintain their weight loss by continuing a low-carb lifestyle, because in the end, as many fat and formerly fat chicks feel, life without starch is no life at all. Those chicks who increased carbs and reduced fat during Maintenance, and adopted a program that looks more like the South Beach plan, stood a better chance of keeping the weight off permanently.

If you're considering a carb-cutting plan, here are some of the questions and answers from our low-carb chicks about what life is really like in the land of no flour or sugar.

meet the atkins chicks

Debra from Illinois

I'm a forty-six-year-old credit support coordinator. I'm divorced with two daughters and a son, and my seventeen-year-old daughter is low-carbing with me. My parents are both diabetic and I'm hoping the Atkins diet will help me avoid that problem in my life. I lost thirty pounds once before on Atkins but picked the weight back up. This time, though, I have my daughter doing the plan with me, we're supporting each other, plus I have the support of my friends at work and at 3FC, which makes all the difference!

Rosie from New Jersey

I need strict rules when it comes to dieting. For me, it's all or nothing. Atkins helps me feel in complete control, especially where trigger foods are concerned. I am eating very healthy, more fish and veggies and I am taking vitamins. I am taking care of myself for once!

Kim from New Jersey

My biggest problem in losing weight has been the biggest problem in my life: I do not know or understand the word moderation. *I'm either all or not at all. And when I put all my effort into something, then other things have to give. So now that I am on Atkins and really trying to follow the program, my house is a mess! I've tasted pretty much everything in my lifetime. Now I need to again taste the feeling of being thin and active with my family. I am finding Atkins really works well with my lifestyle. I just need to keep reminding myself that I have a different metabolism than my husband and children and can't eat like they do. But when I am sixty my family will hopefully care less that I ate differently than they did, especially if they can look back on the bike rides we took together.*

Q: I would trade my right arm for a loaf of bread right now! I thought this diet was supposed to take away my carb cravings. Isn't there anything I can do?

3FC: All you can do is hang in there, baby! It may sound cliché, but that doesn't make it any less true. The Atkins Induction phase is based on the theory that your blood sugar needs to be stabilized in order to cut the carb cravings. If you've only been on Atkins a short time, it may take you a few more days to get past this. You may not be past the cravings until the end of this first two-week phase. So stick with it, and if you don't cheat at all, you'll have fewer cravings and the hard part will be over sooner rather than later, we promise! Nibbles of carbish foods can set you back, so it's important to fill up on protein and fats right now. Try snacking on foods like string cheese and nuts to help cut the craving, or eat smaller but more frequent meals.

The book *Atkins Essentials* says that if you haven't overcome your carb cravings by the end of Induction, you are either cheating or refusing to let go. We can buy the part about cheating—maybe you have eaten some hidden carbs that you didn't realize weren't allowed on Induction—but refusal to let go should be reserved for death or *Oprah* tickets. If you're still craving carbs, it isn't a craving, it is true love. If you're a chick who loves carbs and just can't live without them after two weeks of struggling, maybe you should just mosey on over to another chapter and see what some of the less carb-restrictive diets have to offer. This is a diet, not a chamber of horrors. It's important to remember that and find a way to lose weight that you can enjoy and that you are able to maintain long-term.

Q: Whenever I tell someone I'm following Atkins, they cringe and warn me that it's dangerous to my health. I try to explain that the studies say this is a safe diet, but they won't listen. Do I have to go through the rest of my life defending my diet?

3FC: Just the term *low-carb*, and more specifically *Atkins diet*, can elicit the same disapproving looks that are usually reserved for adultery, embezzlement, or a second slice of chocolate cheesecake. To be frank, we don't know if your friends are right or wrong. There really aren't any studies that show this type of diet to be safe long-term. The only studies that have been conducted so far lasted six months to a year. The Atkins plan and other low-carb diets have been around for a long time, but no one has been keeping score. Sure, they are effective for weight loss, but we don't know if they will increase your chances of heart disease or create other problems down the road.

Beef, for example, is a staple of the average low-carb diet, but recent studies have shown that regular meat consumption can significantly increase the risk of colon cancer. Low-carb diets are higher in fat and usually include high percentages of saturated animal fats. Studies from Cambridge University and from the *Journal of the National Cancer Institute* report that the rate of breast cancer among premenopausal women who ate the most animal fat was one-third higher than that of women who ate the least animal fat. If you are eating more of these products, then it stands to reason that you are increasing your chances of disease later on. The Atkins Foundation offers dissenting opinions about common low-carb concerns on their Web site, but they sound like they were written by a PR rep rather than a doctor. We recommend that you discuss any concerns with your physician and have regular physical exams to make sure you stay healthy.

It may be years before we really know the long-term effects of low-carb dieting. In the meantime, stick to your diet if you feel comfortable with it. Losing weight will certainly improve your health, and a low-carb diet is still a healthier option than staying fat. The next time your friends offer advice, just let them know that you are aware of the health concerns but comfortable with your choices.

Q: I've considered going on a low-carb plan, but I just don't get it. How can you eat all that fatty food and still lose weight?

3FC: That is really a very common question, and it's one that even we still wonder about a little. But the bottom line is, when we tried low-carb dieting, it really did work! Low-carb dieting isn't just butter and bacon. You can eat lean meats, seafood, salads, and plenty of vegetables. And of course, you are allowed cream, cheese, sausages, and other fatty foods, but you can eat or not eat as much saturated fat as you choose. Many experts believe low-carb dieting works because you are actually eating less than you were when you were not dieting. Since your food choices are limited, you don't have as many foods to choose from, so you eat less. Also, the protein you are eating helps keep you full longer. It takes longer to digest, so you don't get the munchies like you do when eating packages of nonfat cookies, for example. You usually end up eating less than you think. If you really can't say good-bye to bread, pick another reduced-calorie plan. The main thing is that you pick a diet you can live with.

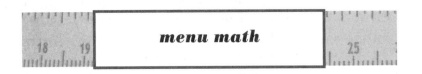

menu math

Why does cutting back on carbs help us lose weight? The answer is not magical properties in fat and protein that get us skinny, it's fewer calories. High-carb foods are often more calorie dense than the same portion of a lower-carb fruit or vegetable.

Here are some comparisons:

1 cup white, long-grain rice: 205 calories
1 cup steamed broccoli: 52 calories

1 medium baked russet potato: 168 calories
1 cup green beans: 44 calories

1 English muffin: 133 calories
1 cup sliced strawberries: 52 calories

1 hamburger bun: 120 calories
2 cups sliced cucumber: 16 calories

1 cup spaghetti: 197 calories
1 cup spaghetti squash: 42 calories

STRUTTING OUR STUFF

I followed the Induction guidelines from www.atkins.com and tried to stick to the plan as closely as possible. I chose foods from the list that I enjoyed and didn't think about the calories at all. At the end of each day, I nervously logged my daily food and assumed I'd eaten over 2,000 calories' worth of fatty foods. I was shocked to see that my average was 1,100 to 1,300 calories each day! Regardless of the lack of carbs, I was still just on another low-calorie diet. I lost about two pounds per week. I couldn't stick to the plan, though, because I thought it was too limited and I didn't think it was healthy enough for me, personally. I don't have any health issues that require me to limit carbs, and my weight is affected more by the calories I consume, and by exercise. —SUZANNE 3FC

Q: *I just started on Atkins and I'm going to a covered dish dinner. What can I take that I am allowed to eat, that doesn't scream, "Look at me; I'm on a low-carb diet!"*

3FC: We live in the South, so every potluck dinner we've ever attended involves a parade of covered dishes, all of which include some combination of rice, cream of mushroom soup, or Ritz crackers. While that would make any Junior League president proud, it doesn't do much for us Atkins chicks, and it can make our own carb-free contributions to the table very unpopular at supper. After all, what nondieter would ever pass up potato chip casserole in favor of crudités? With the proper covered dish accessories, however, you can make the tastiest dish on the table, without blowing your cover.

Low-Carb Tips for Uncertain Chicks

- Vegetables don't have to be drenched with carb-laden sauces to taste good. They can be seasoned with bacon or butter, or you can try adding olive oil and a few simple herbs or spices. Buy fresh or frozen vegetables for the best flavor.
- For crunch, you can add slivered almonds instead of corn flakes or crackers.
- Try topping your casseroles with shredded or grated Parmesan cheese. You can make nearly any vegetable into a tasty casserole by using heavy cream in place of creamy soups. See our Carbless Cauliflower Gratin on page 68.

Q: What do the shades of Ketostix mean? This morning I was deep purple, but I ate a breath mint and now I'm only light purple.

3FC: It's unlikely that your breath mint changed your test strip. Regardless, don't live by the stick. If you are in ketosis, that is good enough. The most popular theory is that color changes with hydration. Drinking extra water can lighten the shade, just as lack of water can make it darker; however, that isn't the only reason the color may change.

The shades of the pad can also change depending on factors such as foods you have recently eaten, your metabolism, recent exercise, medications, or various other medical conditions. A darker shade of purple doesn't necessarily mean you've become more of a fat-burning machine. Continue to test your stick at the same time each day. If you are losing weight, don't worry about it.

clipped wings: ketosis

Those who say you can attract more flies with honey than vinegar obviously have never been in ketosis. Pickled breath isn't your only concern. Other side effects of ketosis can include nausea, weakness, dehydration, fatigue, insomnia, and headaches. As daunting as this may sound, there are a few things you can do to ease the symptoms.

- Drink water, water, and more water!
- For nausea, try diet ginger ale.
- Get a full night's sleep on a regular basis.
- Exercise every day, even if it's only lightly.
- Chew parsley, sugar-free gum, or mints.
- Eat small meals frequently, even if you aren't hungry.
- Don't cut out caffeine all at once.
- Eat all of your available carbs each day.
- Don't be afraid of fat! Higher fat content will keep you satisfied.

Q: I'm not sure I'm getting the right amount of carbs. I'm careful, but I'm not losing weight. I'm confused about total carbs, hidden carbs, net carbs, and Net Atkins Count.

3FC: Nutrition labeling can be confusing, particularly when it comes to carbohydrates. It is possible that you are consuming more carbs and calories than you really need. The Atkins plan tracks net carbs and Net Atkins Count. Net Atkins Count, listed on Atkins products, refers to a patented clinical method that measures the average blood sugar response to individual products. If a product doesn't list a Net Atkins Count, you will have to determine the net carbs of the product. Deduct the grams of fiber from the total carbohydrates, and this will give you the net carbs. If the glycerin and sugar alcohol counts are also on the nutrition label, you can deduct those too. For whole foods and recipes, just consider total carbs minus fiber. To further confuse things, some manufacturers list "net impact carbs" or "effective carbs." Be sure to read the labeling to see exactly what their definition means, as it can vary.

Be aware also that there may be hidden carbs in your food. These could include fillers in deli meats, powdered mixes, the base for artificial sweeteners, or even alcohol. To be safe, choose the freshest whole ingredients that you can, and always read the labels. Cold cuts and packaged seafood could contain sugars as well as starches for texture and preservative purposes. Also try to limit low-carb convenience foods to occasional use, because they may contain excess calories.

more than zero

Why are there portion limits on zero-carb foods? Well, because in the world of food labels, zero doesn't always mean zero. For example, heavy cream has less than 1 carb per tablespoon serving, so the label says 0 carbs. However, two tablespoons contain 1.2 carbs, four tablespoons contain almost 3 carbs, and a pint of cream has 13 carbs! Coffee also has a little more than one carb per cup. Eggs are approximately .5 carb each, and cheese also has .5 to 1 carb per ounce, depending on what type you're eating. Easily, your zero-carb breakfast can have 8 to 10 carbs. To be safe, use a good nutrition software program to see what your true carb counts are, or follow the guidelines and limit these foods.

Q: I've been on Atkins for three weeks and I'm exhausted. With all the protein I eat, shouldn't I have more energy?

3FC: Carbohydrates are the body's main source of quick energy. Protein is converted to energy, but at a much slower pace than carbs. Are you getting enough carbs? It's easy to think that if dropping to twenty carbs is good, dropping to ten is even better, but this isn't actually the case. As carbs are our chief source of quick energy, you need at least twenty carbs a day to function effectively. Double-check your total carb intake and make sure you are getting at least twenty carbs if you are on Induction, or more if you have graduated to OWL. Also, don't eat all of your carbs in one meal. Try spreading those twenty carbs throughout your day. If you exercise a lot, you may even need to increase your carbs just a little. Try taking a multivitamin, and make sure you drink enough water. If you still don't see an improvement, see your physician, in case there is an underlying problem you don't know about.

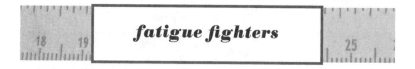

fatigue fighters

- French fries and mashed potatoes aren't the only starch villains to avoid. The couch potato can also foil your dieting efforts. Just sitting around, at the office or at home or in front of

● *Continued on next page* ●

the tube, can leave you feeling lethargic. Now, more than ever, you need to get up and move in order to revitalize yourself!

● Make sure that you're hydrated. Dr. Atkins tells us that even slight dehydration can cause fatigue, so drink up!

● Take a tip from kitty and enjoy a catnap. A short nap can be refreshing and make a huge difference in your energy levels for the rest of your day.

● Try a little afternoon delight to rev your engines. Sex gets the blood flowing and your motor humming!

Q: I only eat low-carb versions of everything. I've not had a full-carb candy bar, snack chip, or sandwich in ages! So if I'm only eating low-carb foods, why aren't I losing weight?

3FC: Many experts believe that low-carb diets work because you elimi-nate entire groups of food and so end up eating fewer calories. Low-carb plans have become so popular that manufacturers are competing for our business. Instead of doing without pasta and candy, we are eat-ing low-carb versions of pasta and candy, and ice cream, snack chips, cakes, and just about anything else you can imagine. The trouble is that we're replacing the calories, and then some. Low-carb diets are like any other diet: you have to eat less than you burn for fuel, and moderation is essential. Try counting your carbs, curbing your snacks, and eating more vegetables or other healthy foods. Pay attention to your list of in-gredients. A snack of almonds is healthier than an "energy" bar with a long list of preservatives, high-calorie fillers, and chemicals.

Q: I'm so tired of the same thing for breakfast, what else can I eat? And please don't say bacon and eggs!

3FC: We've seen some really disgusting recipes for pancakes made out of pork rinds, so we feel your pain. We think pork rinds were made for beer and ballgames, not for sugar-free syrup! We have a few alternative palate-pleasing, nontraditional breakfast ideas.

Try making hash browns using shredded zucchini instead of potatoes. Pair them with sausage for a nice change of pace. You can also try grilling a steak or other juicy meat and top with avocados, or eat leftovers from the night before. Variety is the spice of life, after all, so what's wrong with eating a little dinner for breakfast?

Another interesting idea we've come across is the infamous breakfast burrito. Use a low-carb tortilla, and fill with any combination of cheese, sausage, chopped cilantro, tomato, mushrooms, hamburger, and even bacon and eggs! Or if low-carb bread fits in with your daily carb count, toast a slice and spread with peanut butter or cream cheese and a pinch of cinnamon. In the middle of a carb craving, it'll taste as good as a Reese's cup, we guarantee. If you're really in a pinch, you can keep ready-to-drink low-carb shakes in the fridge, or have meal replacement bars handy. They aren't the best choice, but it's better than going to the Waffle House.

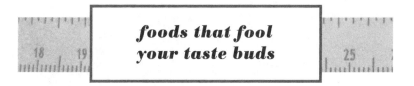

foods that fool your taste buds

We know how difficult it can be to give up your favorite high-carb foods, but there are substitutes, such as our Chocolate Almonds Diablo on page 69, that can fool your taste buds and give you an artificial and completely legal carb rush that's almost as good as the one you get after biscuits and gravy on Sunday morning. Well, almost as good anyway. Here are a few ideas from our Atkins chicks.

- I had the hardest time giving up potatoes and rice, until I discovered how versatile cauliflower was. Cooked, chopped

• *Continued on next page* •

cauliflower is great for a potato salad substitute. Cut raw cauliflower into small, rice-sized pieces, then place in a covered bowl and microwave for a few minutes. It will be mild and just like rice!

● Baking mixes are still wildly expensive and, to be honest, not all that good. If you don't mind the taste of soy flour, you're in luck! Otherwise, try nut flours. Nut flours lose something in texture but gain in taste. New low-carb tortillas and breads on the market are good.

● My downfall has always been pizza. Most low-carb pizza crusts are like disks of flavorless cardboard. I solved my problem by topping low-carb tortillas with pizza toppings and making wraps. I get all of the flavor and the good stuff without having to mentally get past the cardboard barrier.

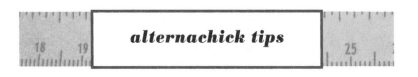

alternachick tips

If you think going low-carb is impossible without including steak, you may be surprised to learn that many vegetarians are also losing weight by following Atkins or other low-carb plans. A few of our vegetarian alternachicks shared their low-carb experiences.

I am a strict vegetarian (not vegan) and am still following the Atkins plan. It was hard at first, but each day I find something that makes it easier. I will never stop being a vegetarian, but I have to get this weight off, so I am in for the long haul. My carb cravings have virtually disappeared, and I am rarely hungry, so that is great. After the first few

*days, I realized that for every meat product on the plan, there is a vege-
tarian substitute, and they usually have low-carb contents as long as
they are not breaded.* — CHRISTY

*I've come to realize that my low-carb diet will never be as low-carb as
everyone else's. Most meat substitutes have some carbs, so it's impossible to
go very low and still get enough protein. I still feel so much better than
when I was on a high-carb diet, and I'm still losing weight.* —JANET

*I've tried the vegetarian versions of a few low-carb plans. I started on
Atkins, then I switched to Carbohydrate Addicts LP, but then I moved
on to Protein Power. I think PP is very vegetarian friendly!* — CELIA

*I tried to do a vegetarian version of Atkins, but it wasn't easy. I spent
more carbs on protein products such as tofu or beans and had to cut
back on other veggie carbs to make up for it. Since I lost some of my veggies, I added a multivitamin daily. I was never able to get a proper balance and eventually realized there was no such thing as a vegetarian
Atkins diet.* — SHELLY

---

*Q: I was drawn to the Atkins plan because of all the meat, cheese, and eggs,
but now I find out I have to eat at least four cups of veggies each day. Even
my mother couldn't get me to eat my vegetables. I can manage an occasional
salad, but anything beyond that is out of the question!*

3FC: You might have come into this diet singing your own personal ren-
dition of "Cheeseburger in Paradise," but your mother was right! It is important to get the fiber and nutrients that vegetables offer, even on a
high-protein, high-fat diet. So if you don't like plain old vegetables, do
what we do, and dress them up a little. Try our Blue Cheese and Pecan
Green Beans recipe on page 71; after all, vegetables can be as bland or as
extravagant as you like. And particularly when it comes to cauliflower
and broccoli, don't forget the power of cheese! Sprinkle everything with

a good cheese and you'll be guaranteed to clean your plate. Grilling vegetables will bring out rich, sweet flavors that will surprise you and leave you craving more. Fill a low-carb tortilla with grilled veggies and cheese for a delicious wrap sandwich. Try a vegetable and beef shish kebab for a change of pace! A little imagination can make vegetables irresistible.

And you need them. Vegetables may be your only good source of fiber while on a low-carb diet. They will help keep you regular, especially important since constipation is a common problem among low-carbers. You'll also benefit from antioxidants, which can protect you from heart disease and certain kinds of cancer.

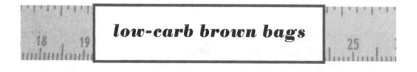

low-carb brown bags

Does your nine to five interfere with your diet? Here are some of the low-carb chicks' best ideas for easy brown bagging the low-carb way. Most of these can be brought to work in an insulated lunch bag.

- peel-and-eat shrimp
- deviled eggs
- homemade soup
- tuna/chicken salad and pork rinds (or Wasa crackers, if your diet permits)
- low-carb yogurt
- antipasto plate
- low-carb wrap rolled with Laughing Cow cheese, ham, and chopped olives
- roast beef rollups with cream cheese and roasted red peppers
- turkey BLT rollups

- veggies and dip
- salad, Caesar or garden
- egg salad on romaine hearts
- leftovers!
- string cheese and nuts

To Market, to Market

Shopping for Atkins-friendly foods can seem like a trip to the farm: you have cattle, a chicken coop, a dairy, and a lettuce patch. This means you never have to go into the potato chip barn or down the cookie row. Almost everything you really need in a supermarket can be found in the perimeter of produce, meat, and dairy. This is good news for Atkins chicks in the midst of a chocolate chip attack. If you don't get near it, you can't eat it.

As manufacturers continue to produce low-carb versions of old favorites, we may find the need to explore the inner aisles of breads, sauces, and pastas in search of labels (undoubtedly with large lettering) proclaiming low-carb status. We've trekked through the dark underbelly of carbohydrate-loaded shelves and emerged with our list of Chick Picks for the Atkins Ongoing Weight Loss stage.

- La Tortilla Factory Low-Carb Tortillas
  www.latortillafactory.com
- LeCarb
- Heinz One Carb Ketchup
  www.heinz.com

● *Continued on next page* ●

- Carbdown Flatout bread
  www.flatoutbread.com
- Atkins Morning Start bars
  www.atkins.com
- Dreamfields pasta
  www.dreamfieldsfoods.com
- Carb Options Asian Teriyaki Sauce
  www.carboptions.com
- Crystal Light Sunrise
  www.crystallight.com
- Hood Carb Countdown milk
  www.hphood.com

Q: Our family has a huge celebration every Fourth of July, complete with grilled burgers, potato salad, and apple pie à la mode. The burger part will be easy—leave off the bun. But how can I resist the potato salad and apple pie? Is it okay to break the diet, just for one day?

3FC: If you can celebrate responsibly, you may be able to go off plan every now and then. Usually, though, you will want to plan ahead and have delicious substitutes available. You have the burger covered; now you just need a side dish and a dessert. Broccoli with cheese sauce is always a hit, even for nondieters. The cheese sauce will also be yummy on the burger!

Nothing hits the spot more on the Fourth of July than a bowl of ice cream. You'll never miss the hot apple pie. Low-carb ice creams are common in every supermarket now, and they're really good! If you want to impress your guests, make our homemade ice cream on page 72 that is so rich and creamy, they'll never believe it's a diet food.

Play hard and get the most out of your holiday. Whether it's a game of touch football or a walk around the block with a loved one, this is one holiday that screams for outdoor activities. Take advantage of it, and forget about the food.

Q: I've been on the Atkins diet for almost three months. I've had a few terrible bouts of constipation, and that isn't like me! What can I do?

3FC: Grab a bottle of Metamucil and repeat after us, "This too shall pass—in twenty-four to forty-eight hours." In the meantime, start working on your water and fiber habits! You should be drinking at least eight 8-ounce glasses of water a day. Stay away from caffeinated beverages. The caffeine can dehydrate your body, making bowel movements slower. Be sure that you are eating your daily allotment of vegetables and fruit, and also try to incorporate nuts into your snacks.

You should also make an effort to fit exercise into your regular schedule. Even a twenty- to thirty-minute daily walk can make a difference in your bowel movements. Don't miss an opportunity to find a bathroom when the urge hits.

 beating the low-carb blues

Low-carbohydrate plans made the headlines again in March 2004, when scientists announced that low-carb diets, such as the Atkins program, could cause depression and mood swings. Researchers at MIT, one of the country's top research universities, discovered that high levels of carbs and low levels of proteins were key to producing enough serotonin to regulate our moods. Low-carb dieters frequently complained of depression or irritability but did not realize that their new lifestyle could be the cause. The effects were not always seen in individuals with normal serotonin levels but were noticeable in people who had had previous problems with depression or had bipolar disorder. New

● *Continued on next page* ●

low-carb dieters were surprised by the news, but some seasoned dieters experienced an "aha" moment.

If you have a history of depression or bipolar disease, you may want to reconsider choosing a low-carb diet. If you choose this route and notice any problems, consult your physician. She may decide to prescribe medication used to treat depression. Another option may be to gradually increase your carbs until you feel more comfortable. Exercise is also important for mitigating depression. One hour of aerobic exercise per day will make you feel much better, plus it will burn more calories so you reach your goal faster!

Q: Does anybody notice that her sex life has improved since starting a low-carb diet? I've been on Atkins for two months now, my sex drive has gone through the roof, and I have much stronger orgasms!

3FC: Okay, all of you fellas out there, don't make any mad dashes to Wal-Mart for a gift copy of *The Atkins Diet* for your wives before you read this, because while there are a couple of different reasons why low carbs could lead to better sex, they may not apply to everybody.

First, there is a connection between high blood sugar, or hormonal imbalances aggravated by excess weight, and low sex drive. It is a not-uncommon side effect in diabetics who have a problem controlling their blood sugar. Low sex drive, fatigue, and other unpleasant symptoms can occur. When you are on a low-carb diet, you're regulating your blood sugar much more than before you went on the diet. These symptoms can be improved by the diet, but only if you had the problems with sugar and/or hormones to begin with.

If your blood sugar and hormones are normal, then you could possibly still experience increased sexual appetite while on Atkins because of an increase in self-esteem. If you've been on a diet for two months, you're probably getting more exercise, which also stimulates libido. Losing a few extra pounds can take stress off your body and improve your confidence in how good you look in your birthday suit.

You'll experience this boost with any weight loss, not just the low-carb kind.

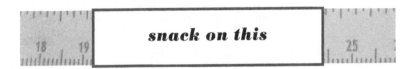

snack on this

If you're aching for some extra snacks but don't want to blow your diet, try a one-carb snack! These snacks have approximately one carb each.

- 2 ounces provolone cheese
- 8 ounces soy milk
- ½ celery stalk with 1 tablespoon of cream cheese
- 1 beef hot dog, no bun
- 6 ounces steamed crab with 2 tablespoons drawn butter
- 2 teaspoons hummus
- 1 deviled egg
- 1 cup peel-and-eat shrimp with 2 tablespoons of tartar sauce
- 1 roasted chicken breast

*atkins in
an eggshell*

Professional Counseling Yes and no. You can call Atkins information agents at a toll-free number if you have questions about

• *Continued on next page* •

the plan. Don't expect a "You go, girl!" or ribbons. This is just for nitty-gritty diet questions.

Support System There is nothing official from Atkins. You won't attend meetings, but there are countless unofficial Atkins support forums on-line, including at www.3fatchicks.com.

Fitness Factor Atkins encourages exercise throughout the program, but there is no specific exercise plan. Also, according to the American Council on Exercise, "carbohydrates are essential for an effective workout."

Family-Friendly Not very! This plan requires additional cooking for the dieter's special meals if a balanced dinner is to be fed to kids. Most pediatricians recommend that children not follow a low-carb diet.

Pros Quick weight loss, particularly in the beginning. You'll be less hungry than on some diets, as protein suppresses appetite.

Cons Restaurant choices are limited and get boring. Can be difficult to stick to long-term. The jury is still out on long-term safety.

$$ Meat and other staples are costly, and low-carb specialty foods are very expensive.

The Person This Diet Is Best For Someone who loves meat and eggs, who doesn't mind taking the extra time needed to prepare menus, and who doesn't get bored easily.

recipes from the front lines

When you're eating foods that are fat- and protein-heavy, try switching out the beef and butter for more healthful options. Here's one of our own recipes that is low in carbs and includes *good* fats from fish and olive oil.

tilapia with slow-roasted grape tomatoes

Serves 4

1 pint grape tomatoes
2 tablespoons olive oil
½ teaspoon kosher salt
2 tablespoons white wine
1 small shallot, minced (1 tablespoon)
Freshly cracked black pepper to taste
4 tilapia fillets (4 ounces each)
4 tablespoons freshly grated or shaved Parmesan cheese

Preheat oven to 325°F. Toss tomatoes with olive oil and salt in the bottom of a 2-quart shallow casserole dish. Roast in oven, uncovered, for 30 minutes. Remove pan from oven; lightly smash tomatoes with back of wooden spoon, stir in wine, shallots, and black pepper; return to oven for additional 20 minutes. Slow roasting brings out the sweetness in the tomatoes;

• *Continued on next page* •

don't be tempted to skip this step. Remove dish from oven and stir mixture. Increase heat to 400°F. Lay tilapia fillets across tomato mixture and dust with additional black pepper to taste. Return to oven for 12 to 15 minutes or until fish flakes easily with a fork. Remove fish to serving platter and spoon tomato mixture across top. Top with freshly grated or thinly shaved Parmesan and serve.

Per serving: 4 grams total carbs (3 net carbs), 198 calories, 9 grams fat, 2 grams saturated fat, 1 gram fiber, 24 grams protein

Here's a cheesy solution that helps our low-carb chicks dance to their own tune, even when everybody around them is doing the mashed potato. This is a very rich and creamy casserole, and it hits the spot when you have a hankering for potatoes.

carbless cauliflower gratin

Serves 4

Nonstick cooking spray
1 bag (16 oz) frozen cauliflower
½ cup chopped onion
¼ teaspoon salt
¼ teaspoon white pepper
1 cup shredded sharp cheddar cheese
¾ cup heavy cream

Preheat oven to 350°F. Spray a 9 × 9-inch pan with cooking spray, and set aside. Thaw cauliflower in a colander under running water. Cut any large florets into bite-sized pieces. Spread cauliflower evenly in pan. Sprinkle onion over cauliflower and season with salt and pepper. Top with the cheddar cheese, then drizzle the cream evenly over the top. Bake for 40 minutes, or until casserole is thick and golden on top.

Per serving: 9 grams total carbs (6 net carbs), 303 calories, 26 grams total fat, 16 grams saturated fat, 3 grams fiber, 10 grams protein

Here's a devilishly sweet solution, guaranteed to fool even the most indulgent sweet tooth without costing you carbs.

chocolate almonds diablo

Serves 8

Butter
3 tablespoons Splenda
1 tablespoon unsweetened cocoa powder
½ teaspoon cinnamon
1 egg white
2 teaspoons heavy cream
1 cup whole almonds

Preheat oven to 300°F. Line a baking sheet with foil and spread with enough butter to coat. Combine Splenda, cocoa, and cinnamon in a small bowl and set aside. Whisk egg white and cream in a small mixing bowl until frothy; stir in almonds. Carefully drain away excess liquid. Add dry ingredients to the almonds and stir to coat. Spread almonds on baking sheet in a

● *Continued on next page* ●

single layer. Bake for 15 to 20 minutes, until almonds are toasted and dry. Use a spatula to loosen any almonds that are stuck to foil, then cool on pan. Remove to a storage container and seal tightly.

Per serving: 7 total carbs (5 net carbs), 184 calories, 16 grams total fat, 2 grams saturated fat, 2 grams fiber, 7 grams protein

When you're deep in the trenches trying to wait out a nacho attack, let this recipe for a nacho casserole take you up over the next hill.

when-you-really-need-nachos pie

Serves 4

8 ounces shredded Monterey jack cheese
½ cup cottage cheese
1 cup chunky salsa
5 eggs
½ cup buttermilk
1 tablespoon cilantro
¼ teaspoon salt
Sour cream for garnish

Preheat oven to 350°F. Spray a pie pan with nonstick cooking spray and set aside. Combine cheeses and salsa in a medium bowl. Spread into pie pan. Add eggs and buttermilk to bowl and blend well. Add cilantro and salt. Stir, then pour over the salsa and cheese mixture. Bake approximately 40 minutes or until lightly browned and puffed in center. Garnish with sour cream.

Per serving: 8 total carbs (7 net carbs), 351 calories, 24 grams total fat, 13 grams saturated fat, 1 gram fiber, 27 grams protein

---

Dressed up with champagne mustard, salty blue cheese, and sweet pecans, these green beans have a little something for everyone.

blue cheese and pecan green beans

Serves 4

1 teaspoon champagne mustard (Dijon will work as well)
2 teaspoons red wine vinegar
1 teaspoon chopped fresh chives
1 tablespoon minced shallots (about 1 small shallot)
2 tablespoons olive oil
12 ounces fresh green beans, trimmed and cut in bite-sized
   pieces
¼ cup blue cheese
½ cup pecans

Fill a medium saucepan with 6 to 8 cups of water. Bring to a boil. Meanwhile, mix mustard, vinegar, chives, shallots, and olive oil together in a small bowl; set aside.

    Add the green beans to the boiling water, and cook at a low

● *Continued on next page* ●

boil until just tender, approximately 5 to 6 minutes. Drain beans and immediately rinse with cold water. Don't rinse for too long or the beans will get cold, and nobody likes cold green beans.

Pour the drained beans back into the saucepan. Add the oil mixture to the beans and toss to coat well. Add blue cheese and pecans and toss again. Serve immediately.

Per serving: 9 total carbs (5 net carbs), 201 calories, 18 grams total fat, 4 grams saturated fat, 4 grams fiber, 4 grams protein

Celebrate your carb independence this Fourth of July with a homemade ice cream that is so yummy, it will give your non-Atkins friends bowl envy!

apple almost ice cream

Serves 8

1 large egg
3 large egg yolks
¾ cup granulated Splenda
1 teaspoon apple pie spice
Pinch salt
3 cups heavy cream
½ teaspoon vanilla extract
1 tablespoon butter
¼ cup chopped pecans

Whisk egg, egg yolks, Splenda, ¾ teaspoon of the apple pie spice, and salt in a small bowl until well blended. Heat cream in a medium, heavy saucepan over medium-low heat, stirring constantly, until cream begins to bubble around edges and is hot. Carefully spoon a little of the hot cream into the egg mixture, whisking constantly to temper the eggs. Add a little more cream and continue to blend well. Slowly pour egg mixture into the saucepan with remaining cream, whisking thoroughly as you go. Continue to cook and stir until mixture coats the back of a spoon, about 2 or 3 minutes. Remove from heat and stir in vanilla extract. Pour mixture into a medium bowl and cover with plastic. Chill at least 4 hours or overnight.

Meanwhile, preheat oven to 325°F. Melt butter in the bottom of a small baking dish. Add pecans, stir, and then sprinkle with the remaining ¼ teaspoon apple pie spice. Toast mixture in oven for about 30 minutes or until lightly browned. Watch carefully that it does not burn. Transfer mixture to a small bowl and allow to cool until you make the ice cream.

To make ice cream: Pour chilled custard mixture into ice cream freezer and freeze according to manufacturer's directions. Add pecans during last few minutes of freezing process and allow mixture to blend evenly.

Per serving: 6 total carbs (6 net carbs), 386 calories, 39 grams fat, 22 grams saturated fat, 0 grams fiber, 4 grams protein

Words to Live By

Stressed *spelled backwards is* desserts. *Coincidence? I think not!*
— AUTHOR UNKNOWN

I worry about scientists' discovering that lettuce has been fattening all along. — ERMA BOMBECK

chicks who count

weight watchers

LET'S JUST CUT to the bottom line. Weight Watchers works. Chicks who count on Weight Watchers (WW) do lose weight, and they keep it off too, over the long haul, in greater numbers than any other dieters and all without ever having to say no to a single food group. No wonder Weight Watchers is by far one of the largest, most well-known, and most effective weight-loss programs in the world.

Weight Watchers just plain takes all the fun out of cheating, because you can eat everything that the carbo-loving heart of Dixie has to offer. You can eat fritters, pies, and yes, even those wicked potatoes, but you have to learn to eat them *in moderation*. That word just keeps cropping up everywhere, doesn't it?

Moderation is an unavoidable element in long-term weight loss, and effectively teaching their clients the art of moderation may be what makes Weight Watchers not only the biggest name but also one of the most successful programs of all time. WW teaches moderation as a life skill and gives you tools that you can use for the rest of your life, not just while you are on your way from a size 18 to a size 6.

Weight Watchers weekly meetings are the backbone of the program and almost as easy to find in Anytown USA as a Starbucks. If by some remote chance you live in a town where they don't have a Weight Watchers, you can join Weight Watchers at Home or Weight Watchers Online. These are very good substitutes for the live meetings; however, you won't be experiencing the personal contact, which is really the hallmark of this diet plan.

Some of our chicks squirmed at the thought of going to the meetings but then learned that there's really nothing to be afraid of. We'll admit that before we went to our first meeting, we half expected to find buzzing fluorescent lights with a bunch of metal chairs in a circle, and a couple of sober-looking judges with pens and clipboards standing in front of the dreaded scale just waiting to mortify us—or even worse, hand us a glass of Crystal Light and force us to sweat to the oldies.

When we finally broke down and went to our first Weight Watchers meeting, the reality couldn't have differed more from our fantasies. Weight Watchers meetings are a little like classes, where you learn all about how to lose weight and keep it off, and where you develop the sense of support and community you need to be successful.

Your Weight Watchers community is a crucial part of the program. They will be there for you when you set your goals, celebrate successes, experience setbacks, or trip over stumbling blocks. And almost as important, you will be there for them too. There is no coercion involved with this process. Nobody is forced to participate or contribute, nobody will see how much you weigh, and you won't be forced into circle time, buddy sessions, or any other involuntary socializing.

If going to the meetings just doesn't float your boat, there are other options. WW Online has duplicated almost the entire WW experience on their Web site, located at www.weightwatchers.com. You can join their program for a reasonable monthly fee. You'll have access to weekly topics and to a multitude of user guides and tips, and you can have weekly weigh-ins from the privacy of your own home, which can be a real relief to many of us shy chicks, who are more comfortable stepping on a scale in their private nest than in front of the whole coop.

If you'd like to attend a meeting, but there isn't one near you, then you can join WW at Home. This option is only for people who do not have a meeting in their area. If you subscribe, you will get all of the guidebooks and basic accessories, plus a subscription to *Weight Watchers Magazine,* along with some extra goodies so you can do everything right in your own home. You won't have a regular leader and meeting mates for support, but you will be able to call WW toll-free for six months.

Weight Watchers' latest program theme is called Turn Around, which is not to be confused with our reaction whenever we pass a sweetshop. This kind of turnaround is about turning your life around and starting off in a new and healthier direction. At Weight Watchers there are two paths, or plans, that lead to a total transformation—the big turnaround in your life.

The first is the ever-popular Flex plan. On the Flex plan you count "points" assigned to each food based on calories, fat, and fiber. All foods have a point value. The number of points that you are allowed each day is based on your weight. As you lose weight, your daily targeted number of points will decrease, since you won't need as many calories.

In addition to the daily allotment of points, you'll get more points to use as you choose throughout the week. You can earn up to twenty-eight extra "activity" points each week, just by exercising. Now that's motivation to get moving! You also get another thirty-five points each week to spend as you please, no matter how little you exercise, just because Weight Watchers loves us. If you want to spend a few points each day for small indulgences, that is perfectly fine, or you may enjoy saving them up all week to spend at one big splurge.

The second plan, the Core plan, is Weight Watchers' answer to carb-limited diets. While this isn't a low-carb plan per se, it brings together the most favorable aspects of today's popular low-carb and "good carb" diets, without sacrificing its value as a balanced diet. On Core, your eating is unlimited, as long as you eat Core-approved foods and as long (and here's that pesky moderation idea again) as you eat only until you are no longer hungry.

Like carb-focused plans, the Core plan requires self-control and discipline on our parts, because we're being trusted to understand that "unlimited" does not mean that you can approach every meal like an all-you-can-eat buffet and stuff yourself silly. In other words, we are being trusted to limit ourselves. This isn't always an easy task for us fat chicks, who still insist that the most important part of any balanced meal is seconds. Core, however, is great for chicks who don't want to be bothered with counting points, or who are comfortable with being restricted to a list of permissible foods, rather than being allowed to choose from the whole candy store.

The Core food list is also more liberal than some of the other carb-focused plans out there. You can eat in moderation potatoes (yes, *potatoes*), popcorn, rice, and other starchy foods that are strictly forbidden on other carb-controlled diets, so you actually can get the best of both worlds. But as we all know, you have to give to get, and you will be giving up some of the Flex plan food options—like sugar, alcohol, and juice—on the Core plan. You can eat these non-Core foods, but you have to use the extra weekly point allowance that is given to all members. Or you can use those activity points that you are earning from exercising each day!

Both the Core and the Flex plans give you a lot of freedom, plus extra privileges for extra effort. There's no other mainstream diet on the market today that gives you daily treats for exercising. Regardless of which Weight Watchers plan you're on, you can earn and spend those points any way your pecan-roll-loving heart desires.

All in all, Weight Watchers has the most satisfied and successful group of dieters that we have surveyed at 3fatchicks.com. The majority of dieters who left Weight Watchers did not go to another diet. Instead, they employed the tools they learned at Weight Watchers to limit their own consumption. When they started to pick up weight, they cut back. It's that simple, once you've learned the method. This is strikingly different from the experience of chicks on the wing from other diets: those chicks left diet programs and flew to another coop as fast as their wings could carry them because their old programs had not taught them the arts of moderation and portion control, as Weight Watchers had taught its fledglings. We think that WW succeeds partly because, basically, everything is allowed, as long as you eat *in moderation!*

We talked to our chicks who count about their questions, suggestions, and concerns, about why they thought they were so successful, or why they failed with this plan, and here is a little of what they had to say.

meet the chicks who count

Carol in Tennessee

I began my life skinny, as a one-pound preemie. I stayed underweight until my thirties, when I finally leveled out at a normal weight. When I reached my forties, everything changed and I became overweight. I weighed 176 when I joined Weight Watchers and then lost 33 pounds, though I regained most of it within a few years. I rejoined Weight Watchers with a new commitment and reached my goal of 135 pounds.

I'm sixty-seven years old now, and I've maintained my loss for three years. I walk four miles on my treadmill every morning, and then I plan my points for the day. I couldn't maintain my weight without either one of those routines. I eat well, and the plan is easy to follow. I know that if I continue with the meetings, I will stay at goal. I go to Weight Watchers every week as a Lifetime Member, and I always will.

The Fat Chicks Air In

Carol in Tennessee is our mom, and we are very proud of her for lots of reasons, but most recently, for her renewed commitment to good health, because we want her around forever. We love you, Mom!

• *Continued on next page* •

Dawny from Chesterfield, England

I'm thirty-five years old, married for twelve and a half years, and have a beautiful little three-year-old boy, AJ. I also have two stepdaughters, one of whom has just given us a gorgeous granddaughter, Ella. I have been attending WW meetings since January '04. It was the one New Year's resolution that I actually managed to stick to! I have lost 53½ pounds so far, with only 2 pounds to go to reach my goal weight. I feel that in some ways it has taken for ever and a day, but I know realistically that the weight is more likely to stay off if I lose it slowly. I have come to the conclusion that I will have to be a member of WW for life now, that this is a weight-loss journey that I will have to follow forever. I will always be a fat person, no matter what size the body is. I could so easily go back to how I was before, but I really have no intention of doing that if I can possibly help it. I wish all new Weight Watchers members all the luck in the world. It really does work, you know; you just have to put in a bit of time and effort.

Jill from Canada

One morning fourteen months ago I finally had an epiphany: if I didn't do something soon, I didn't even want to think about what kind of future (if any) was in store for me. Luckily I had a very caring friend who came to that first WW meeting with me. After the meeting I sat in my car and cried. I hadn't weighed myself for so long, and while I knew it would be bad, the number filled me with despair. It seemed insurmountable, but then I thought, "Well, I've got nothing else planned right now and time's going to pass either way. I might as well try this and see what happens." Before I knew it, a month had gone by with noticeable results, so I kept going . . . and going . . . and eventually it just became a way of life. And other benefits came along with the weight loss: if anyone had told me a year ago that I'd be walking, hiking, and playing tennis every week, I wouldn't have believed them. I applied for and got a wonderful new job that I never would have had the confidence to try for a year ago. You know what the very best thing is about losing this weight? Even more than looking better? It's having a feeling of control. For the first time in my life I'm controlling food instead of let-

ting food control me, and that feels better than anything I've ever tasted!

Karen from Ohio

I joined Weight Watchers in the early fall. I lost 59.8 pounds by the beginning of summer and maintained fairly well until my wedding six months later. Then I got too comfortable and gained 11 pounds back. Yuck. I have since recommitted with renewed vigor to Weight Watchers. You can see the progress in my weight tracker. This new, committed effort is being reinforced by two great friends. One has recommitted as well and the other has made her commitment for the first time. My hubby is a wonderful support and loves the evolving me. I try to keep myself on the Flex plan. I like the bottom line. There's strength for me in numbers.

Q: I'm having a difficult time working in exercise to earn activity points. Is there any other way to get them?

3FC: In a word, *no!* There is no other way to earn than to burn. Sorry. You have to work in your exercise time. It isn't just about the activity points. You need to exercise to burn fat, build muscle, and strengthen the heart. Exercise should be looked at as a permanent part of your life, like showering, eating, or cleaning. Anything you can consider "aerobic" is exercise. A heavy housecleaning session can even do the trick for beginners if you get your heart rate up. Aim for thirty to sixty minutes a day of exercise. Do it in front of the TV if you must multi-task. If you have a busy, stressful life, you may want to try Pilates or power yoga. They can relax and tone you at the same time. With enough determination, almost anybody can squeeze in a little exercise time. If necessary, start on the weekends and work up to including exercise in your busier workdays. Try to be creative, because regular exercise is as important as moderation in any long-term weight-loss plan.

reality bytes

We all know that exercise will help us lose weight, but sometimes reality just isn't enough to get us out of that recliner and onto the stepper. So the next time you're trying to summon a little motivational lift and thrust, try repeating a few of these reasons to exercise, and reach for the sky.

1. Endorphins are a natural high that last for a long time after you climb off the elliptical machine.
2. Exercise is a great stress reliever. If you're feeling wound up after a rough day at the office, work it out with a little kick-boxing cardio!
3. Muscle takes up less room than fat, so you may drop sizes even if you don't lose weight. Just imagine how great that will feel at your next weigh-in.
4. You'll be more energetic, so you won't have to work as hard to get up off the couch next time, plus the more lean muscle mass you have, the more calories you burn, even when you're lying down.
5. Exercise improves the quality of your sleep, and getting proper rest is not only important to your overall well-being but can also help stave off some extra pounds. Studies have shown that when you're tired, you eat more empty calories and store more fat.
6. You'll have less chance of acquiring certain illnesses, such as arthritis, osteoporosis, and some types of cancer.
7. Exercise is a great cure for the blues and may lessen the symptoms of depression or anxiety.
8. Exercise reduces your "bad" cholesterol level.

9. There's nothing like earning a few activity points to make you feel really good about yourself.
10. When you feel fit and toned, you just feel sexier.

i can't believe i ate the whole thing, and other weigh-in nightmares

I was buying refreshments for my son's birthday slumber party. I had bags of chips, a few two-liter bottles of soda, frozen pizzas, cookies, candy bars, and even a box of doughnuts for their breakfast. After I put everything on the belt, I looked up at the person in line behind me, and it was my Weight Watchers leader. — TONYA

When I was on Weight Watchers, I had a book with point values, and the type was so small in the book, I mistook a half of a pizza for being only three points. I ate pizza every day for two weeks. When I couldn't figure out why I was gaining at my weigh-ins, I told my group about the pizza and even showed them in the book where it said it was only three points. It turned out to be three points for one-twelfth of a pizza! — SHANNON

Q: I'm really not into being surrounded by groups of people when I step on the scale. Do I have to weigh in? Isn't there some alternative to this weekly embarrassment?

3FC: We'll give you the bad news first. Yes, you have to weigh in at the meetings. But the good news is that if you're sticking to the plan and losing weight, you're not going to feel embarrassed to step on the scale, you're going to feel proud and excited. It's tough in the beginning, we admit. But you'll be glad to know that it isn't really a public weigh-in, per se. Nobody will see your weight but the weight recorder. The number on the scale is not visible to other members, and it will never be mentioned out loud. In some classes, the scale is even segregated so that nobody even sees you get on it. And you can count on your Weight Watcher leader to be sensitive and compassionate about the process. Your fellow classmates will be too. We've all been there, or are there right now, so you should feel supported, not humiliated, no matter how much you've gained or lost each week.

Many of our Weight Watchers chicks have learned to have a lot of fun with the weigh-ins, and they get a few good laughs with each other to boot, which of course is not only therapeutic but also burns a few calories. You'll be relieved to know that the weigh-ins usually start thirty minutes before the meeting begins, so you can get there early and weigh while nobody is around. If you still really have a problem with the weigh-ins, you might consider joining Weight Watchers Online.

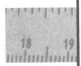 ## conquering the weigh-in jitters

In the early diet stages, when we are still wearing around the middle a few of the doughnuts left over from our former breakfast life, the thought of stepping on a scale in public is enough to send many chicks scurrying back to the coop. We asked our Weight Watchers chicks to share the rituals that they've developed to help them cope with their weigh-in jitters and climb on that scale every week anyway, to face their personal bottom line, and here are some of their thoughts.

- If they'd let me weigh naked, I would! I can't do that, so besides taking off the obvious shoes, I wear shorts under my pants when it's cold out. I always weigh in with the same shirt and shorts. I take off my pants, shoes and socks, watch, etc. No scarves, retainer, or hair pins, and I don't wear a padded or underwire bra to the meetings!
- I have weigh-in panties. I always wear them to each weigh-in, and I always have a loss. It may sound crazy, but it works!
- I exercise as hard as I can the day before the meeting. The extra sweating helps release any water retention that might be building. Of course no liquids the morning of the weigh-in, so I can get on the scale with an empty bladder! I drink coffee as soon as the weigh-in is over.
- I don't eat my extra weekly points allowance until after the meeting. I generally splurge and use them all at once.

Q: I really like the idea of eating Core, but I don't trust myself to limit myself with eating. If I could do that, I would have never gained weight in the first place.

3FC: Try a combination plan we've come up with called "Flore." Follow the Core plan, but count your daily points. You don't have to do this permanently—just until you feel you can fly on your own. What you do with these daily totals is up to you. Some members just journal in their food so they can see what they *might* have spent on points, had they been on the Flex program. Sometimes just writing down what you eat helps you control your portion.

Other members count their points and stick with their target point range from the Flex program while eating the Core foods, because they don't trust themselves with portion control, but they like the idea of the whole-grain goodness of Core. You can count your intake as you would on the Flex plan, rather than adopting the Core method of trying to set your own limits. We've found that many of our chicks don't feel comfortable with the idea of eating until they're satisfied, because satisfied is a relative term, particularly for those of us in the Captain's Platter Club of life. Sometimes a little external structure and accountability is a comforting thing, so if you don't feel you can do without that structure, don't! But as soon as you feel you're ready to try Core without counting on training wheels, we suggest that you give it a try, since you're going to have to learn how to do this eventually, if you expect to keep the weight off long-term. And why complicate a simple system unless you have to? We do need to mention that our "Flore" plan is not recognized or endorsed by Weight Watchers. This is strictly a member idea.

Q: What is the best way to use my weekly allowance points? I don't want to gain weight. That is a lot of points!

3FC: Don't worry! Be happy! Your target points are carefully calculated to accommodate the thirty-five weekly allowance points, so using them will not interfere with your weight loss. Live it up! Use those points in any way you see fit. Some chicks who feel like they don't get enough daily points even add five points to every day without impeding their progress. They might use them to beef up their breakfast, have an extra snack, or fit in a light dessert each night. Some spend points on a glass of wine and a small serving of dark chocolate, so they can indulge and boost their antioxidants at the same time. Chronic snacker chicks may save those precious five points to satisfy a bad case of the midnight munchies. Others save them up for one special dinner. Some chicks save them for a martini on the weekends, or an elaborate dessert. If staying on plan is hard for you, then you might like to use those extra points as a dangling carrot to keep you on plan for the week. If you know you can have that steak, potato, and dessert on the weekend, you have something to work toward.

To Market, to Market

If you have the munchies but don't have any extra calories to spare, try these one-point snacks and live it up without getting weighed down.

Warning Label: The bang you get for your Flex point buck may vary depending on the brand.

- 1 percent cheese single
- café au lait with ¾ cup skim milk and 1 package sweetener
- 1 cup sugar-free Jell-O and 1 tablespoon fat-free whipped topping
- 1 sheet reduced-fat graham crackers
- 1 cup grapes
- 3 cups low-fat microwave popcorn
- 1 mini bagel
- 1 bottle Yoo-hoo Lite
- 1 fresh peach
- 1 Boca Burger patty
- 2 cups vegetable juice
- 1 cup veggie chips and salsa
- 1 sugar-free Fudgsicle
- 1 Light Laughing Cow cheese wedge
- 1 Eggo waffle

Q: My friend does not recommend that I join WW because she said I can fill up the whole day on low-point junk and not get enough nutrition. She suggests I do something stricter, but I love the idea of the freedom I can have on WW. Any ideas?

3FC: Actually, your friend is wrong. There *are* nutritional guidelines to follow, so you won't lose the day to empty calories unless you break the rules. Points are only part of the program. You need to use the points wisely to get the nutrition you need.

You will have freedom on the plan, but some requirements have been laid out for you, such as the minimum number of servings for vegetables, dairy, healthy fats, and protein. Read your materials carefully so that you get as much guidance from your Weight Watchers program as possible. Even without the guidelines, all chicks should learn to be responsible for meeting their nutritional needs. You may be able to work the system to eat candy bars and spinach salads all day on Weight Watchers, but would you want to?

Q: I am going to eat dinner at my new in-laws' for Christmas and I don't want to make a big deal about my diet. How can I make the most of my feast without blowing it too badly?

3FC: By the time the end of December rolls around, after a month of seemingly endless holiday parties, you are probably ready to throw in the towel and dig in deep. You're smart to plan ahead. This one is tricky! Depending on how your new family cooks, there are various possibilities.

Side dishes are usually not light if they are served as a casserole, so try to take a pass on those if you can come away without looking like too much of a calorie grinch in Whoville. Many casseroles contain cheese, crackers, or creamy sauces, or in our neck of the woods, mini marshmallows. If vegetables are cooked without high-calorie sauces, go for the least starchy vegetable you can find, as the starchier vegetables have more calories.

Hopefully, the entrée is a roasted turkey. You can eat a good-sized portion of skinless breast meat without loading up on calories. The protein will help keep you full longer, and if you're lucky, the tryptophan in the turkey will knock you out until dessert is over. If a salad is being served, get a large portion of it and place slices of the roasted meat on top.

Go light on the bread, and skip the rolls entirely if they're drowning in butter or holiday gravy. Try to add cold salads, but limit portions from ones with mayonnaise in the sauce. Avoid desserts as much as possible. You can clear a day's points in one sweep of the dessert table, so if you do want dessert, limit yourself to one piece or bring one like our Chocolate-Covered Cherry Cake on page 100.

Q: We have a food court at my job, but only one restaurant there has nutritional values listed, and I've eaten there until I'm sick of it. What can I brown-bag that doesn't need to be microwaved?

3FC: If you can carry along an insulated lunch bag, you can generally keep things at a tolerable temperature without a microwave. Try some of these suggestions for a different taste treat that's good on the go.

- Salad with chickpeas, sunflower seeds, light dressing
- Chicken or tuna salads wrapped in a tortilla
- Cold roasted chicken, sans skin
- Pita filled with nonfat cream cheese and berries
- Pasta salad
- Salsa and nonfat dip with raw zucchini or squash
- Grapes dipped in low-fat strawberry yogurt
- Hummus with a sliced pita and fresh veggies
- Bagel with nonfat cream cheese and fruit spread

A thermos with vegetarian chili or light soup or one of our salads on pages 96–98 are also easy to bring along. Pack some whole-grain crackers for crunch. If you're tired of standard lunches, try some snack food like baked chips, light granola bars, or low-fat popcorn.

The moral of this story is don't be afraid to experiment. Break out of your comfort zone, and try some new flavors to tempt your taste buds. Variety will help keep you on plan. Take a risk; it beats eating the same thing every day, and you might find a new favorite food!

Q: I just joined Weight Watchers. I read about a plan on the Internet that will help people break a plateau, and in the plan, you cycle your points up and down every day, with one really high-point day each week. I've written down the formula for my target point range. Is it okay to do it even though I'm not on a plateau? I'd like to try and avoid one, if possible.

3FC: Weight Watchers is one of the most successful diets on the market today, and it is very simple. Give the plan a good try before you tweak it. There has been a lot of research done by professionals to come up with the healthiest and most effective program they can bring you.

Here's a little bit about the theory behind your cycling plan. First of all, cycling has been around almost as long as diets have been around. Many diets rely on cycling to help break a plateau. The goal is to trick the body into releasing fat so it won't think it is starving. By giving it a heftier portion of food unexpectedly, you make your body think the famine is over, and it isn't afraid to burn a few calories. Cycling can be done in many ways, so don't feel you need to follow a specific formula. For instance, you can change your exercise program around. If you've been walking, try doing some kickboxing. Start a weight training routine if you haven't done so already. If you've been doing the same exercise video for months, change it to another one. Simple changes like this will not only break the plateau, but it will make things more interesting for you.

Also, if you utilize your Weight Watchers program as intended, you're probably going to see some cycling regardless. You will be getting activity points for your exercise, which will vary the daily points. You will also get that extra thirty-five weekly point allowance. If you take a special meal or dessert for the bulk of that weekly allowance, you'll practically have your cycling system already done for you.

Q: I've almost hit my goal weight and I don't think I need to go to meetings anymore. What can I do that is more convenient? Should I just get an on-line support group?

3FC: Congratulations on your weight loss! We're betting that the weekly weigh-ins and meetings helped you reach your goal. Our mother taught us to not fix something if it isn't broken. If these meetings have helped you reach your goal, then it makes sense to continue so you can stay at your goal.

Our mother also taught us that weekly meetings are as important to maintenance as they are to weight loss. She goes to her meeting every week, and she's been at goal for three years. She is proud of her weight loss and loves getting free meetings as a reward for sticking with it.

We also know people who have reached their goal through gastric bypass and go to Weight Watchers for weekly support, even though they have to alter the eating plan to make it work for them. They know what millions of other dieters know: Weight Watchers has an outstanding support system, and it keeps them on their toes.

If you continue attending meetings, you will still be weighed consistently and be accountable for your gains and losses. You'll have the incentive of free meetings as long as you maintain your goal weight. You'll serve as an example to others who are trying to reach their goal, and that will be a very rewarding feeling. You'll also share good tips with your co-watchers, learn how to make it through any rough patches you might encounter, and even come home with free, tasty recipes.

Q: I stick to my points, but I'm always hungry! This just can't be enough points for me. I try to spend them wisely. I don't eat "diet cookies" or other junk food that might give me the munchies, so it must mean I need more points. Will I get used to this?

3FC: Congratulations on cutting out the junk food, but you still might be spending your points on the wrong foods. The point values are based on calories, fat, and fiber, but not on food volume. Some foods are denser and have more points for a smaller amount of food. Foods with a lot of water content usually take up more space and are more filling. For example, for two points, you could have a quarter cup of raisins or two whole cups of grapes. Differences like this spawned a diet plan called Volumetrics, which was created by Dr. Barbara Rolls, PhD. Volumetrics teaches us how we can eat lots of high-volume, low-

calorie foods and virtually stuff ourselves silly, and all for just a handful of calories or Weight Watchers points. It's easy to apply this logic to
any diet plan, including Weight Watchers. Once you learn how to
choose higher-volume, lower-calorie foods, you can easily satisfy your
appetite and stay within point range.

↗ ↗ ⋀ ⋀ ⇐ | STRUTTING OUR STUFF | ↗ ↗ ⋀ ⋀ ⇐

We asked more than a thousand chicks to talk about their
best and worst experiences with Weight Watchers, and here's
a representative sample of what our chicks are clucking
about.

- I can eat chocolate, have a beer, eat Taco John's, etc.; I just
  have to track my points for the day. I like that it's nonrestric-
  tive and easy to fit into my lifestyle.
- The flexibility is great. There are *no forbidden foods!* I can eat
  what I *like.* I have discovered that portion control is not too
  difficult once you get your mind set right. It has actually
  opened me up to a wider variety of foods than when I wasn't
  dieting. My diet consisted of the same basic foods (either
  massive quantities of unhealthy foods or healthy foods prepared in an unhealthy manner). Weight Watchers has actually opened up my world.
- I like getting weighed in. I know that sounds really weird, but
  if I have a successful week, I'm encouraged by the person
  who is weighing me. If I don't, they make me feel that I can
  still keep going.
- The meetings aren't scheduled at convenient times. They
  don't offer a wide variety of times and days. And they charge
  you even if you don't attend.

- I don't like constantly thinking about points. I wish I were able to "intuitively" know how much I should eat to maintain my weight . . . and then be able to do so!
- The biggest challenge is to not get bored. I find myself eating the same things because I know the points value.
- I hadn't realized what large portions of food I was eating before. It is hard to keep those under control.

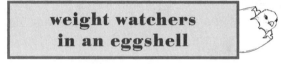

weight watchers in an eggshell

Professional Counseling Weight Watchers leaders are not required to be licensed professionals, but they are chosen very carefully. Leaders must be Lifetime Members, and they are hired and trained by the Weight Watchers organization.

Support System Weight Watchers is our favorite support system, bar none. You will be weighed, receive professionally made materials and presentations, and meet other dieters in a nonintimidating, positive, and motivational environment.

Fitness Factor Members are rewarded for exercise by an increase in the amount of food they can eat each day.

Family-Friendly Very! There are no forbidden foods, so you can eat dinner with the family, as long as you exercise portion control. While there is no child care, some meetings don't mind if you bring the little ones along.

● *Continued on next page* ●

Pros Weight Watchers has a proven method, with demonstrated success and widespread availability; the plans are simple and easy to follow and emphasize the life skill of moderation, which is essential to long-term success. There is also a Weight Watchers program designed specifically for teenagers. You can read more about these programs at www.3fatchicks.com/weightwatchers.

Cons You can eat a lot of junk food and still stay in your point range. Meetings are only once a week and you have to pay for meetings even if you miss them.

$$ Somewhat expensive. Weekly meetings start at eleven dollars and up. Some locations sell books and accessories, at reasonable prices.

The Person This Diet Is Best For A chick who has other people to please at the dinner table, or a chick who doesn't like too many restrictions or external control.

recipes from the front lines

You can put this strata in the oven to reheat before your morning regimen, and it will be hot and ready to go out the door with you to the meeting. Bring one for a friend, or reheat leftovers another time.

blueberry french bread breakfast pudding

Serves 2

1 large slice (1 ½ ounces) French bread
2 teaspoons cream cheese
2 tablespoons blueberries, fresh or frozen
¼ cup egg substitute
2 tablespoons half-and-half
2 tablespoons skim milk
1 tablespoon maple syrup
Liberal dash cinnamon
Dash nutmeg
Nonstick cooking spray
Additional maple syrup or powdered sugar (optional)

The night before serving: Spray 2 (1 cup) ramekins with cooking spray. Cut bread into ½-inch cubes and divide into two portions. Take one portion and divide it evenly between the two

* Continued on next page *

ramekins. Place one teaspoon of cream cheese on top of bread in each dish. Top with remaining bread cubes and set aside.

Combine remaining ingredients in a small bowl and blend well. Pour mixture over the bread in the ramekins, and slightly press mixture down. Cover each dish tightly with aluminum foil that has been sprayed with nonstick cooking spray. Refrigerate overnight.

The next morning: Preheat oven to 350°F. Bake covered dishes 20 minutes; remove foil and bake an additional 20 minutes, or until golden brown and firm to the touch. If desired, sift powdered sugar over tops, or serve with additional maple syrup.

Per serving: 3 WW points, 144 calories, 4 grams fat, 21 grams carbs, 1 gram fiber, 6 grams protein

---

If you can brown-bag your lunch, here are a couple of salad recipes that let mayo take a break without giving up flavor. Your taste buds will feel like you cheated, but your thighs won't!

sour cream chicken salad

Serves 2

2 cups romaine lettuce, chopped
2 chicken breasts without skin, cooked and cubed
½ cup roasted red pepper, chopped
6 tablespoons nonfat sour cream
½ teaspoon lemon juice

Salt and fresh ground pepper, to taste
2 tablespoons almond slivers

Place half the lettuce in a small bowl, or into a plastic container, if packing your lunch.

In a medium bowl, add the cubed chicken and red pepper, and toss until mixed. In a small bowl, add nonfat sour cream and lemon juice, and mix thoroughly. Add sour cream mixture to chicken and pepper mixture. Mix gently, to keep from smashing the chicken cubes. Add salt and pepper to taste.

Place half the chicken salad over each of the two servings of lettuce. Top each with half the almond slivers.

Per serving: 5 WW points, 227 calories, 6 grams fat, 10 grams carbs, 2 grams fiber, 33 grams protein

tuna potato salad

* * * * * * * * * * * * * * *

Serves 4

7 ounces canned tuna in water, drained
16 ounces canned diced potatoes, drained
¼ cup corn kernels, cooked
2 tablespoons roasted red pepper, chopped
2 tablespoons minced onion
1 teaspoon Dijon mustard
1 tablespoon white wine vinegar
2 tablespoons olive oil
2 tablespoons nonfat chicken broth

In a medium bowl, combine tuna, potatoes, corn, roasted red peppers, and onions. In a small bowl, combine remaining in-

● *Continued on next page* ●

gredients to make dressing. Toss dressing with tuna mixture. Good at room temperature or chilled.

Per serving: 4 WW points, 198 calories, 7 grams fat, 18 grams carbs, 3 grams fiber, 15 grams protein

Here's a recipe you can use whether you are on the Core plan or the Flex plan.

salmon cakes with red pepper cream

Serves 4

1 pound salmon fillets
1 teaspoon whole peppercorns
1 wedge lemon
1 medium potato, scrubbed and baked until done
½ cup diced onions
¼ teaspoon salt
Black pepper, to taste
½ teaspoon dried dill
2 egg whites
¼ cup cornmeal
½ cup roasted red pepper
½ cup nonfat sour cream
1-inch piece green onion, white part only

Preheat oven to 425°F. Spray a 9 × 13-inch pan with cooking spray and set aside.

In a large saucepan, bring a few inches of water to a boil. Add peppercorns and lemon wedge and turn down to a simmer; allow to simmer 5 minutes. Add salmon fillets and simmer 10 to 15 minutes, or until done. Remove salmon to a medium mixing bowl and set aside until cool enough to handle. Break salmon into small pieces.

Mash the baked potato in a small bowl. It should yield about one cup. Mix in the onion, salt, pepper, dill, and egg whites. Add mixture to the salmon in other bowl and blend well.

Place cornmeal in a dish. Form salmon mixture into eight patties using about ⅓ cup mixture per patty. Roll in cornmeal, then place in prepared baking pan. Bake for about 20 minutes, then turn patties over. Bake an additional 10 minutes, or until patties are lightly golden brown.

Make Red Pepper Cream:
Combine sour cream, red pepper, green onion, and salt in a food processor or blender. Whirl until well blended.

Serve each patty with a dollop of red pepper cream.

Per serving: 4 WW points, 104 calories, 3 grams fat, 20 grams carbs, 2 grams fiber, 20 grams protein

---

Here's a good recipe that our mother got at her Weight Watchers meeting! Our whole family loves it, even the ones who aren't on a diet.

miss wilma's ambrosia

. . . .

Serves 8

15-ounce can fruit cocktail, packed in light syrup
12-ounce can pineapple tidbits, packed in juice

• *Continued on next page* •

11-ounce can mandarin oranges, packed in juice
2 small boxes Jell-O brand sugar-free instant pudding mix,
    white chocolate flavor
1 cup fat-free sour cream
6 ounces Cool Whip Lite

Drain the liquids from the cans of fruit and reserve 1½ cups juice. Mix the reserved juice with the pudding mix, using a hand mixer. Beat for 30 seconds. Mix in the sour cream until blended, then fold in Cool Whip. Add fruit and stir to combine well. Chill for a few hours before serving.

Per serving: 3 WW points, 168 calories, 3 grams fat, 28 grams carbs, 1 gram fiber, 3 grams protein

---

Here's a dessert you can bring to any holiday party and no one will know you're counting points!

chocolate-covered cherry cake

Serves 16

16 ounces water pack canned cherries, drained
1 box milk chocolate cake mix
¾ cup Egg Beaters
¼ cup applesauce, unsweetened
¼ cup canola oil
½ cup cocoa powder
1 cup brown sugar
1½ cups boiling water

Preheat oven to 350°F. Spray a 9 × 13-inch baking dish with cooking spray. Spread cherries over bottom of dish; set aside.

Combine cake mix, egg substitute, applesauce, and oil in a mixing bowl and blend with electric mixer until well blended. Pour batter over cherries in pan.

Combine cocoa and brown sugar, blending well. Sprinkle mixture evenly over top of cake batter. Carefully and evenly pour the boiling water over the cake mixture. Place in oven and bake about 30 minutes, or until a cake tester inserted near center comes out clean. Do not insert cake tester all the way to bottom. Remove pan and cool slightly before serving.

Cake will make its own chocolate cherry sauce at the bottom! If desired, serve with a dollop of fat-free Cool Whip.

Per serving: 5 WW points, 227 calories, 6 grams fat, 41 grams carbs, 2 grams fiber, 3 grams protein

Words to Live By

Fat is not a moral problem. It's an oral problem.
—JANE THOMAS NOLAND

My doctor told me to stop having intimate dinners for four unless there are three other people. —ORSON WELLES

chicks by the pound

LA weight loss, jenny craig, eDiets

N O CHICK IS really an island, but when it's late at night, and the family is sleeping peacefully in the arms of a blissful sugar coma, while we're trying to fight off yet another chocolate and creamy nougat craving, many of us can start to feel like we're stranded on an uncharted desert isle in the middle of the diet ocean. And it's these isolating, Three Musketeers moments that send many of us rowing frantically back to the comfort and companionship of empty calories.

Dieting can be a lonely experience, and sometimes the most important weapon in our weight-loss arsenal is not a pair of running shoes or a bag of carrot sticks or a diet book, but a community of people who are all on that same uncharted isle with us, who can toss us a calorie-free life vest or remind us that we're not alone.

This kind of support is the basis of subscription diet programs like LA Weight Loss, Jenny Craig, or eDiets. These weight-loss plans offer a built-in cheer squad as part of their program, as well as a coach. Subscription programs will hold your hand through every pound. Some programs offer group meetings; others provide one-on-one support. Some diet services even include prepared food. With subscription programs, you can expect to be encouraged, inspired, and guided through every step of your weight-loss journey. They want you to succeed and will usually pull out all the stops to get you to your goal weight. Of course, all of this goodwill and hand-holding will also involve your letting go of some of your hard-earned money.

Why would you want to pay for help and support while you're losing weight? Can't you just follow a healthy menu and get a little exercise and seek out some support for free? Well, yes, you can. And in fact, this is what actually works best for most people. Research has shown that most people who lose weight and keep it off do so by doing their own thing. They don't sit in rooms confessing their darkest dark chocolate secrets. They don't stand on a scale while Nurse Ratched scrutinizes their progress. They don't have their meals delivered every day.

Some chicks, however, who either have busy lifestyles, find zero support at home, or lack the willpower required to beat those late-night chocolate cravings, need the structure, planning, and support that subscription plans provide in order to be successful. And that kind of success is worth more than money.

Weight-loss centers and services are popping up all over the country. Some are good, some are good and expensive, and others just want to lighten your load by lightening your wallet. It's very important, therefore, to do your research before joining a subscription program. Investigate all your options, and read all the fine print in any contract before forking over your cash. We talked to some of our chicks by the pound who have tried some or all of these programs, to find out what they had to say about the good, the bad, and the ugly sides of subscription diet programs.

meet the chicks by the pound

Jennifer from Ohio

I wasn't heavy as a kid, just kind of a bigger girl. When I finished school, I tried several times to get rid of the excess weight, but nothing seemed to work for me. I had limited success with Weight Watchers but didn't learn how to eat properly. I finally got up to 234 pounds and decided enough was enough. I had a friend at work who had amazing success with LA Weight Loss, so I decided to give it a try. I started the program in September, and I lost nearly 40 pounds by Christmas, although I've been a little stalled since then—partially because I exercise too much, and partially because sometimes I cheat. This is a plan and program I feel I can live on for the rest of my life, a true lifestyle change that I haven't been able to make in the past.

Samantha from Ohio

The Jenny Craig program may seem expensive at first, but what you get in return is priceless. Let them take over, and you will lose the weight! Having a personal consultant made all the difference for me. I never succeeded at dieting before, because I needed someone to push me along. I got that with Jenny Craig.

Leslie from Massachusetts

I absolutely love the articles on eDiets, and the best part of this diet program is that you can chat on-line with members from anywhere. At Weight Watchers you have to go to meetings once a week, but with eDiets you can talk to other members anytime you want. I find that solid support has been the biggest factor in my weight loss. In two months I have lost ten pounds safely and without starvation diets or

● *Continued on next page* ●

strenuous exercise. It is also more personal and confidential chatting with someone on-line as opposed to going to a meeting where I might feel judged or where I might compare myself to other people.

Marie from California

I like eDiets because it is much more focused than other on-line support resources; it feels more like a community than just a random bunch of people thrown together. I got involved in one of the Challenges they offer and became a team captain. It was my commitment to the team that led to a deeper commitment to the diet/exercise plan and resulted in my losing thirty pounds that I've kept off for a year now.

Marilyn from Colorado

I find eDiets has helped me tremendously to stay focused and obtain my goal. I love not having to go out in rain or snow to be weighed each week, and I can check in on a daily basis versus once a week at a meeting. I have met many interesting people who keep me on track daily. I also love the option to try their various diets and switch plans at any time. If I reach a plateau, I just try switching plans. They also have an excellent support and maintenance board.

LA WEIGHT LOSS

LA Weight Loss Centers are one of the fastest-growing franchises in America. Glitzy advertising campaigns promise an 85 percent success rate and weight losses averaging in the neighborhood of two pounds per week until you reach your goal weight. Who could ask for anything more? But yet, there is more.

LA Weight Loss offers several basic low-fat, calorie-controlled diet plans to choose from, based on your current weight as well as your weight goals. Members receive one-on-one support from a consultant three times a week at their local center. And the plan will work if you can stick to it. Sound too good to be true? Well, here's the fly in the pie. LA Weight Loss is one of the most expensive diet programs available, and it generates more negative feedback than any other diet plan in our henhouse. Here's why.

Expensive program fees and the high-pressure sales of protein bars and other products make this diet hard for a lot of our chicks to swallow. Furthermore, LAWL bases their success rates on "internal audits" not available to the public, so we don't really know what their criteria are. There are no published studies to prove their claims.

LAWL offers six weight-loss plans, called "color plans"—orange, red, blue, purple, yellow, and green—which vary in total daily calories. Food choices are based on an exchange system. You can have a certain number of servings of proteins, vegetables, fruits, dairy, fats, and starches. You are provided with lists of acceptable foods for each food exchange, so you never have to wonder what you can eat—as long as you prepare your own meals. You are also given a list of frozen dinners and selected fast-food items, along with their corresponding exchanges. On the plus side, the LAWL program calls for regular supermarket foods, and includes a detailed manual with a food list that leaves nothing in question. So far, so good, right? Well, just wait. Along with the normal foods, you are also encouraged to purchase LA Lites protein bars and other products, which can really add up. This is where they get you. The bars cost $14 per box of seven bars, and you are supposed to eat two boxes each week.

LA Weight Loss fees average $7 per week. This may sound very affordable, especially since Weight Watchers charges around $13 per week and you don't even get one-on-one counseling. The crucial difference is that you pay Weight Watchers one week at a time, and you choose how long you wish to remain a member. If you don't like the plan, you can leave and find something that suits your lifestyle better.

LAWL takes the opposite approach. You may pay only $7 per week, but you pay the entire amount up front. Your sales rep (aka consultant) will help you determine a goal weight and how many pounds you should lose. They assume you will lose two pounds per week. If you need to lose fifty pounds over twenty-five weeks, you will be charged $175 up front. *Plus* you will also be pressured to purchase a six-week stabilization period and a one-year maintenance period, also for the same $7 per week. Your $7-a-week program now will cost you a nonrefundable $581. But wait, there's more!

Your LA Lites protein bars will run you $1,596, which includes the two boxes per week until maintenance, when you drop to one box per week. You may be offered a discount on the bars if you buy in bulk. Total cost to lose fifty pounds is actually $2,177 plus the cost of groceries.

The average weight loss with Weight Watchers is also two pounds per week. At $13 per week, your total cost to lose fifty pounds would be $325 plus the cost of groceries. Once you reach and maintain your goal weight, you can attend meetings for free as a Lifetime Member.

Has the sticker shock hit yet? Then you're probably coming to your senses and wondering why anyone would choose LA Weight Loss over Weight Watchers. It wouldn't be our first choice, that's for sure. Some of the LA Weight Loss chicks on our forum liked the constant encouragement they received from the thrice-weekly meetings. Some feel that if they pay such a large amount of money in advance, they will be motivated to live up to their commitment. Many chicks really enjoy the one-on-one counseling and learn how to just say no to those pricey protein bars. Other chicks were taken by surprise by the high fees and then couldn't back out or felt so pressured they couldn't say no to the costly frills.

We talked with current and former LAWL members to get the scoop on why they love or hate programs like LA Weight Loss.

7 7 ⋏ ⋀ ⇐ | STRUTTING OUR STUFF | 7 7 ⋏ ⋀ ⇐

The Chicks Sound Off on Subscription Diet Programs

THE BEST THINGS ABOUT SUBSCRIPTION DIET PROGRAMS
- You will always have a support system at your disposal, whether in a group meeting or one-on-one.

- Professional dietitians create the meal plans, so you know you will be eating a balanced diet.
- Support sessions can be a lot of fun and make dieting less stressful and less lonely.
- Some programs include all of your food. Zap it in the microwave, toss the dish in the trash, and you're done. What could be easier?
- You are not pushed out of the nest as soon as you reach goal. Most programs walk you through a maintenance period so you will be prepared to keep the weight off.

What to watch out for

- Some plans call for long-term, very expensive contracts.
- Additional purchases of foods or products may be required and can be costly. Always check the fine print.
- Don't put too much stock in the white coats. Most counselors are not health professionals but can be former clients or any Jane or Joe who walked in off the street. Make sure you are comfortable with that, and save your health questions for your physician.
- If the plan isn't for you, it may be difficult to get out of your contract or receive a refund.
- You may not like to be weighed by other people.
- Even without a long-term contract, these programs require a regular flow of cash. If you can't afford to keep it up, you may fail the program.
- If you don't like your counselor, you may not be able to switch to a new one.
- Exercise is an important part of any weight-loss program. Some programs never even mention the word. Find out how exercise fits into your new plan before you begin.

Q: I like the counseling and the LAWL plan, but I'm going to have to tap into my kids' college fund to pay for the LA Lites bars! Can I still join this program?

3FC: If you can't afford the bars, or just plain don't want them, then by all means, don't buy them! This is a free-market economy after all, and you don't need the bars to make progress toward your goal weight. There is nothing special in those bars that will speed up your weight loss. We promise. We've talked to quite a few LAWL members who do just fine without the bars. Others choose alternate, less-expensive protein bars that are available in health food stores and supermarkets. Luna Bars seem to be a favorite replacement. They are very similar to LA Lites in nutritional value but cost just a fraction of the price. Another option is to check out eBay, where LAWL expatriates go to unload their surplus supplies. Stand up to the peer pressure, and tell your consultant to mark your file so they don't try to sell products to you again.

To Market, to Market

LA Lites Alternatives

If you don't want to buy the LA Lites but still want to include protein bars in your diet, you can buy less-expensive bars at your nearest health food store or on-line. The general rule of thumb for choosing substitutes is to look for approximately 180 calories, four grams fat, at least eight grams protein, and less than thirty grams carbohydrates. Come as close as you can to these numbers in the substitute bars that you buy, and you will be fine. Our LAWL chicks suggested these as possible alternate bars for you to choose from. Browse your health food store for more options. Most of these bars cost about half the price of LA Lites.

- Luna Bars
- AdvantEdge Morning Energy Bars
- Myoplex Lite Bars
- Powerhouse Nutrition Lean Brownie
- Sugar Free PowerBar Protein Plus
- Optimum Nutrition Complete Protein Diet Bars
- Slim-Fast Low Carb Diet Breakfast Bars

Q: I've started exercising and lifting weights and love the results! I'm losing inches, but the scale is barely budging. My consultant is upset that I'm not meeting my two-pound weekly goal. Should I stop exercising?

3FC: The rules on exercising while on LAWL seem to vary from center to center. Some members tell us they are encouraged to exercise in order to accelerate their weight loss. Others told us they were specifically told not to exercise, because any muscle gain could keep them from meeting their weekly goal. No one should dispute that exercise is good for you. It not only helps tone you during your weight loss and therefore burn more calories, but it helps you to keep the weight off later. Many LAWL chicks tell us that their success is judged by the scale only and not by inches or body fat percentage. We think you should insist that you be allowed to exercise. No one wants to be a flabby chick, no matter what the number on the scale says!

Q: I'm miserable after only four weeks on LAWL, and I want to jump ship. I need a plan that offers more flexibility, which I know I can stick to. What if I can't get out of my contract?

3FC: This is the reason prepaid diet plans are never a good idea. You probably don't know what is going to work best for *you* until you try it. It will probably be very difficult to get out of your contract with LAWL. If you paid with a credit card, you might be able to request a chargeback. Otherwise, you are stuck. You might try the plan again, but allow yourself a few healthy cheats. More than 60 percent of the LAWL members we surveyed said they cheated sometimes and still lost weight. Some people have told us that they couldn't stick with the diet plan and tried a different diet with more success, but continued to keep their appointments with their consultants since they paid for them already and positive support is always helpful. Keep in mind, though, that the consultants are not health professionals but sales reps who are paid commissions based on products they sell to you. If they are not selling anything, they lose some of the motivation to help you. Hopefully, your personal experience and your LAWL support system will be a positive one, and you can combine the consultations with your own diet for your success.

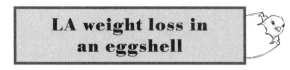

LA weight loss in an eggshell

Professional Counseling Far from it. Your counselors are usually trained in sales, not support, and may have never had to lose a pound.

Support System Regular one-on-one support with your counselor.

Fitness Factor Varies depending on your center. Some push it, some discourage it.

Family-Friendly Yes. The meals are balanced and you can use regular supermarket foods to create family-friendly recipes.

Pros The diet plan is nutritionally balanced, though nothing special.

Cons More focus on high-pressure sales than on support. Reps are encouraged to sell you something every time you walk through the door.

$$ Mind-numbingly expensive.

The Person This Diet Is Best For A chick who needs constant encouragement or pushing to stay on plan, and who has money to burn.

JENNY CRAIG

Just like Joy Behar and Kirstie Alley will tell you, Jenny Craig does it all for you. And she really does. Jenny plans. She cooks. She'll even deliver your meals right to your front door. Jenny tracks your weight, encourages you to stay on plan, and is there 24/7 when you need a little extra support. When it comes to weight loss, many chicks feel that you just can't find a better friend than Jenny.

With the Jenny Craig plan, you can visit your consultant and purchase your food in your local center. If you don't have a center near you, you can use Jenny Direct, which ships your food and offers unlimited counseling by phone. Basically, the only thing Jenny won't do is wash your fork after your meals. In fact, the only difficult part about the Jenny Craig program is paying for it. Food, products, and service plan fees make this program suitable mostly for chicks who have very thick wallets to go with their thick waists.

Food costs average between $80 and $120 per week for the full plan, which includes three meals and three snacks every day. If you have your meals delivered through Jenny Direct, you will also pay a delivery fee. Individual entrées can cost up to $6 each, which is about double the cost of a Lean Cuisine meal at your local supermarket. Satisfaction with food quality seems to vary widely from chick to chick.

Variety also seems to be an issue, as many Jenny chicks get bored after the first month. Jenny Craig introduces an average of three new dishes every year and retires less-popular options at the same time. You will supplement your Jenny meals with fresh fruits, vegetables, and dairy products that you provide. When you are about halfway to your goal weight, you can start providing your own meals one or two days a week, so that you learn how to feed yourself properly. But for the most part, you'll eat strictly Jenny Craig foods.

We have never joined Jenny Craig, but we wondered what "a day in the life of" would be like, so we ordered a trial package. Breakfast was a handful of multigrain cereal, which was tasty but not filling. Thank goodness Jenny recommends supplementing meals with fresh fruit and vegetables. We thought the cheese curl snacks were pretty good; they were lightly seasoned, not greasy, and didn't turn our fingers orange. We also tried a soup and a vegetarian dinner. The potato and garlic soup received mixed reviews. Our Jennifer shuddered and couldn't get past the second bite, believing it tasted too artificial. Suzanne enjoyed hers and thought it was definitely a step up from supermarket soup. The pasta fagioli contained a vegetarian sausage, soybeans, kidney beans, a small amount of pasta, and a specially seasoned tomato sauce. It sounded good, but it also received mixed reviews. Jennifer, transported to her childhood, smiled from fond memories that she couldn't quite place or describe. Suzanne cleared that up for her in three words: Chef Boyardee Beefaroni. Dessert was a small bag of tiny cookies that looked like they came straight out of a Happy Meal. Overall, we thought the food was okay, but it did not convince us to give up our regular diets and convert to Jennyism.

The fees for Jenny Craig are high, and this is a crucial factor for many prospective Jenny chicks. You will pay for a support plan, plus the cost of food. The Gold Plan is the lower-priced option, around $200, and covers support for six months. The Platinum Plan is the more expensive program, about $365, and lasts either a lifetime or three years, depending on the rules in your state. Both plans include one-on-one support from your consultant, either in a center or over the phone. There are no group meetings, à la Weight Watchers. You get personal attention from your consultant, who will offer suggestions and encouragement to help you reach your goals. And Jenny frequently offers short trial memberships at a low cost, so you can try them out before you commit to anything long-term.

For the most part, the Jenny Craig program is well planned and leaves little room for error. They literally do everything for you, from meal planning and cooking to cheering you along. This plan is appealing for anyone who needs strict structure or convenience. Most people probably won't need this level of hand-holding. Those who do need it and can afford the program usually stick it out long enough to see some significant weight loss.

The number one complaint we've noticed is the expense of the food. Most Jenny Craig members are very happy with the program, though there are a few out there who have less than positive experiences to share.

Q: I just started the Jenny Craig program but am not sure I can afford the meals. Lean Cuisine dinners cost about half of what Jenny meals cost. Can I buy my own food and still be successful?

3FC: Part of the success of the Jenny Craig program stems from the fact that they control your food for you, until you learn how to make better food choices on your own. Plus, because Jenny provides in advance only as many meals and snacks as you'll need, you don't have an unlimited supply and are not likely to overeat. Besides, at these prices, who can afford seconds? Being on Jenny Craig is a little like being stranded on an island: you know the next airdrop of food will not come for two more weeks, so you make your supply last. If you know you can hop on a raft and go to the next island for more supplies, you may be more inclined to eat additional foods that you don't need. The high price you pay is not just for the food but also for the external portion control and the peace of mind that comes from letting somebody else make the hard decisions for you.

When you are halfway through the program, you can move to Halfway Days, where you buy only part of your food from Jenny, the rest from your local supermarket. By then you will have learned enough about self-control to be in charge. You will also be motivated by the weight you've lost to stay on track, but until then it's a good idea to stick with Jenny.

If your budget or your appetite truly can't wait, try buying a small quantity of frozen dinners to keep on hand, and see how you do. Your Jenny Craig counselor understands budget issues and will work with you. You will also need to be aware of the exchange system and make sure the new meals fit in your program. Your counselor will help you to gradually increase the frequency of your own meals until you feel comfortable that you are in charge and are not going to hop on a raft and row in the direction of the nearest all-you-can-eat luau.

Q: I joined Jenny Craig to lose weight for my class reunion, and I worked hard to reach my goal. I ignored the advice of my consultant and ate strictly Jenny Craig food the entire time to make sure I met my goal quickly. It paid off when all of my classmates were surprised by how hot I looked! Now that the reunion has passed, I've tried to keep the weight off, but I can't seem to make the right choices. I'm quickly regaining the weight. Will I have to re-join Jenny for life just to keep the weight off?

3FC: The Jenny Craig program makes it easy to lose weight, because they do everything for you. At some point, though, you have to learn how to take control of your eating, and this is where the Halfway Days come in. Jenny teaches you how to eat, but you have to do your part too. You skipped a crucial phase in your weight-loss journey, which would have prepared you for maintenance. Talk to your counselor about going back, and don't take any shortcuts this time.

Consider rethinking your goals, as well. Reunions, weddings, and other special dates are fine for smaller short-term goals, but they don't keep you motivated after that magical date has passed. Think about how much healthier you feel now. Make it your goal to keep that feeling long-term. Above all else, don't let go of the wonderful feeling that you had at your reunion. You were a hot chick then, and you can stay that way!

Q: I love the packaged entrées and soups, but my whole family hates vegetables and we never eat them. Even President George H. W. Bush refused to eat broccoli! My counselor says I need to change my habits and eat more veggies because the entrées alone are not enough.

3FC: It may not have been the broccoli that moved President Bush to ban it from White House menus and even Air Force One; it might have been his broccoli chef. Bland, overcooked veggies are certainly not a meal for a president, or a fat chick on a diet! But if you experiment with cooking techniques and seasonings, you may be surprised with what you come up with. Many of our members have shared tips for improving on Mother Nature when it comes to vegetables. We *love* oven-roasted vegetables and veggies cooked on the grill. These methods bring out new, richer flavors that you didn't know were there. Condiments such as soy sauce or some of the Jenny Craig sauces are also perfect for adding new depth to the flavors in everything from broccoli to zucchini. Don't be afraid to experiment!

Q: I'm bored with the food selections in Jenny's kitchen. It's becoming more and more difficult to stick to the program. What should I do?

3FC: Boredom can be a real diet buster! There are several things you can do to add variety to your meals without straying from plan. It's better for you to keep eating the Jenny Craig foods, but you can change them somewhat by seasoning with spices or Jenny-approved sauces. Make use of the list of unlimited free foods; for instance, add some roasted red peppers to the JC chili, to add sweetness and additional flavor. Consider using a Jenny Craig cookbook to prepare, with your consultant's advice, recipes that will fit into your plan. Freeze leftovers to liven up another boring day. If you think more creatively in the kitchen and the market, you will eat more creatively.

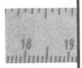

> ## *jenny craig recipe for success*

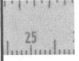

Since Jenny cooks all of your meals for you, you'll never have to don an apron in the kitchen. So instead of offering a recipe for this diet plan, we thought we'd share a few ingredients to help make this plan a success!

- If the meals become monotonous after a while, try changing your environment instead. Buy a few special dishes, a new tablecloth, and even pull out the candles and music. Make your meals seem like special treats, even if this is the seventh time you've had Jenny's Personal Pizza this month!
- Take advantage of your counselor—in a good way. Never skip a session, use all the time you have available, and don't be afraid to open up about your diet concerns or slipups. Your counselor's goal is to help you succeed, so let her.
- While Jenny doesn't offer an exercise plan, you can try an online program like www.eFitness.com, join a gym, or just get out and stroll the neighborhood. The important thing is to get moving and not just depend on the diet to get you to goal.
- Birds of a feather flock together. Look locally or on-line for other Jenny Craig members and make new diet buddies. You can share insider tips and advice that you won't find anywhere else.

Q: I'm apprehensive about joining a plan where I will have to see a personal counselor, but I also think I need someone to seriously kick me in my 4X pants. This is embarrassing. I don't even want anyone to know how much I weigh. Will I have to share my weight and eating habits with a lot of people?

3FC: Don't worry; you won't have to weigh in with a group of people on Jenny Craig, just your consultant. You can also ask to see the same consultant every time if it makes you more comfortable. Don't think twice about letting them know how much you weigh. They can probably make a good guess just by looking at you, anyway. Many JC consultants are former clients, so chances are that they were once a 4X too! The first weigh-in is always the hardest. You'll come to look forward to future weigh-ins because it's an opportunity to see the pounds drop off. Don't be afraid to jump in there. Take off your shoes, jacket, jewelry, and spit out your gum, then hop on that scale! Get to know your consultant and make her your best friend away from home. Blurt it all out, honey, and make the most of it, because you're paying for it, and Jenny's one-on-one support doesn't come cheap. Try to overcome your fears and take full advantage, so you are sure to get your money's worth.

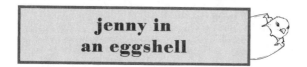

jenny in an eggshell

Professional Counseling Sort of. You can see your counselor any time or have access to a counselor 24/7 by phone. However, they are not health professionals; they are usually people just like you who have lost weight and know the Jenny Craig system inside and out.

Support System Just the one-on-one support from your counselor. You can join their free on-line forum if you want support from other members. You can find more Jenny Craig resources at www.3fatchicks.com/jennycraig.

Fitness Factor Exercise is encouraged, but they do not offer a specific exercise plan. You're on your own.

● *Continued on next page* ●

Family-Friendly No. All meals come in little single-serving packages. You'll still have to cook for the rest of your family.

Pros Meals are prepackaged, so you can't overeat. You never have to worry about what you should or can eat.

Cons You don't learn how to make your own choices until you are halfway to goal, when you are allowed to have occasional meals on your own. Meanwhile, what will you do if your FedEx shipment of food gets diverted to Alaska? Additionally, the food isn't all so fabulous.

$$ Very expensive. The food costs make Jenny Craig one of the most expensive diet plans available.

The Person This Diet Is Best For The chick who doesn't like or need to cook, doesn't want to worry about planning meals, and doesn't mind paying for the luxury.

eDIETS

The eDiets plan is an interactive on-line dieting program that you can mold to fit your lifestyle. It is totally Internet-based, which is handy for many of us who are shy about stepping on a scale in front of a crowd each week. The eDiets system has a well-rounded approach to healthy weight loss, including menu plans, recipes, support groups, and fitness plans. Their Web site can be overwhelming at first thanks to the massive amount of content available; however, if you give it a little time, you'll be finding your way around quickly. This program simplifies much of your diet, whether you initially choose a program that works for you or you need to switch diets. If you want to eat vegetarian, low-carb, or low-fat, or even just delete a certain species from your diet, you can let eDiets do the work for you. You can choose from eDiets' own programs, or you can choose a commercial plan that they have incorporated into their program, such as Atkins, Eating for Life, or Bob Greene's Total Body Makeover. We've been waiting patiently for eDiets to include a Krispy Kreme or a Burger King plan, but that hasn't happened yet.

The great part about eDiets is that you can change your diet plan anytime, as often as you want. It's a very flexible approach to dieting. If you check out a menu and see that it isn't for you, just click to another diet plan to find a menu you can live with.

The core of eDiets is the total nutrition planning that they create for the dieter. The dieter inputs her weight, goal weight, height, activity level, and a few more pertinent items, and then chooses from one of the many diets that are suggested. Based on your weight-loss goals, a plan will be developed for you with the proper amount of calories. Then eDiets creates your entire menu and even a shopping list for the next week, based on your individual practical and physical requirements, including satisfaction and convenience. You can even choose meals from fast-food restaurants for any meal of the week. Sounds easy, but what if you don't like what they plan for you? Just click a button and you can choose from a list of substitutes. Just print your shopping list and you're all set!

Like all good diet plans, eDiets recommends regular exercise. Their fitness section will help you plan a workout regimen based on your goals and abilities. It also shows you how to do exercises with a virtual trainer. And take it from us, he's really inspirational. We accidentally left our screen on, and when we came back three hours later, he was still doing sit-ups. Just imagine the virtual abs he must have! If you don't like or cannot do one of the prescribed exercises, you can trade it for another one. Just like the eMenus, the exercise routines offer great flexibility.

On eDiets you can also get a full-course support system. If you subscribe to this section, you will have access to message boards for all of the plans they offer, plus special boards created for group efforts, motivation, exercise, recipes, and more. Chat rooms are also available, and eDiets has chats scheduled several times a day so you can chat with the eDiets staff and guest speakers on various subjects.

Finally, there is an exhaustive recipe area on eDiets. If you subscribe, you will have access to over 2,000 diet-approved recipes. Here you can print recipes and compile grocery lists for your chosen dishes. This is a big time saver, so you can more easily fit in all those exercise sessions you've been putting off!

The eDiets program is going to cost you anywhere from approximately two to ten dollars a week, depending on how many extras you choose. We've all been spoiled at some point by freebies on the Internet, but sometimes you really do get what you pay for.

Q: I just signed up to eDiets, but there is no way I can afford to eat like this. The cost of produce and all of the extra meat is just too high for my budget.

3FC: If lean meat, fruit, and vegetables seem too expensive, then perhaps you need to take a closer look at your household budget. If you've been feeding your family boxed dinners and family-sized budget frozen dinners, then yes, maybe you will wind up spending a little more for fresh, quality food, but consider what you'll be eliminating from your budget each week. No longer will you have to dip into your wallet for indulgences like chips, ice cream, cakes, burgers, pizza, soft drinks, candy, alcoholic beverages, or frozen snack foods. And because healthier food means healthier bodies, you will probably spend less in medical costs. Besides, health is always a sound investment and can mean the difference between paying the grocery store now or the cardiologist later. And cardiologists cost a lot more than broccoli.

how to eDiet without going eBroke

Here's a few tips from our eChicks about how to stay on plan, and on budget.

1. Pick one snack from your menu and repeat that through the week. It's cheaper to buy one or two items to split for several days than to buy five cartons and barely touch them.

2. Buy your vegetables at a farmers' market or roadside stand. Save money and get fresher ingredients.

3. Purchase frozen produce when possible. Stock up during sales and cut your produce expenses in half compared to fresh produce.

4. Choose recipes that use beans and tofu for a meat replacement. You can save up to 75 percent of your entrée expenses by doing this.

5. Buy the Sunday paper each week to check the sale pages. Find the one grocery store that has the best overall savings based on your grocery list.

6. After you print your shopping list, go through your cabinets and see what you already have, then mark that off your list.

7. Buy spices in bulk at a co-op or your local health food store. A small scoop in a baggie can be bought for mere cents, compared to several dollars for a full jar.

8. Buy large quantities of freezable foods when on sale. To keep organized, date each item with a freezer marker before placing in the freezer, and mark it again when you thaw it.

9. Don't buy specialty products. Bars, shakes, candy, or "diet" brands can often be replaced by similar products.

10. Experiment with substitutions. If raspberries are four dollars a pint, try two-dollar strawberries instead.

Q: I can use free message boards all over the Internet. Why should I pay extra here to chat at eDiets?

3FC: You are right, there are many large, free message boards on the Internet, including 3fatchicks.com! Personally, we three chicks are as happy as pigs in mud at 3FC, however, with eDiets you will have the convenience of having this message board at your fingertips while you are checking your menu, entering your statistics, or choosing a workout routine. You may be more inclined to visit them, and participate in them, if you are a paying customer. We've always found at 3FC that more involvement with our support group helps us stick with our program in the hard times.

Unlike many free support systems, eDiets has several chats each day with professionals from various fields, like registered dietitians, psychologists, and fitness trainers. We've found that these chat rooms are not utilized nearly as much as they could be. In many circumstances, the chat rooms are nearly empty, and sometimes chats are even canceled for lack of attendance. These are prime opportunities to pick the brains of the minds that can help you succeed. The eDiets site has a paid staff, so you are paying for their licensure and knowledge. Free sites, such as ours at 3fatchicks.com, have volunteer administrators and moderators, who are less likely to cut your meat for you before you eat it.

Q: I find eDiets always has something for sale, and the last time I bought something, I got a lot more than I bargained for. This was kind of a turnoff. Are they really interested in helping me drop my pounds or just my money?

3FC: Certainly eDiets can seem a lot like a virtual shopping mall, and there are plenty of ways to click away your hard-earned cash. This is, after all, an extensive site with many licensed professionals on staff to pay for. Weight loss is a billion-dollar industry, and people who are in this business are in it to make a profit. But that doesn't necessarily mean that they aren't offering a valuable service, and of course, moderation isn't a bad idea when it comes to shopping either.

The program's one-stop shopping design, which allows you to do all your diet-related business in one place, is part of what makes eDiets so popular. The eDiet "mall" includes not only support and planning, but a store offering diet foods, snacks, exercise equipment, videos, books, supplements, and beauty products. This is ultraconvenient for busy chicks who just don't have the time to shop around and don't mind paying a little more for the convenience.

And, of course, dieters are prone to impulse shopping for diet products, so we make great customers. Just be cautious and, as you're learning to do during a Big Mac attack, try to control your impulses. There may be fifty ways to lose your blubber, but you only need to try them one at a time. Just because you signed up for a new diet doesn't mean you need to buy multiple diet foods, exercise videos, magazines, supplements, and cookbooks. Take it one step at a time and don't burn up your resolve—or your budget—in the first two weeks.

buyer beware

Seventy-one percent of chicks who left eDiets did not think it was worth the fee or were unhappy with other financial practices; however, when we sampled eDiets ourselves, we found it to be rather straightforward regarding costs, and we had no surprises when the credit card bill came. With any on-line purchase, though, you need to read what you are buying. The most common complaints among our eChicks:

- The initial fee is $1.99 a week, but subscribers did not read that it was billed quarterly and were unpleasantly surprised to find $25 on the credit card statement.
- Dieters signed up for the main plan only, but when checking out, found the premium plans in the shopping cart. These plans had to be deselected or would be purchased. Some di-

● *Continued on next page* ●

eters clicked through without paying attention and unintentionally bought the larger packages.

- Some dieters were not happy that all of the programs were billed separately. The plans looked inexpensive, but they added up when purchased.
- Some felt that they were tempted with diet candy or similar products while searching the site for support to get past their sweet tooth and snacking issues.
- Dieters felt that it was too easy to buy the extra products because their billing information was stored in their account; in a weak moment they could make impulse purchases without ever leaving their chair.

Q: Why shouldn't I just print my menus or buy frozen dinners and quit? I can do the same thing on my own.

3FC: One of the things that we eChicks love most about eDiets is the convenience of having meals that are readily available and easily changed. You can make changes right up to mealtime. You can even change the whole diet plan right up to mealtime. Having such a flexible program, which will conform to fluctuating moods, helps you cater to the finicky chick in us all and makes it less likely that we will quit. In our view, that is worth every penny we spent. After you have been on eDiets for a few weeks, you just might get the hang of it and be ready to start doing things on your own. If you do, just be aware that you've lost a solid support system, accountability with weigh-ins, the assurance that your daily calories are balanced and nutritious, along with all of the multiple resources that were at your fingertips on eDiets. Make sure you can find replacements for these as well, or you may find you aren't as successful with your weight loss as you had hoped.

eDiets recipe for success

We tried to come up with a smashing meal for eDiets, but the only recipe we could find that was acceptable on all plans was boiling water. Instead, here are our best tips for using eDiets to help you succeed at weight loss:

1. Utilize the meal plans for restricted diets. Sometimes when we don't have a lot to choose from, meal planning can look bleak, even though we have many possibilities before us. For instance, when Suzanne tried Atkins, even though she had a fridge full of acceptable foods, she could only manage to come up with salad for breakfast one morning. If she had had eDiets, she might have had mock French toast or a basil frittata!

2. Maximize your fitness possibilities through on-line chats with eDiets' own personal trainers. Are you stuck in an exercise rut? Don't know the difference between a Swiss ball and a medicine ball? You can get a fresh new approach to fitness and find answers to any question you may have in one of eDiets' scheduled chats.

3. Do you need a helping hand to keep you on your diet? Sign up for a mentor. You'll have somebody to help you through the rough patches and cheer you along the way. After you are on the road to success, sign up to pay it forward and mentor someone who was once in your shoes.

Q: When it comes to helping me make good choices at fast-food joints, eDiets is really great, but what can I order when I'm going out to a fancier place?

3FC: You're right, eDiets does a great job helping you to work fast-food restaurants into your meal plan, but they don't list many full-service restaurants, so here are a few pointers from our eChicks, to help you dine out without bombing out.

1. Arm yourself with a restaurant nutrition guide to make your best choices for the plan you are on. Most chain restaurants offer nutritional information if you ask.

2. Go all the way and eat at an elegant restaurant. It will be harder to overeat with ornate stemware and fancy dishes.

3. Keep a couple of small pieces of chocolate by the plate. When you feel satisfied, push your plate back and eat the chocolate. This gets the taste for dinner out of your mouth, and the dessert signals the body that it is through eating.

4. Want seconds? Make it a dinner salad with light dressing, and hold the cheese.

5. Score your plate into halves. When you've finished your half, pop a strong mint or cinnamon gum into your mouth and kill those pesky taste buds for a few minutes. When it comes to eating moderately, Altoids can be your best friend.

6. Find the best-looking waiter in the place, then ask to sit in his station. Stud muffins have zero calories.

7. Ask for vegetables on the side instead of potatoes or pasta. Unless it is a casserole, you are almost guaranteed fewer calories.

8. Ask if the baked potatoes are oiled or buttered before they are baked, and avoid them if they're swimming in fat.

9. Remember that condiments are an accent, not an entrée!

10. Ask your server to bring half your meal on the plate and pack the other half to go.

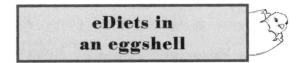

**eDiets in
an eggshell**

Professional Counseling With your paid subscription, you will have access to dietitians, personal trainers, psychologists, and more.

Support System The program has an excellent chat network and message forum, for an additional fee. You can read more about what eDiets has to offer at www.3fatchicks.com/ediets.

Fitness Factor Motivation and instruction are available to get your body moving, as well as an interactive fitness system that will teach you to exercise.

Family-Friendly Yes. You can pick and choose your menu, plus switch out meal plans for other dishes your family can eat.

Pros A wide variety of diets to choose from. Great daily menus with instant shopping lists.

Cons Everything has a price tag. Advertisements for their extra services at every corner.

$$ It is reasonably priced for the basic program, but all of the options are extra, which can be expensive in the end.

The Person This Diet Is Best For The impatient dieter who hops around to different diets, or the person who spends a lot of time at the computer.

recipes from the front lines

The LA Weight Loss plan calls for a lot of simple but healthy foods, such as lots of vegetables and lean meats, but it can get boring. Here's something to spice up your life—or at least your dinner!

hot and spicy buzzard

Serves 2

½ cup low-carb ketchup (we like Heinz)
¼ cup Worcestershire sauce
¼ teaspoon crushed garlic
4 teaspoons finely minced sweet onion
¼ teaspoon dry mustard powder
1 teaspoon dried thyme
¼ teaspoon coarse fresh cracked black pepper
1 extra-large buzzard breast (may substitute 1 pound boneless, skinless chicken breasts if buzzard is not available)

Preheat oven to 350°F. Combine all ingredients, except buzzard, in a small bowl. Place buzzard in a glass baking dish and rub half of sauce over the breast, turning to coat, and reserve remaining sauce. Cover dish with foil and bake for 20 minutes. Remove foil, turn buzzard over, and continue to bake for an additional 20 to 30 minutes or until breast tests done. Spoon remaining sauce over breast and serve. Be careful, it bites!

Words to Live By

I haven't trusted polls since I read that 62 percent of women had affairs during their lunch hour. I've never met a woman in my life who would give up lunch for sex. —ERMA BOMBECK

A positive attitude may not solve all your problems, but it will annoy enough people to make it worth the effort. —HERM ALBRIGHT

fit chicks

8 minutes in the morning,
body for life, curves

EVER SINCE JANE FONDA encouraged us in her *Complete Work-out* series to "feel the burn," some of us chicks have been pulling out the spandex and the leg warmers and the color-coordinated sweatbands to start programs that emphasize exercise, rather than diet, as the main focus of our weight-loss strategy.

Most other diet plans focus on the food and build in enough activity to make sure you don't eat more than you can burn. Exercise-driven weight-loss programs, however, take exercise to a new level; they help you lose weight through targeted and regular activity, accompanied by diet guidelines.

When you actually put down the remote control and go to select an exercise-driven diet plan, though, things can get kind of confusing. When you first enter the world of commercial fitness, you can feel like you've just landed on Planet Infomercial, full of enthusiastic bumper stickers that promise everything from radically improved health to instant beauty to spiritual enlightenment in no time flat. "Work out for just thirty minutes, three times a week, and realize your wildest weight-loss goals!" "Transform your body, your mind, your spirit, inside and out, in just twelve easy weeks!" All these glowing promises can really make a fat chick's head spin. So how do you determine who is telling the truth and who is trying to sell you some prime swamp land in Florida?

We've found that when it comes to the glowing adjectives and purple promises of the weight-loss industry, it's best to take a step back and look at "just the facts, ma'am." And fact number one is that regardless of the weight-loss plan you choose, you are going to have to exercise. Yes, it's true; you have to move to lose. And we've heard all the excuses, so don't even bother. We know it's difficult to work all day, cook, clean, take care of kids, shop, run errands, and do all the other things that life calls for. However, the fundamental laws of physics say that if we don't exercise, we aren't going to live as long, as happily, or as healthfully as we could.

We three were never too crazy about exercise. And that is an understatement. Until just a few years ago, our experience with exercise was limited to two items. One was a pink spring-loaded contraption we squeezed while we chanted, "We must, we must, we must increase our bust!" The other was a stylish brown nylon rope thingy connected with pulleys that hung on our doorknob. We attached all of our limbs at once, and "toned" ourselves by pulling them back and forth. We mostly just got our heart rate up by screaming, "Don't open the door!" whenever anyone walked by.

This must sound like the typical "When we were your age, we had to walk ten miles to school barefoot!" And, in fact, that's not far off, because we really are living in a new and improved fitness world. These days, fortunately, there are plenty of programs and devices that are exciting, convenient, efficient, and effective, and you won't wind up on the wrong side of a door jamb.

For one thing, gyms aren't the high-pressure scenes that they used to be. There have also been a lot of improvements in gym culture, which is good news for all of us timid gym bunnies who have been shying away from fitness centers because we remember the high-pressure social clubs of the eighties. There is still some socializing, and some pretty staggering six-pack abs, but overall, people in gyms are answering a health alert these days, and not a booty call.

There are also women-only facilities now, and hospitals now feature wellness centers frequented by doctors and other health-related employees, who are there, by and large, for the health benefits. What safer place to test your limits on a treadmill than surrounded by cardiologists! And of course, there are great programs you can do right in the privacy of your own home.

Whether you are selecting an exercise-driven weight-loss program or just an exercise program that will complement your diet-driven program, here are some things we think are important to consider:

- Pick a program that emphasizes fat burning, not just weight loss.
- It's best to find a regimen that is designed or at least has been tweaked for a woman.
- Some programs offer options or solutions for larger women with special fitness needs.
- If you're just starting out on a fitness regimen, pick a program that's good for beginners but offers room to grow.
- It's important to find a plan that emphasizes balanced nutrition for overall fitness and energy levels.
- Always consult with your doctor before beginning any fitness regimen.

And bear in mind . . .

- Results are not always quick.
- Fitness requires dedication and perseverance. If you slack off too soon, you will lose any benefits you gained and end up at square one again.
- Be patient. You may have to experiment to find the right combination of diet and exercise to be effective for you.

- Some plans, like Curves, may not grow with you as you lose weight and increase your fitness level, so you may need to change programs or join a traditional gym.
- Since you will be building muscle as you burn fat, you may not see a dramatic drop in pounds, but you will lose inches. If you want to see progress, instead of stepping on a scale, check yourself with a tape measure or watch your clothing sizes drop.
- Reaching your goal weight doesn't mean that you're finished. Maintaining a fit body with exercise is a lifelong commitment. Use it or lose it.

In this chapter, we will guide you through some of the most popular weight-loss fitness programs available today: 8 Minutes in the Morning, Body for Life, Body for Life for Women, and Curves. To help us get our finger on the pulse of these popular programs, we asked our fit chicks to share some of their thoughts and experiences about what worked and what didn't work for them.

Although there are positives and negatives to all exercise-driven weight-loss programs, one thing is true no matter which regimen you choose: when it comes to exercise, there are no excuses! Some studies show that around 90 percent of women who lose weight and keep it off long-term do so by incorporating exercise into their diet programs. Those who stop dieting and exercising after they reach goal often regain their weight. Exercise isn't a temporary solution, it is a commitment, and the benefits are countless! So the good news is that much of the hype you hear and read is true. You really can protect your bones, fight your flab, boost your metabolism, burn calories, help ward off disease, improve your sex life, and find greater peace of mind, all through regular exercise. And all you have to do is get up off that couch and start moving to the music!

meet the fit chicks

Ilene from Ontario

At forty-eight, I am in better shape than I was in my late twenties, when I first discovered exercising after quitting smoking. Presently I run and weight-train three to four times a week. In the summer I bike and Rollerblade too. Exercise, along with eating five to six healthy meals per day, has kept my weight stable. I love to see people starting an exercise plan and I am especially happy when I see that they enjoy it and are eventually hooked! I'm an exercise junkie now and I want everyone else to be one too. Make sure the exercise you do is fun though, because it is for a lifetime!

Tiki from Michigan

I've had success in the past doing just cardio, but I ended up with a smaller, squishier version of me and that isn't what I want. I want nice leg muscles that can help me teach my cheer team their jumps, strong arms so I can do push-ups with my son, and the exercise that builds my muscles will also help to build my bones and protect them from osteoporosis. With strength training, I'm down from the 170s to 156. The goal is a solid 135. I like having some curves on my body.

Jo from Wyoming

I was overweight simply because I got too busy doing other things and failed to pay attention to what I ate. I am finding maintenance difficult since old habits die hard. It is nice to be a smaller size, to be able to do more things, and to be able to shop in the ladies department rather than the XXX sizes. And above all things, I do not want to regain any of the weight I have lost. I joined Curves for Women and am enjoying it. This past year I went through a series of radiation treatments. I am convinced that eating properly and exercising regularly helped me through it all. I formed the habit of going directly to Curves for my exer-

● *Continued on next page* ●

cise right after each radiation treatment. That was a good stress buster. At seventy-nine years of age, I believe that we can lose weight and maintain that loss at any age, and we can keep smiling along the way.

Melanie from Pennsylvania

I'd heard of a program called Body for Life, which was based on heavy lifting and eating six small meals a day. The before-after pictures promised me exactly what I wanted. We had plenty of weights at home, so I started. A few weeks into Body for Life, I realized I was probably going to maim myself doing this at home without proper gym equipment. I found a fantastic trainer, now my boss, who at fifty-seven years old is a true testament to the fact that the fountain of youth is found in a gym. He taught me how to eat, how to work out, how to design my workouts for specific goals, and how to just keep on doing it, day after day, year after year. After four months of my new program, my weight was still 135, but I'd dropped from a size 8/10 to a size 6. My body fat dropped from 27 to 22 percent. My trainer suggested I get my certification and come work for him. Me? The ex–fat lady? I've been working as a personal trainer now for two years and love it. I wear a size 2 to 4, my body fat is 15 to 16 percent, and I've maintained my weight at 125 pounds.

STRUTTING OUR STUFF

Melanie Gumerman is a certified personal trainer. She is also a part of the 3FC team and moderates our fitness forums. We asked Melanie what we could gain from hiring a personal trainer.

Melanie

I love seeing my clients succeed. I train women, men, older adults, weight-loss clients, athletes, rehab clients, fibromyalgia patients. Picking goals and milestones is crucial to success and to long-term success-

ful maintenance. If I didn't keep setting goals and doing something I enjoy, I wouldn't still be doing this. I've learned through the years that a trainer can help in so many more ways than the obvious ones. Here are just a few of the benefits you gain from working with a personal trainer:

- Education about the proper technique and form for an exercise so that you don't get hurt and you do work the muscles that you think you are working.
- A program that is specifically designed to meet your individual goals.
- An understanding of how to put together your own workouts with alternate exercises if you don't want to or can't afford to always work with a trainer.
- The ability to set realistic long-term goals and plan how to get there.
- Accountability and a reason to show up at the gym.
- Ongoing support and new exercises and training modalities as your fitness level or interest changes during your fitness journey.

We have learned that personal trainers are not only more affordable than we thought but often crucial to keeping their clients on an exercise program. A short-term contract with a trainer, or even occasional sessions, could mean the difference in success or stalling. An experienced trainer can accelerate your weight loss!

JORGE CRUISE: 8 MINUTES IN THE MORNING AND THE 3-HOUR DIET

For all of us busy chicks who don't exercise because we don't have time, the Jorge Cruise program claims we don't have to put off the inevitable any longer. Because after all, who doesn't have just eight minutes in the morning to devote to better health?

Okay, we know this sounds a little far-fetched, and in fact, we were a little skeptical ourselves and probably never would have even tried this plan if Mr. Cruise hadn't been such a hottie. As it turns out, Mr. Cruise's theory does make sense and does work, although once you read between the lines, you will see that there is more to the program than those golden eight minutes in the morning.

This plan works best for newly hatched fit chicks who don't exercise at all. It's a palatable program that helps start fitness beginners on the road to better health. On this program, you will start each day with a quick, energizing "Cruise Move," tone your muscles, and boost your metabolism to burn more calories all day long. What isn't emphasized in the title, however, is the considerably longer time you'll spend power walking three times a week to maximize your weight loss.

Mr. Cruise's diet plan is not very well delineated. We are given general guidelines and a few basic nutritional dos and don'ts. After that, you're left to fend for yourself. Most of the 8 Minute chicks we surveyed thought the plan wasn't specific enough with regard to diet. Cruise has since solved that problem with the addition of another book, *The 3-Hour Diet,* which encourages you to eat healthy foods every three hours.

The book *8 Minutes in the Morning* isn't intimidating, as other fitness books can be. The photographs inside are not of skinny, superfit chicks. Cruise promotes not getting skinny but getting healthy and feeling better, which are more positive and realistic goals.

Unlike many other diet and exercise programs, Cruise helps us to deal with the emotional aspects of dieting and weight loss as well. You are encouraged to love yourself and cultivate a positive self-image. Cruise considers self-esteem to be the key to the success of his program, and we agree that every dieter should pay more attention to the self-love aspects of the weight-loss process, because when you feel better about yourself, you just automatically start to look better.

The core of 8 Minutes in the Morning is the exercise program called "Cruise Moves." Cruise Moves are designed to help firm your muscles as well as boost your metabolism when you're at rest. According to Cruise, lean muscle mass is what controls your metabolism. Your body burns between 20 and 50 calories for each pound of muscle, every day. So, his theory goes, if you increase your lean muscle mass, you burn more calories. If the Cruise Moves firm up five pounds of lean muscle within the first few weeks, you could burn an extra 250 calories per day. This equals more than twenty-five pounds of fat loss per year. This is a good tip, no matter what diet and exercise plan you follow! During this phase of the daily program, you will exercise for eight minutes every morning. Each day you will focus on a different body part, so that your whole body has had a good workout by the end of the week. Eight minutes of exercise is definitely doable, but if you are using the Cruise plan as your weight-loss program, don't start whistling "Dixie" yet. Cruise also suggests thirty minutes of power walking three times a week, to exercise your heart and burn even more calories. Realistically, we all need sixty minutes of exercise a day to maintain and ninety minutes a day to lose, but many people can't commit to that kind of time without any previous exercise experience.

The 8 Minutes in the Morning program seems to work great for our fitness newbies because it's quick and easy and not intimidating. And let's face it, eight minutes of exercise a day is better than nothing, and hopefully it will give newbies a positive taste for exercise and push them to do more. Some of our more seasoned chicks felt that this program didn't hold up too well for them over the long haul and felt that they needed more exercise after the first few months. A whopping 34 percent of the chicks we surveyed didn't lose any weight at all on this plan and left for another program, such as Weight Watchers or Curves.

So to get the real skinny on the 8 Minutes in the Morning program, we asked our fit chicks to air in on their experiences with the charismatic Mr. Cruise.

Q: My first month doing 8 Minutes was great. I actually lost weight! Months two and three were not so good. I'm still cruising but not getting anywhere. I do my eight minutes every morning; I follow the Cruise Down Plate and just eat the foods in the book. Is this program just for beginners?

3FC: Yes and no. Many of our members felt that this program was best for starting out, and they later moved on to join gyms or other fitness programs that pushed them more. That's not a bad thing. Getting in shape is a positive lifestyle change, no matter which way you slice it. And just as sitting on the couch only leads to lying down on the couch, exercising generally leads to the desire to do more exercise. So try to do a little more and see if it boosts your weight loss. Maybe you aren't exercising as much as you could be right now. You didn't mention power walking, and Cruise suggests a good half hour three times a week. This may be the boost your body needs to start burning more weight.

Another suggestion would be to look more closely at your food intake. If you follow the guidelines in the book, you should be right on track. However, eyeballing portion sizes isn't for everyone. A "fistful" of anything is a relative term. For one thing, whose fist are we talking about, Shania Twain's or Shaquille O'Neal's? It can't hurt to add up your calories every day to make sure you are eating enough, but not too much. Fit Day is a great Web site where you can track your diet and exercise. Go to www.fitday.com and sign up for a free account for logging your food, and take a few minutes each day to use it. You might be surprised!

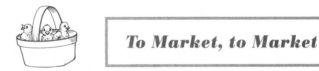

To Market, to Market

Best Food and Fitness Trackers

If you feel that keeping track of calories every day is about as much fun for you as math class, you might consider nutrition software that tracks your daily intake. These newfangled programs can make dieting fun and easy, and you're sure to make a perfect score every day. Many even let you enter your activities so you know how many calories you burn. Most offer free trial periods, so you can try before you buy.

- FitDay, www.fitday.com. Choose between a basic, free on-line version and a deluxe software program to purchase and install on your own computer.
- Diet Power, www.dietpower.com.
- ProTrack, www.dakotafit.com.
- Balance Log, www.healthetech.com.
- Check out www.3fatchicks.com/onlinetools for reviews of the newest diet and fitness software.

Q: I'm having trouble with the portion control approach in the Cruise Down Plate program. I know how to count calories. How do you know how much is too much?

3FC: Cruise suggests that we practice portion control, because it's a natural way to control consumption. Once you learn how much is too much and how little is too little for your body, eating moderately becomes a lot easier than counting every calorie every day for the rest of your life. But it can be a little difficult getting a handle on this new approach at first. Here's how it finally boiled down for us. Take a standard nine-inch dinner plate and mentally divide it in half. Fill the upper half with vegetables. Then mentally split the lower half into two sections. Fill one of those with meat or other high-protein food, and the other with carbohydrate foods. Cruise offers suggestions for each food group. Add a fat, preferably flaxseed oil, which helps your body to function and also helps curb your appetite. Now, clean your plate! If you are still hungry, eat more vegetables. It's not as easy as it sounds, though. There *are* foods that need to be measured, but you can quickly learn to eyeball those amounts too. Cruise recommends eating three meals and two snacks per day, which is typical of most balanced diet plans. He also recommends finishing each day with a delicious dessert. You'll always be full, and you'll never feel deprived.

If you need something more structured, Cruise's new book, *The 3-Hour Diet*, fills the bill. Unlike his *8 Minute* series, this book focuses on diet rather than exercise. This time we are told to eat every three hours, and we can have snacks such as candy bars and potato chips and have fast food for dinner. You are encouraged to eat *something* every three hours, to keep the metabolism revved and burn more calories, even if that something is one sugar-free cookie or fifteen fat-free potato chips. However, this is still very much a diet. Recommendations include small portions, fat-free cheese, and sugar-free gelatin. Fast foods include grilled chicken, plain burgers, and salads with lemon juice or nonfat dressings.

Q: I understand the fitness part of the 8 Minutes program, but there isn't enough info on the diet. I'm so confused about what to eat! Can I just follow another diet plan, like Weight Watchers, and do the fitness part according to the book?

3FC: Absolutely! It is recommended that you follow the diet guidelines in the book, but it's not required. Of course, if your vegetable for the day is a piece of sweet potato pie swimming in brown sugar and marshmallows, you're not going to lose weight. But if you're reasonable about your diet, you will see the benefits of exercise as long as you are consistent with the fitness portion of the program. Don't stress yourself out over the diet plan in the book. If you haven't looked at *The 3-Hour Diet*, you may find it easier to follow than the guidelines in the *8 Minute* books. The important thing is to find a diet that you are comfortable with, so you'll stick with it.

Q: The 3-Hour Diet includes a treat such as candy every day so we don't feel deprived. My problem is that I don't trust myself to have it in the house because I'll eat it. I could make a bag of cookies disappear in only eight minutes!

3FC: You aren't alone. It's difficult to keep candy and other treats in the house, considering that overeating and even a little lack of control is what got most of us fat to begin with. If the book recommends one quarter of a bag of M&Ms, how easy is it to resist eating the rest of the bag? First of all, it's okay to choose a snack that isn't so tempting to overeat, such as yogurt, fruit, or veggies. If you want a cookie or one Reese's Cup, we suggest you store the rest in the freezer. If you do sneak into the bag, you might change your mind before the extra portion thaws out. Better yet, don't even buy it in bulk packages. Take the time to drive or walk to a local convenience store and buy just one single-serving-sized snack. The extra trip may be annoying at first, but it will pay off in the end.

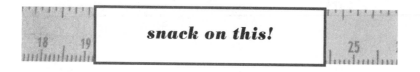

snack on this!

The 3-Hour Diet and 8 Minutes in the Morning allow two snacks a day that could be sweet or salty treats that you probably thought you had to give up entirely. If you don't trust yourself not to overeat, try these snack ideas that offer easy portion control.

- Browse the snack aisle for kid-sized snack packs. You'll find treats, such as gummi-bears, in small packages designed for packing in lunch boxes.
- Bake your own brownies using a low-fat brownie mix or one of the delicious recipes from www.3fatchicks.com. As soon as they are cool, cut into small squares, wrap tightly in plastic, and put them in the back of the freezer.
- Don't be put off by the extra cost of individually wrapped portions. They're usually cheaper than a binge.
- Go ahead and buy a full-sized candy bar from a vending machine at work. Score points with a coworker by cutting it in half and sharing.

Q: My 8 Minute Moves are the perfect thing to get me started each morning, but I fizzle out pretty quickly. I work in an office all day and don't have time to eat. I'm tired and hungry when I get home, and just the thought of a power walk leaves me exhausted. Am I destined for the slow lane?

3FC: It doesn't matter what diet plan you are following, you need to eat during the day. You can't cruise on empty! All of Jorge's books recommend three meals and at least two snacks for a reason. It may not be convenient to eat an apple or go out for a salad, but there are a lot of quick and easy foods that will sustain you until you get home. Snack on nuts, Pria bars, or other fast snacks suggested in the books. Lunch doesn't have to be time-consuming, as long as you prepare it before you even leave the house. Pack a cooler with everything you need to quickly assemble a sandwich or salad at your desk. It's easier than you think. Within a few days, you'll find that you have so much energy, you may even want to power walk all the way home! Pita sandwiches make the perfect lunch on the go. One pita half has just seventy calories! Stuff with a garden salad, peanut butter and jelly, fruit and cream cheese, or even scrambled eggs and bacon. Pack any wet fillings in a small plastic container, and fill your pita at lunchtime.

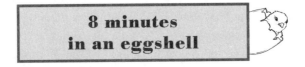

8 minutes in an eggshell

Professional Counseling Limited. You can subscribe to the online service and pay for premium support. You won't get one-on-one counseling, but you may get to join a live chat with Jorge himself!

Support System Paid subscription to on-line service includes community support forums where you can get encouragement and advice.

Fitness Factor Absolutely! You'll exercise every day and learn the importance of fitness in the weight-loss equation.

Family-Friendly Not really. Most of the meal ideas are designed for one person. Fitness is also often a solo experience.

Pros Doesn't require much time, plus everything about exercise is spelled out for you. The diet is vague, however, which was a problem for some chicks.

Cons You may outgrow the exercise routine quickly, though that isn't exactly a con in the big picture!

$$ Cheap! Other than the cost of the book and maybe a pair of dumbbells, you don't need any special equipment. Suggested meals are very affordable. If you opt for the on-line service or premium support, though, the cost can quickly add up.

The Person This Diet Is Best For The fitness newbie, the single person, or anyone with very little time to devote to fitness.

↗ ↗ ⋀ ⋀ ⇐ STRUTTING OUR STUFF ↗ ↗ ⋀ ⋀ ⇐

The Heavy Hens Air In on Fitness

Let's face it: exercising while obese is not easy! You may not be able to do the same exercises as thinner women. You may have problems bending over and getting up quickly, and your

● *Continued on next page* ●

joints may hurt from the extra weight. You may have difficulty using some kinds of exercise equipment. You may also feel self-conscious exercising around other people. But it can be done, and you really will be glad later. We've been there, and we will share our best tips, and those of the heavy hens in our community, to help you get started.

- Check with your doctor before starting. If you are obese, you have a higher risk of heart disease or high blood pressure, so you may need to be monitored during an exercise program.
- Don't worry about starting slow. You can graduate to more traditional exercises as you gain strength and lose weight.
- If you can't walk for a full half hour, try ten-minute walks, three times a day.
- If weight-bearing exercises, such as walking, are too hard on your joints, try swimming or water workouts. If you feel too self-conscious for the pool, check your local wellness center. Some offer water classes just for overweight women.
- Do push-ups against a wall or the back of a chair.
- If chafing from exercise is a problem, try one of the new body lubricants, such as Body Glide or Soothing Care Chafing Relief by Monistat, to prevent friction.
- Leakage may be a problem, because of the extra padding pressing down on the bladder when you do sit-ups or other exercises. Use a panty liner for now, and rest assured that this problem will probably go away as you lose weight.
- If sit-ups put too much pressure on your back when you do them on the floor, try doing crunches while lying on a balance ball.
- When choosing fitness equipment, be sure to ask about the weight limit, especially on budget-priced models. Many treadmills and elliptical machines were not designed to hold more than 250 pounds. There are a lot of better-quality machines that will hold you now and will provide many years of

fitness. You might even try a Gazelle or other glider. These machines are very low-impact and great for getting started.

BODY FOR LIFE

Body for Life (BFL) is a body-sculpting and weight-loss program that is adaptable to almost anybody. The program is led by Bill Phillips, a formerly overweight man who is now sporting a dramatically healthy and chiseled body. BFL, which recently had a makeover, now has a version exclusively for chicks, called Body for Life for Women, led by our new hero, Dr. Pamela Peeke, who understands that fitness really can be feminine.

Body for Life, promising "12 Weeks to Mental and Physical Strength," encompasses positive thinking, a balanced eating plan, and a cardio and weight training program. Keep reading! Don't let the weights turn you off. BFL is one of the most intensive "weight lifting for weight loss" plans, and it will build muscle, but having muscle tone doesn't mean you're going to be bulky. Trust us. Fat rolls feel a lot bulkier than strong muscles do.

The point of the Body for Life plan is to lose fat, not muscle. According to Bill, half of the weight lost in a typical diet is muscle tissue. By lifting weights, you save and develop muscle tone, which means you lose more pure fat.

The Body for Life program is broken down into a few major components. First we learn how to Cross the Abyss. Don't be worried if you're afraid of heights. This abyss is a psychological one, and it represents our need for a mental transformation to change our mind-set if we are to achieve our goals. This section of the book is probably not the most popular one with impatient chicks, but stick with it, because it will greatly increase your chances of achieving your goal and making it stick.

Here in the abyss, you will identify what your goals are, what you need to do to get there, and what bad habits you have that are likely to hold you back. Talk about a reality check! You'll have to be totally honest with yourself, before you can safely reach the other side.

Be sure you pick goals that are attainable. Climbing to the top of Mount Kilimanjaro before you touch your next Twinkie is perhaps a bit of a stretch, but making a commitment to exercise a little more every day and cutting down on your Twinkies whenever you can is perhaps a little more attainable. Achievable goals are important because you'll be spending a lot of time writing them down, reading them back, and saying them over and over to yourself every night for the next twelve weeks. You don't want to spend the next three months thinking about how you're falling short.

BFL has a wham-bam-thank-you-ma'am approach to exercise. The plan includes twenty minutes of intense cardio three times a week, alternating with three days of forty-five-minute weight-training sessions. That's it. This leaves time for more important things in life, like a little afternoon delight under the spreading magnolias.

We love the Eating for Life section. Here's why: you get to eat six times a day. That's right, six times a day! What's the catch? These are small, low-fat meals, and you have to keep them balanced with carbs and protein. Most meals can be made by measuring a fist-sized portion of carbs and a palm-sized portion of protein, prepared in a low-fat manner. There is no calorie counting. Many of the meals are quick fixes, and the book lists many examples of acceptable foods. You'll choose a protein and a carb for each meal, and you'll add a vegetable to two of the meals. Your meals can be as simple as cottage cheese and an apple or a meal replacement shake. You can also cook regular meals with lean meats, healthy grains, and vegetables. You'll do this for six days, and then once a week you get a free day when you can eat anything you like.

Yes, you read that correctly! We three chicks live in the land of milk and honey-glazed ribs, so we like the idea of being free to indulge in the richness of our culinary heritage without having to pack our bags and go on a guilt trip afterward. You can eat anything you like on free days, but remember, you need a calorie deficit to lose weight, so don't go overboard. Choose foods you can't eat during the week and limit yourself to one serving. Don't go hog wild. Eat just one Moon Pie. Have a half cup of fried okra, not the whole pan full.

We'd be a lot happier if there was a video to accompany this book to show the fluid movement of the weight-lifting moves for those of us who are new to strength training. We also think the program could be improved with a scorching butt routine and more emphasis on food portions, but to get the real skinny on Body for Life, we went to the fit chicks on this program, and here's what they have to say:

Q: *I've been on this for four weeks and haven't lost weight. What is wrong? Am I building muscle?*

3FC: Although you are building muscle, you aren't seeing results on the scale at this point. It is possible that your muscles are retaining water since they are new at training. This is perfectly normal and healthy. If you aren't losing weight, measure your success in other ways. Are you getting stronger? Were you once topping off with five-pound weights, but find yourself lifting eight- or ten-pound weights now? You should also take your measurements, and take an updated photo of yourself to compare with your starting photo. The scale isn't the only tool to measure perfection. A snapshot can show more results than the numbers between our big toes. When it comes to before and after, a picture really is worth a thousand calories!

If your pictures or measurements aren't very impressive, take another look at your portion sizes. Do you have too many yolks in your omelet? How thick is your palm-sized protein portion? Are you mixing your protein shakes with milk or water? Are your meals more than 20 percent fat? Is your free day sucking up all of the good work you've done the rest of the week? Keep tabs on every bite you eat, and count your calories. Make sure you are eating six balanced meals, spaced apart as directed in the BFL book. Make necessary adjustments and by week eight you should see a big difference.

You might also consider adding extra cardio to the plan to burn more calories. Some of our fit chicks do feel that they don't get enough cardio on this plan, and they incorporate extra cardio sessions throughout the week. We suggest that if you add cardio, don't add more of the high-intensity sessions as outlined in BFL. Instead, add less intensive, but longer, fat-scorching sessions.

STRUTTING OUR STUFF

Our Chicks Air In on Portion Control

Does your hand grow when it is time to measure your fist-sized portion of pasta? While some BFL chicks use measuring cups just to be safe, there are some more creative options. Here are a few tips from our chicks to prevent portion overload.

Try baked spaghetti squash in place of pasta. It's awesome and you can eat a ton of it for very few calories! — MEG

Slice or shred cabbage very fine (like you would for coleslaw) and sauté it in a bit of olive oil or pan spray. You can have heaps of it with tomato sauce and browned ground turkey breast or lowfat ground beef, with a sprinkle of Romano or Parmesan cheese. It tastes wonderful and you get a helping that fills your plate and stomach. You can mix in a half cup of whole-wheat pasta if you really want the pasta, but I don't miss it at all. — MEL

I add cannellini beans or black beans and canned artichokes (in water) to pasta to make a full bowl for an "American" pasta meal. I get the taste of the pasta and some extra fiber. I find that a quarter cup of pasta, a quarter cup of beans, three artichokes, plus sauce, is a good meal for me! — ELLEN

Q: I feel like all I eat is oatmeal, apples, and eggs. When my free day comes, I go wild and enjoy myself, but I spend the next few days battling cravings. Is there a happy medium?

3FC: Don't take Free Day too literally. It might be guilt-free because free days are permitted on the diet, but you'll still pay for it in the end. This is your day to eat what you want, but excess calories *will* affect your bottom line. Period. No ifs, ands, or bigger butts. So, if you're about to tuck into some southern-fried comfort food, think twice. Don't go overboard and find yourself with a sugar hangover that lasts for days and makes your diet days that much harder.

As for eating oatmeal, apples, and eggs all the time, you can remedy that by buying Bill Phillips's book *Eating for Life*. There are many great recipes in the book, as well as ideas and tips to help you come up with your own meals. You know you can have a palm-sized portion of meat and a fist-sized carb, so all you need to do is add the spices and condiments and you can come up with a multitude of combinations. One great recipe to try is our Shrimp with Asparagus and Couscous on page 175. If you can conjure up your creativity, then you won't have to rely on Free Day to get you through the week. You can eat satisfying meals all week long and still lose weight.

As you progress through the Body for Life program, your body will become more accustomed to this healthier way of eating, and most fit chicks actually prefer good nutrition and eventually forget Free Day altogether.

tips for avoiding a calorie blowout on free day

If you're focusing on Free Day all week long, you're liable to snort cocoa when the big day finally comes. Your first Free Day is the most exciting. You're going to eat whatever you want because, by golly, you've *earned* it. By the end of the day, the sugar coma you've fallen into will help kill the chocolate-induced endorphins—until, of course, next week's Free Day!

Free Day is a wonderful concept, but you don't want one day to untie all of the hard work you've done all week. Remember that calories count! Here are some tips from our fit chicks to help you keep your Free Day fantasies under control.

- Limit Free Day to only one meal instead of a whole day.
- Make a list of what you crave the most through the week. Choose only from that list when Free Day comes around so those foods won't haunt you for another week.
- Don't eat for the sake of it. If what you really want is the french fries, don't buy the burger.
- Eat what you want, but journal every bite and count the calories at the end of the day.
- Don't eat seconds at any meals.
- Weigh in the morning of Free Day.
- Eat six small meals as usual, but eat in any combination you choose. Double up your carbs or add some fat.
- Don't buy bags of Free Day supplies. You don't want them teasing you from the cabinet for the next six days.
- Wear tight-waisted pants while you eat.

- Still drink plenty of water on Free Day, and have a tall, cold glass before each meal or snack.

Q: I'm just not physically strong enough to do this. It's a waste of time, and I can't imagine that I'll ever be able to get results. I even had a hard time getting the dumbbells into the shopping cart.

3FC: Not all chicks were born with golden biceps, but that doesn't mean that trying to work the program is a waste of time! Be more patient with yourself, and work your way in gradually. Start with a set of weights as light as you need. You don't have to start out with fifteen-, ten-, or even five-pound weights. If you need ones and threes, that is a start! It really is okay: you want to challenge yourself but not hurt yourself. You need to build with each set to hit your max on the intensity scale. That will require focus and honesty. Your max will float from one day to the next, especially when you're just beginning. If you can't hit the same weight you did the session before, that's okay. Some days you'll be stronger than others; just keep your focus, and be sure to log in your activity on the journals included in the book.

Jumping from a five-pound weight to an eight-pound weight or from a fifteen-pound weight to a twenty-pound weight can be difficult, particularly across an entire set. If advancing to the next weight seems too hard, buy some single-pound magnetic plates for metal dumbbells from a sporting goods store. Instead of jumping several pounds at once, you can increase one pound at a time and keep steadily advancing.

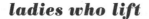

ladies who lift

I added yoga to my plan, and I now feel like I get a better range with my weights. I was never a flexible person, but yoga has allowed me to get in touch with my body and realize how far I can take it. —PAULINE

When I first started going to the gym, I didn't ask the other people for advice. They are impressive and look good because they concentrate on the weights and don't small-talk much. The talkers are the gym bunnies, and you don't want to be one, no matter how cute the name is. If they see you're serious, they'll offer help where needed. —DANIELLE

I can't get the most out of my workout unless I get plenty of sleep. If I sleep less than seven hours the night before I lift weights, I can't reach my potential. —SANDY

I keep motivational pictures on the wall where I lift weights. I get them from muscle-chick magazines. If I'm having a tough time lifting, all it takes is a glance at the muscles on the wall to keep me going. I also have pictures on the inside of the door to the snack cabinet, which has proven to be very handy! —MARYANNE

Q: I just don't believe it. There's no way I'm going to lose weight with three twenty-minute cardio sessions a week. It's just too incredible to be true. Isn't it?

3FC: Okay, we can understand how you might have misgivings about the extraordinary claims this program makes, but we're here to tell you, this program is *not* too good to be true. The twenty-minute Aerobic Solution is high-intensity interval training (HIIT). It's only twenty minutes, but it is one hellfire session. We three chicks prefer what we call "sorta high-intensity interval training" (SHIIT), but that isn't on this program.

You can tweak the cardio if you feel it will work for you, but if you are not experienced, be careful. Bill has done his homework and has a proven program. If you overtrain, you can actually impede your weight-loss efforts. The general consensus is to not add to the number of intense cardio sessions. Instead, try adding longer, less intense workouts, either in separate sessions or as add-ons to the HIIT sessions. With such a small amount of required cardio, you have plenty of time to explore more activities, such as swimming, belly dancing, kick-boxing, or power yoga.

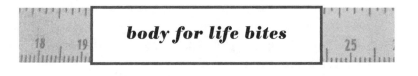

body for life bites

Here's a sample day in the life of a fit chick on Body for Life:

Meal 1 • Oatmeal and scrambled eggs and whites
Meal 2 • Myoplex shake
Meal 3 • Cottage cheese and strawberries
Meal 4 • Turkey and Swiss wrap with fresh green beans
Meal 5 • Grilled marinated chicken breast, baked potato, and
steamed asparagus
Meal 6 • Myoplex shake

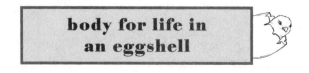

body for life in an eggshell

Professional Counseling None.

Support System Nothing formal. There are various support groups on the Internet, including the forum at 3FC. Check out www.bodyforlife.com for good tips in the guestbook.

Fitness Factor Exercise is intense but time-efficient. Cardio twenty minutes, three times a week, and strength training for forty-five minutes, three times a week.

Family-Friendly Not very. Most of the meals can be eaten by any member of the family, but you'll be eating smaller amounts of food six days a week. This can be difficult when you're cooking normal-sized meals for a family.

Pros You don't have to cook much on this plan. Super simple to follow.

Cons Video to show form in exercises would be helpful. We've heard many requests to increase cardio in the program.

$$ If you drink ready-to-drink shakes and take supplements, at least your wallet is going to lose weight. Otherwise, the food is cheap.

The Person This Diet Is Best For A single chick or anyone who brown-bags her lunch. Also great for the person who wants to get in shape and doesn't know how.

> ## *alternachick tips for getting fit*

Are you looking for a nontraditional form of exercise to wake up your senses and explore your alternative side? Try these tips from our alternachicks, for new and enlightening ways to get in shape.

- Belly dance. If exotic, sensual dance is more your style than hip-hop aerobics, you might try belly dancing as great way to burn calories and get in shape. Follow a video or join a class to shimmy into shape.
- Dance Dance Revolution. Attach a special dance pad to your video game console, hang a disco ball from your ceiling, then follow along for the most fun fitness workout since *American Bandstand!*
- Yourself Fitness. Computerized personal trainer via PlayStation or your PC. Work out your inner alternageek!
- Martial Arts. From kung fu to Tae Bo, the martial arts offer head-to-toe fitness and extreme calorie burning. *Kee-yah!*
- Yoga. Connect with your body on a deeper level, and intensify your inner motivation while you get more flexible. Try power yoga for more calorie burning and better circulation.

BODY FOR LIFE FOR WOMEN

This chickcentric version of BFL takes everything we learned in Body for Life but zeros in on the uniquely female weight-loss experience, which sounded just fine by us! Dr. Pam Peeke, who is obviously a woman, understands that we chicks can get to feeling overwhelmed with the amount of responsibility in our lives. And what chaos doesn't take care of, hormones will. The plan is somewhere between Jane Fonda and hard-core weight training. It's a great mix for any woman, and later on, if you're interested in more weight training or less hard lifting, you can decide which direction you'd like to take. We think this is one of the most sensible and well-rounded diets available.

The book goes through the four hormonal "milestones" of life with us. The doctor's ingenious mantra of "Mind, Mouth, and Muscle" helps us tackle the obstacles we all face during each hormonal milestone.

"Mind" is all about managing stress, taking care of a busy life, and making time for ourselves. It includes ten Power Mind Principles, which will help motivate you, empower you, and build your confidence.

"Mouth" is your new way of eating. The book goes over how to eat, what to eat, and when to eat it, yet the diet makes so much sense, it feels totally unrestrictive. It's very simple. You'll eat three meals and two snacks a day, and the book includes a list of acceptable foods. At meals you will have a portion from the protein list and a portion from the carb list. At least twice daily you'll add in a nonstarchy vegetable, and you are free to add more. You'll use good fats, in low-fat proportions. For snacks, a list of options and portion sizes are available to you.

"Muscle" is the physical portion of the plan. The plan recommends thirty minutes of cardio, at least three to five times per week. You are encouraged to give it your all and to rotate activities. You will also do resistance training three times a week, and the workout is a simple program to follow. You can do the entire program at home, using as little equipment as a few sets of dumbbells. You can round off the cardio and weights with Pilates and yoga.

The driving principle behind this plan is to build up your muscle so you can burn more calories in future workouts. Muscle burns more calories than fat, and if you increase your muscle mass, you will shed more weight by merely existing. How great is that?

One of the best parts about starting Body for Life for Women is that all of these components don't have to be changed at once. Dr. Peeke says that if you want to concentrate on one part at a time, then that is fine with her, although to be successful on this plan, you really do have to get around to reading the whole book at some point. Reading the food and exercise appendix off the Internet isn't going to make this a successful plan. Doing the whole program, you will eventually get mind, mouth, and muscle all working together in perfect harmony!

Q: Is this diet low-glycemic? I am so over low-carb/good-carb. The only thing I lost on those diets was money.

3FC: This is not a low-glycemic diet, but there are "smart carbs" that you will be allowed to eat. You may not have lost weight before because you didn't practice portion control. We love juicy steaks and whole-grain bread, and we are all for any diet that allows these delicious foods, but we also remember that we can't lose weight if we eat a two-pound sirloin and a whole fresh loaf of pumpernickel.

With this plan, you will have a list of smart carbs to choose from. These are carbs that have more nutrients and fiber than their high-glycemic counterparts, such as the whole-wheat pasta in our Seafood Stuffed Peppers recipe on page 176. Brown rice, sweet potatoes, and whole-grain bread are chosen for their nutritional value. As you eat balanced meals with reasonable portions, your goal is to get more bang for your buck with smart choices in foods.

Unlike most popular diet plans on the market, Body for Life for Women encourages you to count calories if you are not losing weight, or if you have a difficult time with weight loss. Serving sizes are given on your food list, so much of the guesswork is eliminated and you don't have to count calories to be successful.

Q: Do I get Free Day on BFL for Women? That was the most enticing part of BFL. The exercise chart says Free Day, but I don't see it anywhere else.

3FC: Yes and no. You will have an exercise Free Day, but as for a total day off from your eating plan, no. Instead of full free days, you are allowed what are called "mini-chills," small nibbles of off-plan foods that you can take to keep yourself in sync without feeling guilty about it.

Peeke says that although you may indulge in many mini-chills at the start of the program, you will probably find yourself going for much longer periods without them later on. There is not a specified amount that you can have, but be aware that whatever calories go in must come out. If you want to lose weight, reserve your mini-chills for those times when if you don't have a cookie or a scoop of ice cream, you are going to begin peeling the wallpaper off the walls. Satisfy yourself with a small portion of forbidden food, and then move on with the plan guilt-free.

tips for boosting your get-up-and-go

We only get one day free of exercise per week. What can we do for motivation those other six days? Here are our top five motivators to keep us exercising when we really want to hit the snooze button:

1. Pencil yourself in. If you schedule your time to exercise, you've made it an important part of your day and you are more likely to stick with it, or at least work harder to think of an excuse.
2. Leave your workout clothes on the dresser. We keep a complete set of exercise gear ready and waiting at bedside so we don't have to search before dawn.
3. Keep a small album of your goal pictures in your gym bag or over the alarm clock. Tack inspirational pictures around the exercise equipment.

4. Announce your victories! Try marking a bright red *V* on your wall calendar on days you stick with the program.
5. Mix it up! Tired of spinning? Try African dance, kickboxing, salsa, or circuit training. Keep it interesting, and keep your muscles guessing.

Q: I've never lifted weights before and I imagine I can't lift very much. I also don't want to look "ripped." Is this program too advanced for me? I looked into BFL before and I didn't think I could keep up.

3FC: This program is made for you! Body for Life for Women is very user-friendly and easily modified for the beginner. One nice thing about the plan is that Dr. Peeke recommends starting with just one element of the program at a time, until you feel you are ready to move on and add the next element.

Muscle, the weight-lifting portion of this program, is as intense or low-impact as you want it to be. So if you're dumbbell-challenged, there is still hope for you. One-, three-, and five-pound weights are okay to start with. You can even repeat one-, three-, and five-pound weights if you want. As long as you are doing all you can do, and truly advancing the weights as you are able, you will still see progress.

And don't worry about looking ripped. A lot of hard work is involved in achieving a body that will make people confuse you with Arnold Schwarzenegger, which is the physique most people think of when they hear "ripped." You will attain a healthy look while on BFL for Women. Just keep going until you get the body you want, and then maintain a holding pattern. The beautiful part is it's all up to you!

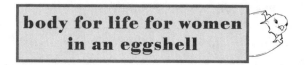

body for life for women in an eggshell

Support System Nothing formal. There are various support groups on the Internet, including the forum at 3FC. Check out www.drpeeke.com for additional information.

Fitness Factor Time-efficient and easily modified. Exercise is an important portion of the plan. Cardio is recommended three to five times a week, weights three times a week.

Family-Friendly Fairly easy to do with a family. Meals are smaller than what the rest of the family may eat. You'll have three meals and two snacks a day.

Pros Plan is simple to follow. It's clearly explained in the book, without vague areas. It can all be performed at home.

Cons There are still off-limit foods, like white potatoes and white rice. No videos to follow along with for the novice.

$$ The food can be bought as cheaply as any other plan. Meat choices may be more expensive, but cheaper items, such as cottage cheese, eggs, and oatmeal can make up the difference.

The Person This Diet Is Best For The woman who would like to get into a solid exercise program or who has had problems sticking to a diet. The Mind portion of this plan overcomes a multitude of obstacles and focuses on positive thinking. This is particularly good for women whose weight loss progress tends to be sluggish.

CURVES

Twenty years ago, gyms were as much about socializing as they were about fitness. The gym bunny trend has scared away many a chick who would like to work out but is afraid of being the chunky chick in the middle of a Victoria's Secret or Abercrombie and Fitch ad. Although the gyms of this century are different, chicks across America are finding comfort and safety in Curves, a women's-only workout facility. We understand that no matter how relaxed today's gyms are, some women just feel intimidated by a gym. We surveyed our chicks and found that the most popular reason for choosing Curves, hands down, was its nonintimidating, all-female environment.

Curves offers clients a diet program as well as an exercise regimen. You are not, however, obligated to follow both elements of the Curves program. You can do either or both at any local Curves facility, or you can buy the book *Curves: Permanent Results Without Permanent Dieting* and do the program right at home.

Curves Diet Plans

Curves offers two types of diets—the Carbohydrate Sensitive Plan and the Calorie Sensitive Plan. Both diets are low-carb; one involves counting calories. You'll take a test to see which diet you need to follow.

The Carbohydrate Sensitive Plan looks eerily like one other low-carb plan that we know of that begins with a scarlet *A*. This diet starts out with a beginner's phase, where you will get to eat twenty carbs (minus fiber) a day. After Phase 1, you'll move to Phase 2 and raise your carbs to forty to sixty per day. You'll stay at this level until you reach your goal.

The Calorie Sensitive Plan allows for a few more carbs up front, but it adds calorie counting to the mix. In Phase 1, you can have twelve hundred calories and sixty grams of carbs per day. After Phase 1, you'll move to Phase 2 and raise your calories to sixteen hundred per day. The carbs stay at sixty grams. Your calories will not increase or decrease based on your weight.

The Curves diet has a "free foods" list valid for both plans. The list includes one protein shake a day, plus a choice of other "foods." At first glance the list looks long, but it does include garnishes and foods you won't eat much of, like parsley, garlic, mustard, and bean sprouts. Still, it's nice to know there is an arsenal of foods that you can eat that won't be tallied against your daily limits.

Either diet plan should get you to your weight loss goal, which is called Phase 3. The plan is to have your metabolism stoked enough that you will be able to eat twenty-five hundred to three thousand calories a day. You will eat normally (if three thousand calories a day feels normal), weigh in every day, and go back to Phase 1 briefly when and if you notice that you're gaining a few pounds. With this cycling, the diet promises that you will eventually build your metabolism to the point that you can always eat normally if you just go on Phase 1 for two days a month.

Exercise

If you're not into socializing with the whole henhouse while you exercise, then this plan may not be for you. At the Curves centers, you'll exercise on hydraulic machines. Depending on how large the center is, you'll have between eight and twelve machines to choose from. The machines are placed in a circle, with wooden boards between them. You will exercise for thirty-second intervals as hard as you can on a machine. Then a signal will announce that it is time to rotate. Get off your machine and walk in place on the wooden board between machines before getting on the next machine. You'll repeat the entire aerobic and strength-training circuit two to three times, depending on the number of machines the facility has. The goal is to do this thirty-minute workout three days a week.

The Curves at Home workout is also a combination strength-training and cardio workout. In this workout, though, you will alternate strength training via exercise tubes with the cardio of your choice, for forty-second intervals.

The whole plan is very simple and supereasy to follow. At only thirty minutes a day, it seems as though anybody could fit this into her schedule. Surprisingly, though, one of the top reasons our fit chicks left Curves was that they couldn't fit it into their schedule. This may not be just an excuse. Curves does not offer day care, and it generally has limited hours, which was a stumbling block for many of our working women and mothers. But here are a few thoughts from our fit chicks in the Curves program:

Q: Can I go to Curves every day? I read that new government guidelines called for sixty to ninety minutes of exercise a day, but Curves recommends much less—thirty minutes, three times a week.

3FC: Yes, you can go more than the three days a week that Curves recommends, but you should not do the full workout each time. It's easy to assume that if three times a week is good, then five times a week must be even better! But this isn't actually the case. Sometimes, especially when it comes to health, less is more. Your muscles need time to heal between workouts—at least one day of rest between sessions. The book suggests that if you want to go every day, then on alternate days you should work at 50 percent or less of your maximum ability. This means you should just go through the motions on the machines for your light days, and concentrate on a cardio workout, which happens every time you switch machines.

The American Council on Exercise has found that you burn 184 calories during the regular thirty-minute workout at Curves. If you cut down the intensity on your off days at Curves, you will be burning a minimal amount of calories in those sessions. Instead of doing extra days at Curves, consider joining a larger gym with more intense cardio choices, or try supplementing with some cardio videos at home so you'll make the most of your exercise time and burn the calories you need to in order to lose the weight.

Q: I get bored and give up every diet that I try. What makes Curves any different?

3FC: The folks at Curves try very hard to make their workout regimen fun for their members. It may not be as good as a bag of popcorn and *Sex and the City* reruns, but they try. First, they specialize in quick workouts. You only have to stick with it for thirty minutes a day, three times a week. While you are there, you're in a circle facing other members. Regulars get to know each other and look forward to spending time there with their workout buddies. Additionally, the staff usually tries to make it fun. They may play games, give away prizes, or have "brag boards" where they post accomplishments for everyone to read. Activities vary from club to club since franchises are independently owned.

So if you're a chick who loves people but hates to exercise, Curves might be a great choice for you. But not everybody is a social butterfly, so if you don't like to chat and play bingo while you work out, look for another plan. Many of the clubs play music tracks that are made specially for Curves. These are, in general, songs you are familiar with, rerecorded by different artists.

If you try Curves and like it, buy a few months' worth of membership at a time, and you may find you are more committed to the process. Stick with it until you've made exercise a habit. Some people just don't have the discipline to stick to a program at home because they haven't made an investment, and they don't have somebody with a clipboard holding them accountable. We don't recommend going to Curves more than the prescribed three times a week if you are prone to burnout, and we don't recommend buying long-term contracts. While some chicks love it and stick with it for years, some prefer to move on to an exercise regimen that offers more variation.

Q: What kind of food can I have on this diet? I've heard different stories about the fruit—berries only, and others say berries and melon. Does this change if I don't exercise?

3FC: We totally understand your confusion. Many people confuse or mesh this program with other low-carb plans. This plan is completely distinct, however, from any other low-carb plan that is on the market. You can have any food you want as long as you do not exceed the daily carb limit. Some foods will be limited or not allowed based on the daily requirement. For instance, a piece of rhubarb cobbler will have more carbs than are allowed in a day, so you won't be eating one of those. A banana will have a lot of carbs, but if you plan it into your day, you can have it. Nobody is going to gasp if you sprinkle some flour into a sauce, or if you use a splash of teriyaki sauce. As long as you don't exceed your daily carb requirement, you are free to eat what you like.

You can do the Curves diet plan without exercising, but we recommend that you do not count your protein shake as free if you are not doing some sort of strength training. You will probably also have to follow the Calorie Sensitive Plan since you will be burning fewer calories. If you want the full benefits from this plan, you'll have to exercise.

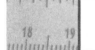

curve balls

The chicks we surveyed had strong opinions about Curves both for and against. Here are the curve balls that made the difference for our Curves chicks between striking out and hitting a home run.

Music Some chicks loved the energizing, upbeat tempo that carried them through the workout. Others had problems with some of the clubs' playing their own line of Christian-based exercise music. Members of other faiths were not comfortable or inspired.

Staff Some chicks felt like family at their Curves. They had involved, dedicated instructors who tried to make their exercise

● *Continued on next page* ●

a positive and enjoyable experience. Others were bothered by a lack of exercise and fitness knowledge on the part of the staff.

Facility The small, intimate atmosphere is a big hit with some chicks. Others didn't like the fact that the club didn't have showers or facilities for clients to clean up after exercising on the go.

Results Curves has helped many chicks lose weight who failed in the past. Other chicks who had some experience with other exercise programs felt that Curves was a step back, and they didn't get the results they hoped for.

 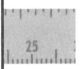

a day in the food life of a curves chick

This is a sample day on Phase 2, where you will spend most of your time on the Curves program. Be careful, though; your mileage may vary as brands and recipes may have different carb and calorie counts.

Meal 1 • 1 egg scrambled with 2 egg whites, mushrooms, and scallions

Meal 2 • Free shake

Meal 3 • 2 deviled egg halves, turkey sandwich on reduced-carb bread

Meal 4 • Grilled chicken breast, salad with free toppings, plus cherry tomatoes, 1 serving of ranch dressing, steamed green beans

Meal 5 • Tuna salad with ½ cup grapes

Meal 6 • Sugar-free hot cocoa and sugar-free raspberry Jell-O

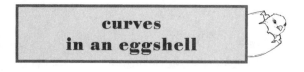

curves in an eggshell

Professional Counseling The instructors at Curves are there to make sure you do the exercises correctly, and they will help you diagnose problems you might have with your weight loss, but they are generally not trained professionals. The franchise owners complete a training session, and they train the staff.

Support System Curves has a wonderful support system through employees and clientele. The equipment is laid out for strong interaction, and many of the Curves play games or recognize "losers" in some way.

Fitness Factor Curves strongly suggests their signature thirty-minute workouts. However, the exercise doesn't grow with you, and you may hit a fitness standstill when you want to take it to the next level.

Family-Friendly The diet portion is fairly easy to follow if you are cooking for a family. With limited facility hours and no day

● *Continued on next page* ●

care, Curves is much more family-friendly to the employees than to the patrons.

Pros The environment is nonintimidating and can get many women into a regular exercise routine who might not have done it otherwise. The diet is easy to follow, without a lot of fine print.

Cons The workout maxes out early on, not giving much room to take fitness to a higher level, and offers little variety.

$$ Varies from location to location. Memberships can be found as cheaply as $29 per month. Discounts are given if contracts are signed. Beware of high-cost supplements for sale at the facilities. The home workout is inexpensive. The diet portion is average, depending on your taste in protein.

The Person This Diet Is Best For Someone starting out in fitness and open to socializing while exercising. Not everyone wants to be chatting while sweating off the pounds!

recipes from the front lines

JORGE CRUISE: 8 MINUTES IN THE MORNING AND THE 3-HOUR DIET

We lightened our version of muffuletta by replacing some of the olives with diced fresh zucchini squash. As the mixture marinates, the zucchini absorbs all of the salty flavors of the salad, and you'll never know the difference! We chose to pair it with a reduced-fat Swiss and extra-lean ham, leaving out the higher-fat cheeses and meats.

mighty muffuletta

Serves 4

¼ cup chopped onion
¼ cup chopped black olives
¼ cup chopped green olives
½ cup diced zucchini (¼-inch dice)
¼ cup chopped roasted red bell peppers
2 pepperoncini peppers, minced
1 tablespoon olive oil
1 tablespoon red wine vinegar
Few cracks of freshly ground black pepper, to taste
4 ounces extra-lean ham, shaved
2 ounces reduced-fat Swiss cheese, sliced thin
4 whole-wheat pita bread halves, split open

● *Continued on next page* ●

In a small mixing bowl, combine onions, olives, zucchini, red bell peppers, pepperoncini, olive oil, vinegar, and black pepper. Cover and chill for several hours or overnight.

To prepare sandwich: Line pita halves with ham and the slices of cheese. Stuff with the olive mixture and enjoy!

Per serving: 192 calories, 7 grams fat, 20 grams carbs, 3 grams fiber, 13 grams protein

---

You'll find all of the distinctive flavors of Buffalo chicken in our easy salad, and it couldn't be more perfect for a pita.

buffalo chicken salad pita

Serves 6

1 can (12 ounces) chicken breast chunks
1 teaspoon hot sauce
¼ cup light mayonnaise
¼ cup light sour cream
¼ cup crumbled blue cheese
1 stalk celery, finely chopped
½ cup grape tomatoes, cut in half
Freshly cracked black pepper to taste
3 pita rounds, cut in half
1 cup lettuce leaves

Drain canned chicken and add to medium mixing bowl. Sprinkle with hot sauce and toss well; set aside. In small mixing bowl, combine mayonnaise, sour cream, and blue cheese; blend well. Add mayonnaise mixture to chicken and toss to coat. Stir in celery and tomatoes, and add pepper to taste. Line pita halves with a few lettuce leaves, then fill with the chicken salad to serve.

Per serving: 291 calories, 9 grams fat, 28 grams carbs, 3 grams fiber, 22 grams protein

---

BODY FOR LIFE

Here's a fit chicks fav that makes Body for Life that much tastier. With recipes like this, you won't be longing for Free Day to have dinner with flavor.

shrimp with asparagus and couscous

Serves 4

1 box Near East couscous, Parmesan flavor
1 tablespoon olive oil
1 pound shrimp, peeled and deveined
2 cups asparagus tips
1 medium tomato, diced

Prepare couscous according to package directions. Meanwhile heat olive oil in a nonstick skillet over medium heat. Add asparagus tips and shrimp; stir until shrimp is done. Add chopped tomato and stir briefly to heat through. Combine shrimp mixture with couscous to serve.

Per serving: 309 calories, 8 grams fat, 35 grams carbs, 3 grams fiber, 26 grams protein

BODY FOR LIFE FOR WOMEN

We like to buy frozen chopped spinach in the loose-pack bags and toss a handful into many recipes to sneak in more veggies.

seafood stuffed peppers

Serves 2

1 cup frozen spinach, loose pack
½ cup whole-wheat pasta (dry), tiny shells or elbows
1 teaspoon oil
2 tablespoons finely chopped onion
½ cup low-fat cottage cheese
2 ounces surimi crab, chopped, or use chopped shrimp
1 ounce reduced-fat Swiss cheese, shredded or cut into small
   pieces
Salt and pepper to taste
2 large, sweet red bell peppers, tops and seed core removed

Preheat oven to 350°F. Allow spinach to thaw, then squeeze out moisture. Set aside.

Prepare pasta according to package directions, but remove from water just before done. Pasta will continue to cook in the oven, so you don't want it to get mushy. Drain and place in a medium mixing bowl and set aside.

Meanwhile, heat oil in a nonstick skillet and sauté onion until just translucent. Add thawed and squeezed spinach to skillet and stir to combine. Remove from heat and add to mixing bowl with pasta.

Place cottage cheese in bowl of food processor, and process

until creamy. Combine pasta, seafood, spinach and onions, cottage cheese, Swiss cheese, and salt and pepper to taste. Stuff mixture into bell peppers. Place in a small baking dish and cover with foil. Bake for one hour or until peppers are tender.

Per serving: 262 calories, 5 grams fat, 34 grams carbs, 7 grams fiber, 24 grams protein

---

Nonstarchy vegetables are allowed almost endlessly. So when you're in the mood for some quantity, try this recipe for a delicious addition to your lean protein choice!

savory roasted green beans

Serves 4

1 bag (16 ounces) frozen whole green beans (do not thaw)
4 teaspoons olive oil
1 tablespoon Worcestershire sauce
Kosher salt to taste
Freshly cracked black pepper (use plenty!)

Preheat oven to 425°F. Toss all ingredients in the bottom of a jelly roll pan, and spread out in single layer. Roast in the oven for 12 to 17 minutes, depending on the thickness of the beans, until they begin to shrivel and become slightly dark.

Per serving: 80 calories, 5 grams fat, 1 gram saturated fat, 9 carbs, 3 grams fiber, 2 grams protein

CURVES

These "free shakes" are free as long as they contain less than twenty carbs and more than twenty grams of protein. So the chicks make them with plain, unflavored protein powder. It's definitely an acquired taste.

apple pie free shake

Serves 1

¼ cup unsweetened applesauce
3 tablespoons nonfat vanilla yogurt, no sugar added
¾ cup skim milk
1 scoop plain, unflavored protein powder (15 g protein per
  scoop)
Hefty dash cinnamon or apple pie spice
2 or 3 ice cubes

Combine all ingredients in a blender and blend until smooth. Pour in a tall glass to serve.

Per serving: 178 calories, 1 gram fat, 20 grams carbs, 1 gram fiber, 23 grams protein

Words to Live By

I often take exercise. Why, only yesterday I had my breakfast in bed.
— Oscar Wilde

I keep trying to lose weight . . . but it keeps finding me!
— Author Unknown

chicks in the zone
the zone diet

I F YOU'RE INTO losing weight while maintaining a round-the-clock natural high that makes taking the pounds off painless, then the Zone diet from Dr. Barry Sears may be a plan that will work for you. In essence, the Zone is a well-balanced diet plan that restricts starchy carbs, which, admittedly, are the only carbs worth talking about for many of us. However, rather than just cutting out carbs, the Zone emphasizes a perfect balance of protein, fat, and carbs. This plan is roughly 40 percent protein, 30 percent carbs, and 30 percent fat.

The Zone is commonly referred to as a low-carb diet, which seems to be a real pet peeve of Dr. Sears. And comparing it to traditional low-carb diets, we would have to agree that it isn't just a fancy version of Atkins, but it could still be considered a *reduced*-carb diet. The National Institutes of Health considers the average diet to be 45 to 65 percent carbohydrates. At 30 percent carbs, this plan is at about the third rung on the low-carb limbo stick, not the floor-rubbing bottom rung that Atkins chicks play at.

Before you run out to stock up on corn on the cob and crescent rolls to go with your rib-eye steak, take a minute to read the fine print. The Zone plan calls for mostly lean protein and nonstarchy carbs, like grilled chicken, steamed green beans, bowls of fruit, and other foods that won't heavily impact your glucose levels.

If you manage to maintain this nutritional balance, Dr. Sears tells us, you will enter a state of hormonal bliss called "the Zone." The Zone is a physical state of harmony that we achieve when we maintain the correct level of insulin (affectionately known as the fat storage hormone), in our bloodstreams.

Dr. Sears claims that if you can keep your insulin from becoming either too high or too low, you will not only lose weight without being hungry, but your health and overall sense of well-being will be drastically improved and you will achieve something called "SuperHealth." Who could ask for anything more?

One easy way to enter the Zone and stay there: before each meal, you must mentally divide your plate into three equal sections. In one section you will have a portion of lean protein. Then you will fill up the rest of the plate with Zone-friendly veggies and fruit, with a dab of good fat, like olive oil, or almond slices. You'll do this for three meals a day.

For snacks, you will follow the same ratio, but with a smaller plate. How much you are allowed to put on your plate depends on your activity level and your lean body mass, which Dr. Sears teaches you how to calculate. This is called your "protein prescription."

The alternate method to counting on the Zone diet is relatively easy to master. You'll be eating a prescribed number of "blocks," depending on your body composition and activity level. The average woman will get three block meals a day. At each meal you can have three blocks each of protein, carbs, and fat. A block of protein is generally equal to an ounce of lean protein. A block of carbs can range from several cups of chopped spinach to one-third cup of mashed potatoes. Clearly, the more advance planning you do, the more bang you can get for your Zone buck. There are numerous books on the Zone, including *Zone Blocks*, which has lists of block portions for every kind of food imaginable. If you want bacon and eggs for breakfast, you can look it up in the book and see, for instance, that two egg whites equal a block, and so does one whole egg or three slices of turkey bacon. If, like most women, you eat three blocks per meal, you can have, for example, nine slices of turkey bacon or six egg whites or any other three-block calculation of protein at your meal. While you're at it, you can look up your fats and carbs and round out your whole plate, Zone style.

While it may sound easy enough to look up your foods and pick individual ingredients, it isn't always easy to make an actual recipe. The majority of your family recipes are not going to be Zone ready, and many just can't be converted at all. It's not much fun to pick apart your meal to try to come out with the correct portions. You'll find it much easier to stick to Zone recipes.

Are you still with us? Now comes the hard part—which is to say, the carbohydrate part. The Zone recommends very few grains; most of your carbohydrates will come in the form of low-density carbs like broccoli, cauliflower, cabbage, or greens. Bread, pasta, and rice should be eaten sparingly, much like a garnish. Grains are high in calories and carbohydrates, and they also have a high impact on insulin, which is the enemy of SuperHealth.

According to Dr. Sears, though, all those starchy carbohydrates like mashed potatoes and cinnamon rolls won't be hard to give up, because within a few days you will enter the Zone, where there is no such thing as a Big Mac attack, and Krispy Kreme doughnuts will never again whisper to you across a crowded room.

Dr. Sears contends that by keeping your insulin in balance, you will be able to lose weight and keep it off. To maintain this balance, you need to eat at regular intervals. You will be eating up to five times a day. While the diet is essentially a low-calorie diet, you can eat a large volume of food, so you shouldn't get hungry. You can access more Zone resources and read more examples of food combinations at www.3fatchicks.com/thezone.

So is there really a magical place called SuperHealth where you can give up cookies and cakes and cream puffs and lose weight without even a twinge of a craving? Well, that depends upon whom you ask.

When the Zone was at its peak in popularity back in the nineties, we didn't give it much of a chance. For us, it was too much of a hassle to tabulate 40 percent protein, 30 percent carbs, and 30 percent fat. It seemed like a diet for mathletes. Also, while it's a wonderful idea to get your body into a hormonal state that will give you superhealth and allow you to lose weight painlessly, we're not entirely sure that any of those claims are true. We're not scientists and we don't know of any independent research done on this question other than by the Zone folks. We do know that the calculations are ridiculously thought-intensive for meal planning, and we're not too sure we'd ever be happy with three ounces of chicken, three cups of green beans, and a sprinkle of almonds at mealtime. Also, the strict balance of foods that needs to be adhered to on this diet can be difficult. You could potentially have to eat a whole package of tofu and thirty-six spears of asparagus for dinner to balance the six cashews you nibbled while you were cooking, or risk falling out of the Zone. And all measurements have to be precise; one teaspoon too much of this ingredient or the other could damage your biochemical euphoria. Trying to make recipes that actually mesh well is even harder, so this is a good diet if you are somebody who is happy with simple mixes and combinations. But for most of us, eating in the Zone can get a little boring.

We never personally knew anybody on the Zone, but obviously, this diet has worked for a lot of people out there, so we recently asked our on-line chicks in the Zone what they thought about Barry Sears's plan, and here are some of the questions and comments that they shared.

meet the chicks in the zone

Marion from California

I've tried a few diets but never stayed on them because I hate to cook and I hate most frozen dinners. What else was left but restaurants! I heard about local delivery of fresh Zone meals. They cook a meal fresh and bring it right to you. It's almost like having my own personal chef.

And since portions are controlled, I can't overeat. It's pricey, but it's worth it. I don't think I've ever been so excited about losing weight!

Sarah from Colorado

I finally broke my plateau since starting the Zone! I weighed in at 139 pounds this morning—the first time I have been below 140 pounds in well over a year! This is so exciting! I think completely giving up rice, pasta, and bread gave me the extra "shove" I needed to break through. For the past week, I have been getting all of my carbs from fruits and veggies, and I'm not the least bit hungry.

Rachel from Florida

I've been counting calories for a few weeks and just recently decided to eat fewer carbs and more protein. So I tweaked my plan a little and it turns out that I had adjusted it close to a 40/30/30 ratio, which I remembered from a Zone book I had read a while back. I pulled the book back out and reread it, and now I'm hooked! The plan makes so much sense and it's so much easier than all the extreme low-carb plans. The Zone seems like just the right amount of everything.

Sue from Tennessee

My husband has been packing on the pounds lately. I don't need to lose weight, but I've been preparing Zone meals for both of us. I don't think he even realizes it, and I haven't told him. We've been eating healthier foods like chicken and salmon. I finally asked him to weigh himself, and he's lost seven pounds so far!

Q: I am hardly losing weight. I'm eating the correct blocks of food and exercising every day, but I'm only losing about half a pound per week. What am I doing wrong?

3FC: You're not doing anything wrong. The Zone does not produce quick results. This is not a thin-thighs-in-thirty-days program. The Zone is a fat-burning diet, and therefore you don't drop quick water weight or lean muscle tissue as on the Atkins diet. You should be losing weight at the rate of no more than one to one and a half pounds per week. Depending on how much you have to lose, you may already be losing weight at a very reasonable rate.

You may want to double-check your lean body mass. It's possible that your lean body mass is rising, which means you are losing fat but gaining lean muscle tissue, which in turn can make you heavier, even though you are looking and feeling more fit. Look at the big picture and don't rely on the scale. Your tape measure should show some results.

If not, look again at the rules of the plan. Are you drinking enough water? Are you measuring your food, or trying to eyeball the portion sizes? Maybe your eyes are bigger than your portion restrictions. Read *The Zone* again to refresh your memory, and make double sure that you are counting your blocks correctly. Not all carbs are created equal. For instance, one block of strawberries is equal to one-third cup of oatmeal.

One more thing you can try—revisit your activity level categories. This may also be a good time to check your exercise level and see if you can add anything to your program. And don't forget to leave enough time between meals so that you can keep your insulin steady and stay in the Zone.

To Market, to Market

If you're taking it on the lam, it's a good idea to bring along some emergency rations so that you can stay in the Zone even though you're away from home. Here are some ideas for what to pack in your brown bag. Mix and match as necessary to make a Zone-ready meal or snack.

1. Tuna or chicken in pouches or tins
2. Reduced-fat cheese sticks

3. Ready-to-drink shakes
4. Protein shake mix and canned milk
5. Applesauce cups
6. An orange or other fresh fruit
7. Chopped raw veggies, like cucumber and broccoli, with cherry tomatoes
8. Almonds and peanuts
9. Hershey SmartZone bars
10. Cash for a fast-food grilled chicken salad

Q: All I ever eat for breakfast are egg white omelets, and I can't take another one. Any suggestions, besides sleeping until lunch?

3FC: You're in luck. Although egg whites are optimal choices, they can get old quick. So break a few rules that won't cost you calories, and have lunch for breakfast. Try eating our salad on page 192, protein-fortified pudding, cottage cheese and fruit, or even a meal replacement shake, such as a ready-to-drink ZonePerfect shake. There are Zone-authorized meals and snacks available; you'll find a current list at www.3fatchicks.com/thezone.

If you prefer strictly breakfast foods for breakfast, you might try making a quiche—chock-full of vegetables—or boiled eggs, protein pancakes, crepes, or even oatmeal and turkey bacon. Try to incorporate fresh fruit into your meal for a more invigorating breakfast. A meal of almond-sprinkled oatmeal, strawberries, and scrambled egg substitute is right on target.

Q: I'm confused. I thought bananas were okay, but now I've heard they are unfavorable carbs. Am I not supposed to be eating them? I'm not sure I can do without my banana in the morning.

3FC: You can eat unfavorable carbs, which unfortunately include bananas, but it is best that you limit them as much as you can. Keep unfavorable carbs to 25 percent of your total carb intake. This means if you get four blocks per meal, one of your blocks can be an unfavorable carb. However, if you have a three-block meal, that's a little harder to calculate! You'll be able to eat more food if you restrict unfavorable carbs, and you won't risk falling out of the Zone because of fluctuating insulin levels.

So the answer is yes, you can enjoy a banana every now and again, but you should try to eat fewer of them, which can be hard at first, we know. As you get used to the program and enjoy the feeling of Super-Health, you'll be happier doing without the foods you currently crave. In fact, Dr. Sears recommends eating a carb-rich meal once a month. This is so the carb hangover will remind you how being out of the Zone feels. This lesson will both help keep you focused and give you a chance to enjoy the foods you miss!

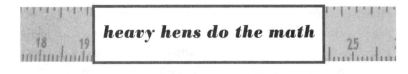

heavy hens do the math

We asked our heavy hens to crunch their numbers, and here are some of the sobering figures they came up with.

- 67 percent were overweight as children.
- 84 percent have immediate family members who are also overweight.
- 32 percent have been on more than twenty diets.
- 80 percent have *not* been diagnosed with a health condition that affected their weight.
- 87 percent felt lack of motivation because their goal weights were so far away and did not seem attainable.

- 20 percent said they walk for exercise because it is easier for them than other activities.
- 21 percent had joined a gym.
- 12 percent were not able to exercise yet, because of their size.
- Only 8 percent felt embarrassed to exercise in front of others. The rest exercise in various ways at home.
- 24 percent said the fear of sagging, excess skin deterred them from losing weight.

Q: I am able to stick to this plan really well, but I'm having a problem on the weekends when I'm off work. I get wild snack attacks, and I occasionally give in. It's just so difficult sometimes!

3FC: If you are truly in the Zone, a hormonal state that lasts around the clock, you should not be experiencing hunger. You may experience difficulties if you spread your meals too far apart or if you are eating the incorrect volumes or ratios. Double-check your weekend food against the acceptable food list, and make sure you are eating meals or snacks no more than five hours apart.

If you're sure that you're eating correctly, your problem may be a case of head hunger. It's fairly common for people to reach for food when stressed, tired, or anxious. It might help to switch the order of your meals and snacks. Try a protein shake for your next meal. It will be balanced and sweet enough that, hopefully, your cravings will subside.

Q: I'm interested in lower-carb diets, but I'm a vegetarian. I tried Atkins once and it was a disaster. Can I do the Zone without eating a block of tofu for every meal? My regular diet is primarily grains, veggie burgers, and tofu.

3FC: The Zone is very soy-friendly. Dr. Sears says that the vegetarian version may even be the healthiest version available. You can have tofu, soy meat substitutes, eggs, and some dairy products to fill your portion of daily protein.

It is easier to be a vegetarian on the Zone than it is on Atkins. On Atkins, you eat mostly protein and fat, with a much smaller portion of vegetables. That doesn't leave a lot of choices for a vegetarian. On the Zone, you eat lower fat, with a much closer ratio of carbs and protein. This means you can have plenty of vegetables on your plate and even some grains once in a while, not just a brick of tofu.

Q: I'm having problems with constipation. If I take fiber supplements, do I have to count them as carb blocks? I'd rather eat my carbs than dissolve them in a glass of water.

3FC: Fiber supplements do not count as carbohydrate blocks as long as they are just straight fiber. "Fiber cookies" would count as a carb, as they also have flour and sugar. Dr. Sears says he first used the phrase "net carbs" in 1995 for calculating carbs. His definition of net carbs is carbohydrates minus fiber, and that is what should be counted for your carb block. When the low carb-craze hit, the phrase "net carbs for Atkins" became very popular; it also included subtracting sugar alcohols from the total. On the Zone, you will subtract only fiber. So, as long as your fiber is straight fiber, you are free to use it. You should also try to incorporate more fiber into your diet so you will not need to use supplements.

Q: There is so much technical information in the book, and honestly, I just don't get it. How do the blocks work, simply speaking? I can't stick to this plan if I have to struggle to plan a meal.

3FC: Originally, meals were described as comprising 40 percent protein, 30 percent carbohydrates, and 30 percent fat. This was just a general idea; it has been refined over the years. An updated version of this formula is the block method. This way of counting will save you from having to carry a nutritional guide and a calculator to the dinner table.

Each meal is divided into Zone blocks. The number of blocks you get to eat is based on factors such as your activity level. Blocks consist of mini-blocks for each group of fat, carbs, and protein. For example, if you get to eat three blocks at mealtime, you'll have three blocks of protein, three blocks of carbs, and three blocks of fat. If you get one block at snack time, that means one block of protein, one block of carbohydrates, and one block of fat.

You must always include all three groups. Portion size depends on the type of food you choose. A block of protein equals one ounce of lean meat. Some protein blocks give you larger portions, like two ounces of shrimp. Carbohydrates vary widely, from several cups of chopped spinach, to a quarter cup of pasta. Fats range from one-third of a teaspoon for oils to six peanuts. You can mix and match from the lists to build your perfect Zone meal.

Complete lists of the portions are included on the Zone Web site and in recent Zone books, such as *Mastering the Zone, The Top 100 Zone Foods,* and *What to Eat in the Zone.*

Dr. Sears actually recommends eyeballing the portions. He says to eat a palm-sized portion of meat, which will take up one-third of your plate. You can fill up the rest of the plate with nonstarchy vegetables and add a splash of good fat. We have to admit it sounds easier than it is. We're not sure how eyeballing the portion sizes can be that helpful if it takes just the right balance to enter the Zone. When portions such as one-third teaspoon oil are involved, or carbohydrate portions that vary from one-third cup peas to four cups cucumbers, it just seems smarter to have a handbook and some measuring spoons handy.

Q: I'm thinking about leaving my low-carb diet and entering the Zone. Am I still going to lose weight? I've lost twenty pounds on low-carb, but I'm ready for some more variety.

3FC: If you are on a strict low-carb diet, then you may very well gain a few pounds as you reintroduce carbs. This isn't fat, however. You'll be regaining water weight you lost at the start of your low-carb diet. Relax, it will come off again on the Zone, only this time you should be losing fat instead of just water!

Q: The Zone recommends fish oil every day. Can I use something else, like flaxseed oil? The fish oil capsules are huge, and sometimes I burp fish through the day.

3FC: The fish oil has been chosen not just for the omega-3 oils but also for the essential acids EPA and DHA. Taking other oils might be helpful, but not as effective for the purposes that Dr. Sears has outlined in his book.

If you can't take a large capsule, you can burst the capsules and take the liquid straight, or mix it in with cottage cheese or a nutritional shake—not a very appetizing thought. You can also look for smaller capsules and increase the number of capsules you take to reach the dose you need.

If you haven't taken fish oil recently, you might be happy to know that there are newer brands on the market that may not give you indigestion. They are more expensive, but they are purer, and will have fewer side effects. Look for an ultrarefined fish oil, commonly advertised as having "no fishy aftertaste." Mmm, what more could a girl ask for? You can also explore vegetarian supplement options at your local health food store.

We would like to note that you should not take fish oil supplements without speaking to your doctor first. Fish oil can interact with and worsen the effects of certain medications or medical conditions.

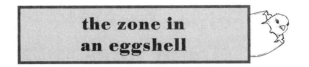

the zone in an eggshell

Professional Counseling None.

Support System There is a forum at the official site and various forums across the Internet.

Fitness Factor There is no official guideline for exercise, but the amount of food you eat is based on your activity level.

Family-Friendly You can feed the whole family on Zone foods. All you have to do is measure out your own portions.

Pros Wholesome foods and a balanced diet. You're less likely to get hungry on this plan than on plans like the South Beach diet.

Cons Very few convenience foods. Might be monotonous for the traveler because of the lack of fast-food options. Measuring can be tedious until you get skilled at eyeballing portions. Non-Zone recipes with multiple ingredients can be hard to convert to Zone portions.

$$ Can be somewhat expensive with more meat and veggies; however, the reduction in junk food helps to compensate, so you probably won't notice a difference in your budget.

The Person This Diet Is Best For Somebody who doesn't mind measuring and having specific guidelines on how to eat. Also vegetarians.

recipes from the front lines

This untraditional breakfast is a great way to get out of the "I'm bored with breakfast" blues. You should note that this recipe does include the unfavorable carb maple syrup. Keep an eye on your unfavorable carb list, and don't overindulge too often.

"i'm bored with breakfast" salad

Serves 1

3 cups spring mix, or other leafy lettuce
3 slices turkey bacon, cooked and torn in bite-sized pieces
½ teaspoon canola oil
½ teaspoon red wine vinegar
½ teaspoon Dijon mustard
¼ teaspoon coarsely ground black pepper
4 teaspoons reduced-sugar maple syrup
Cooking spray
1 egg plus 2 egg whites

Place lettuce mixture in salad bowl and mix with turkey bacon. Set aside. In small bowl, add oil, vinegar, mustard, pepper, and syrup. Mix thoroughly and drizzle over the lettuce and bacon mixture. Toss to cover all the lettuce and bacon.

Spray warm skillet with cooking spray and add the whole

egg and egg whites. Puncture yolk so it spreads across egg whites. When egg sets, turn over and cook the other side. When egg is completely cooked, chop into bite-sized pieces with the edge of the egg turner. Pour chopped egg onto salad mixture and serve immediately.

Per serving: 314 calories, 15 grams fat, 24 grams carbs, 2 grams fiber, 21 grams protein

---

Here's a recipe that keeps the precious balance you need in order to stay in the Zone!

chicken cashew stir fry

Serves 1

1½ teaspoons soy sauce
1 teaspoon cornstarch (1 carb block)
1 teaspoon broth or cold water
½ cup nonfat chicken broth
3 ounces chicken breast, skinless, cut into thin strips (3 protein blocks)
¼ teaspoon freshly grated ginger
1 clove garlic, minced
½ cup broccoli, cut up (⅓ carb block)
1 red bell pepper, cored and chopped (⅓ carb block)
½ cup sliced onion (⅓ carb block)
⅓ cup sliced water chestnuts (1 carb block)
9 whole cashews, split in half (3 fat blocks)

● *Continued on next page* ●

In a small bowl, combine soy sauce, cornstarch, and water or broth. Stir until smooth and set aside.

Heat ¼ cup of the chicken broth in a nonstick skillet over medium high heat, and add chicken strips, garlic, and ginger. Stir for a couple of minutes until chicken is done. Add remaining ¼-cup broth, the vegetables, and cashews, and continue to stir and cook until crisp tender, or to the degree of doneness that you prefer. Add reserved cornstarch mixture and stir quickly until all is coated and sauce is slightly thickened.

Words to Live By

My whole life, I've wanted to feel comfortable in my skin. It's the most liberating thing in the world. —DREW BARRYMORE

Avoid any diet that discourages the use of hot fudge.

—DON KARDONG

grand ole oprah chicks

bob greene,
oprah's boot camp,
dr. phil

FROM THE THIGH MASTER to the Ab Roller to Trimspa Baby! we fat chicks are fascinated with celebrity fitness products, plans, and endorsements. We rush out in droves to buy the latest craze, convinced that after only ten minutes each day, we too can have thighs, buns, and six-pack abs like the stars. Unfortunately, most of us discover that our celebrity fitness miracle is a more useful clothes hanger than a makeover machine. But in the world of Tinseltown trim-downs, there is one role model who for us is worth her weight in gold.

Oprah is the be-all and end-all of weight-loss queens. When Oprah lost weight, we cheered and we loved her, and were never jealous. When she gained weight, we felt her pain, and we understood, because we had been there. When Oprah climbed back up on the diet horse, we hung on to every pound through every episode. We chatted about how chiseled her cheekbones looked, how her hips were getting smaller, and how tiny her waistline had become. When she wheeled out the wagon o' fat to show how much weight she had lost, flashing her skinny jeans to the cameras, we vowed to pass the story down to our children and their children, for years to come. Meanwhile, Calvin Klein jeans flew off the shelves all over the planet.

Looking at the competition, nobody else comes close to being our weight-loss guru. Suzanne Somers, the trim, perky pigtailed blonde who kept us company throughout the seventies, struggled to lose a mere fifteen pounds, but it was lost and documented before we ever knew it happened. Marilu Henner lost around fifty pounds and invested more blood, sweat, and tears in her weight-loss process, but she wasn't in our living rooms every afternoon loving us like Oprah was. And Anna "Trimspa, Baby!" Nicole Smith, well . . . we'll let Anna speak for herself.

So why has Oprah been able to influence hundreds of thousands, if not millions, of us fat chicks to actually do something about our health? After all, she isn't really just one of the girls. The woman is a gazillionaire. Oprah has mansions, trainers, personal gyms, assistants, maids, cooks, and chauffeurs. She can pay someone to lift her legs, cook her meals, and then wipe her brow when she's done. Oprah is one of the most powerful people in America, and definitely one of the richest. So why does Oprah inspire us to lose weight, even though she obviously has a whole lot more help reaching her goal than we ever will?

Well, because Oprah lets us take a peek at the real struggle of weight loss. Oprah took responsibility for every bite that went in her mouth, and she didn't try to make the process look simple or slick. She wanted french fries, damn it, and we understood! She resisted exercise, got frustrated, and told us about where she was going wrong. She shared her bad experiences as well as her joys, and women all over the country who had ridden the same roller-coaster fell in love with her.

We also fell in love with her trainers. Bob Greene became a fitness guru because he and his Make the Connection program helped Oprah get in shape. We 3 fat chicks bought the "Make the Connection" video and all piled up together and watched it from beginning to end, armed with a box of Kleenex. From that day forward, we got together for Fat Chick Day once a week. This was a day we devoted to our futures. We discussed diet and exercise and talked about what we really wanted to do for our health. We each bought copies of Bob's book and journal, and we followed his tips and lost weight, just so we could follow in Oprah's footsteps.

We also fell in love with Dr. Phil, who helped Oprah triumph in her infamous Texas beef court battle. And although he was not connected to the fitness world at that time, it was enough for us that he got Oprah into the right mind-set to triumph over all those angry Texans. He taught Oprah how to put mind over meat, and so it was inevitable that Dr. Phil would eventually adapt his pull-yourself-up-by-your-bootstraps approach to life to the weight-loss world. Now chicks from sea to shining sea are chanting his Seven Keys to Weight Loss Freedom, and counting down their dress sizes too, we hope.

Oprah plays a big role in our personal diet histories. She was a celebrity who had the courage to let us know that she was no different from the rest of us. Oprah got fat just like us, lost weight with difficulty just like us, and put the weight back on afterward—*just like us.* But along the way she taught us that if we don't give up, we can achieve our goals. She reminded us that two steps forward and one step back is better than no steps forward at all. Oprah helped us understand that while the battle of the bulge never really ends, if we hold our ground and keep charging up over that hill, we really can trade our potbelly for a pot of gold at the end of our personal rainbow.

So in a book where we have tried to take a look beneath the surface glimmer of diet and fitness plans, and shy away from celebrity, we felt it was important to include the one school of celebrity fitness thinking that really has made a difference to the waistlines of the world.

meet the grand ole oprah chicks

Megan from Kentucky

I could have never lost weight without Oprah. I tried so many diets, and I always failed. Oprah put aside her vanity and she showed us sweat, and she showed us determination, and she showed us victory. I never see celebrities struggle; they hide it from us—but not Oprah. She's got the same weaknesses that we all do, but thanks to her I know that just because I have a weak side, it doesn't mean that I'm not strong. *I am strong, I fought the battle, and I won. Thank you, Oprah, for helping me get my life back.*

Kery from France

I am a twenty-six-year-old graphic designer. I've had this problem with "bad foods" for a long, long time. I didn't crave vegetables and fruits, but I could go a whole week eating pizza, potatoes, pasta, fast food, cookies, and other junky stuff without even blinking. What caused me to really think about it and make the *decision to lose weight was partly reading Dr. Phil McGraw's book; it may seem like "only a book," but it spoke to me in a way that no friend or family member had ever done, and helped me think and understand why I had many "bad" food behaviors—as well as giving me ideas about how to correct them. Granted, it's not a fairy tale, and it's not easy every day. It's been two months now. I wouldn't say it's a struggle for me; it's more like getting slowly accustomed, and once I am, things seem easier and more pleasant.*

Keli from Pennsylvania

I recently read the Bob Greene Total Body Makeover. *I've read these types of books before but mostly skimmed over parts, and actually doing them was hit or miss. I really read the first chapter on "building a solid emotional foundation." I started looking at why weight loss worked in the past and why it got away from me. I lost sixty-five pounds on Weight Watchers years ago and gained it all back. Bob Greene's concept of "conscious eating," which is really paying attention to what you're eating and why, is helping me. I'm trying to eat for nutrition now, and not for comfort. It's amazing how many times, especially at work, I would eat something that was offered just because it was offered and without even thinking. I found the book enlightening. In fact I'm going to read it again.*

BOB GREENE MAKES THE CONNECTION

Oprah's trainer Bob Greene first brought his program to the world when he published his first book, *Make the Connection*, in 1996. Few weight-loss books have been as moving or as willing to bring a new attitude and approach to weight loss. The central idea was a simple one: if Oprah could do it, we could too.

Make the Connection started the whole Oprah/diet movement. It was a book, video, and companion journal all wrapped up tightly so that even mere mortals like us could lose weight the same way that Oprah did. The book, written by Bob and Oprah, sold millions of copies, and we wish we knew just how many pounds of fat were lost around the world because of it.

Make the Connection was popular not just because of Oprah but also because it was a sound, reasonable approach to weight loss that didn't include a fad diet. The book is still available on Amazon, though the video can only be found on eBay now.

Make the Connection is a multistep approach to weight loss. Here are the steps:

- Do aerobic exercise five to seven days a week, at least twenty to sixty minutes each session.
- Eat three meals and two snacks daily, consisting of a low-fat, balanced diet. Include at least two fruits and three vegetables each day.

- Limit or eliminate alcohol, and drink six to eight glasses of water daily.
- Stop eating two to three hours before bedtime.
- Renew your commitment to a healthy lifestyle each day.

Simple, right? So simple, in fact, that we don't understand why this program isn't still as popular as it was when it first came out. It makes sense, it's easy to follow, and it works. We have even found that our own diet efforts have been more successful when we incorporated these guidelines. But sometimes a chick just needs more. And when we needed more, Bob gave it to us in his second book, *The Total Body Makeover.*

The Total Body Makeover takes a different approach to weight loss and has a stronger focus on exercise than diet. In *Make the Connection,* we did aerobics five to seven times a week. This time Bob added weight training and other exercises for a more complete body workout. The goal is not just to burn off the fat but to tone up the muscles as well so we can look buff in our workout gear!

The most interesting part of *The Total Body Makeover* is that we are advised not to go on a diet, other than to follow a few basic eating guidelines. We should eat three meals and two snacks every day, and we should never skip breakfast. In fact, Bob puts as much emphasis on starting each day with a nutritious breakfast as Mom did! You should also end each day on the right note. Pick a cutoff point and never eat past that time, period. This one tip has helped many chicks lose a few pounds. The food we eat at night isn't metabolized any differently; it's our food choices late at night that are the true culprit. How many of us pig out on celery sticks while watching Letterman? We're more likely to eat chips or ice cream late at night. Remove the option to eat, and you eliminate the bad foods. It really is a lot easier than it sounds.

In *Make the Connection,* we were advised to go on a low-fat diet. In *The Total Body Makeover,* Bob tells us it is in our best interest not to cut calories too much and to give exercise a chance to help us lose weight first. Don't get too excited just yet. We still have to follow common-sense rules at the kitchen table. A nutritious breakfast doesn't include honey buns or anything floating in gravy. However, you won't have to cut out bread, count points, or refer to a forbidden foods list. If you don't feel comfortable with your progress after the first twelve-week round, then you can go on a more structured, formal diet. What diet would you follow? Any one you want. Bob includes a basic rundown of all the popular diets, from Atkins to Weight Watchers, and invites you to choose the one you like best. Or don't follow a diet at all, just eat healthier foods and don't pig out. If you think that this sounds like the perfect program for the chick who hates to diet but loves to exercise, you would be right! Here are the plan basics:

Total Body Makeover Plan Basics

Five Simple Eating Rules
- Have an eating cutoff time.
- Eat a nourishing breakfast.
- Drink at least six 8-ounce glasses of water each day.
- Eliminate alcohol.
- Make eating a conscious act (eat for the right reasons).

Twelve-Week Exercise Plan
- Functional exercises six times per week
- Strength-training exercises three times per week
- Aerobic exercise five days per week
- Double aerobic exercise on sixth day each week
- Rest on seventh day

Bob Greene has routines for beginning, intermediate, and advanced levels, so you can jump in wherever feels right. The program grows with you, as you graduate to each new level. The total beginner will have no trouble getting started. A good half of the book is just photos of exercises and a twelve-week chart so you know exactly what to do on which days. Bob calls this Boot Camp, and for good reason. It is an intensive exercise program, and you will have to be devoted and work hard. The payoff, though, will be more energy, long-term weight loss, and buns of steel. If you need a little inspiration, we recommend that you rent a copy of *G.I. Jane* and envision yourself as Demi Moore in training.

Whether you choose the original *Make the Connection* or the newer *Total Body Makeover*, you are going to exercise a lot every day, including doing cardio and weights. A lot of people are going to do well with this plan, because you see results right away, which is a great motivator. Besides, we are getting to the point in society where everything goes to extremes, fitness included, so there are a lot of fitness plans out there that are more extreme than these. But the *Total Body Makeover* is going to take more dedication than the other fitness and diet programs we've reviewed in this book. We think that *Make the Connection* takes a slightly gentler approach, even though it requires just as much dedication. It is easy to follow, makes a lot of sense, and could be applied to anyone's life, no matter how much or how little time someone has to devote to a fitness plan. To get a more rounded picture of this program, we asked our Oprah chicks to air in with some of their questions and concerns.

Q: The word aerobics *gives me traumatic flashbacks to the eighties, and I get visions of pink tights and frantic dance movements in time to the soundtrack of* Footloose. *Can I do this program without reliving these unpleasant memories?*

3FC: Aerobics does not necessarily equal doing Kevin Bacon–inspired buck-and-wings dressed in a spandex bodysuit. The term covers a wide range of activities, from running to spinning, or even in-line skating. You can choose the activities that you enjoy the most. In fact, you should choose several aerobic activities so you don't get burned out. Variety keeps your exercise routine interesting every day, and you'll be more motivated to continue. Most of the activities are free and can be done in the privacy of your own home. If you do feel a little footloose, you are still free to head to your nearest fitness center and sign up for a dance aerobics class.

Q: There's no way I can eat breakfast every day. I'm not hungry, I don't have time, and I don't even like breakfast food. Can't I just get a big snack later?

3FC: Isn't it funny how breakfast can elicit opposite reactions from people? Some people can't even open their eyes in the morning unless their heads are hovering over a plate of flapjacks, grits, and sausage. Other people consider breakfast a burden and the most expendable of meals. We're told time and time again that if we aren't hungry, just don't eat. This rule doesn't apply at breakfast. Even if you do not feel hungry, have something light, such as our Tomato Basil Eggs on page 218. You'll be less likely to overeat later too. Breakfast doesn't have to include eggs or other traditional foods. Pick a food you really like, so you'll enjoy it. Try a sandwich or a smoothie or a high-protein pizza, such as the frozen South Beach diet pizzas. They are all quick solutions and the beginning of a good habit.

Q: I'm a habitual late-night muncher. I can't watch TV unless I'm eating or go to sleep without a snack. Sometimes I sneak and nibble after the family has gone to bed. I've tried establishing a cutoff time for eating, but I keep slipping back into my habit, and sometimes I "forget" about it. What can I do?

3FC: Late-night munching is a very common problem. Sometimes we eat out of boredom or habit, but rarely out of true hunger. Make a deliberate, conscious effort to break this habit. Set an alarm clock for your cutoff time, so you have a loud reminder to stop eating. Don't rely on your memory if you have the convenient ability to lose track of the time. If necessary, enlist the help of a friend or family member to remind you that your eating day has finished. It won't take long before it feels natural to you.

beating the midnight munchies

There's an old saying that idle hands are the devil's tools—definitely true when it comes to late-night snacking. If we can stay busy, we are less likely to slip our hands into the cookie jar. Here are some ideas our chicks shared to help avoid late-night nibbling.

Buy yourself a nice manicure set so you can pamper your fingers at night. You'd never dream of interrupting the polishing and buffing to muss them up with cheese doodle dust! Pedicures are also a good deterrent. You don't want to slide around on the kitchen floor with wet tootsies, so a good soak and shine can help keep you in one place. —DOREEN

Fill your magazine stand with fitness magazines. When the urge hits to reach for a snack, grab a magazine and remind yourself what your goals are. —MARYBETH

Read anything. No, wait, read about sex. Better yet, have sex! —LAURA

Before you reach your eating cutoff time, make sure you take the time to thoroughly enjoy your last snack or meal. It's easy to get distracted and finish your food without noticing a bite, and then you are left craving more food even if you are not physically hungry. Sit down at your table and eat off a pretty dish. Get rid of any distractions, and just savor the moment. You'll find it so satisfying that you probably won't want anything else later. —ANDREA

Let your cell phone help curb nighttime snacking. Take advantage of the free nighttime calls and phone your diet buddies around the country! This is much better than eating! —JACQUELINE

Use teeth-whitening strips at night, to brighten your smile. You can't eat while using them, and you won't want to eat afterwards! —CATHY

Instead of food, try a gourmet tea from vendors such as www.adagio.com. It's flavorful, comforting, and calorie-free, and some people think green tea can even help with weight loss. —DIANA

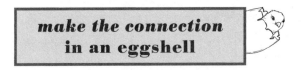

Professional counseling None.

Support System None.

Fitness Factor Regular aerobic exercise is required almost daily.

Family-Friendly Very. You do not have to buy special diet foods, just need to make lower-fat versions of your usual, balanced meals.

Pros Guidelines are very clear and make it easy to stay focused. A companion journal helps you to keep track.

Cons Not as much emphasis on overall fitness as in *The Total Body Makeover.*

● *Continued on next page* ●

$$ Just the cost of the book and the optional companion journal.

The Person This Diet Is Best For Someone who is dedicated, likes a low-fat diet, is willing to exercise daily, and likes having her routine spelled out for her.

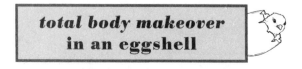

total body makeover in an eggshell

Professional Counseling None.

Support System Bob offers a support forum on his Web site, www.getwiththeprogram.org, but it is limited and slow, and there doesn't seem to be any official interaction. This program is also supported at eDiets, for a small subscription fee.

Fitness Factor It's all about the fitness. Expect to be dedicated six days a week for this intensive workout program.

Family-Friendly Yes! You are not on a diet with this plan, so you can feed your family your usual meals and not feel left out. If you do opt to diet, your plan will be as family-friendly as the diet you choose.

Pros You don't have to go on a diet plan, just focus on the exercise. It's flexible enough for any fitness level. The book goes into great detail to make sure you understand the exercises and routines.

Cons Some people may have difficulty adapting their lifestyle to this plan, especially if they don't like to eat breakfast or have trouble with the eating cutoff time. It can be hard to fit in all the exercise.

$$ Very affordable! You may need to purchase dumbbells or good walking shoes. You can choose aerobic activities that are not free, such as spinning classes or fitness videos, or you can just put on your shoes and hit the pavement.

The Person This Diet Is Best For Anyone who hates to diet but doesn't mind getting her rear in gear and working out.

OPRAH'S BOOT CAMP

We think that Oprah must have been a Marine drill sergeant in her former life. No one else could expect us to go through such a grueling routine as Oprah's Boot Camp. In this program, Oprah started with Bob Greene's *Total Body Makeover* and kicked it up a notch—and we don't mean like Emeril does. Instead of seven workouts per week, we get eight. We are supposed to do aerobics once a day for four days, twice a day for two days, and rest on the seventh. If you think that's tough, wait until you see what you'll eat!

Oprah stresses the elimination of all the white stuff from our diets. That means no rice, no flour, and no sugar. Ouch! But if you can get past the pain principle, you'll realize that whole grains are healthier, and sugar never gave anyone smoother skin or a better sex life. You are permitted two fruits daily and all the green vegetables you want. You can eat lean proteins and include just a little bit of good fat daily.

For the first four weeks, this is all you'll eat. You don't even get whole grains—no oatmeal, whole-grain bread, not even a grain of brown rice. Assuming you make it through the first four weeks, you can gradually add the whole grains back into your diet.

Now, we know what you are thinking. At first glance, Oprah's Boot Camp sounds really difficult, and a whole lot like Dr. Atkins. And the first part of the diet doesn't seem balanced, so why would Oprah suggest that we do something so restrictive? We thought she loved us! Maybe it's tough love, because while the plan does start out difficult, it gets easier, and ultimately, it really works. If you can survive, you really will feel better, and you really will lose weight. One of our own members had this to say after she completed the twelve-week program:

> *This plan would work great if we, like those featured on Oprah's show, had a boss who worked out with us and would get mad at us if we cheated (I mean who wants to make Oprah mad?), had gym equipment at work, and time set aside to exercise. And like Oprah, had people to prepare meals and personal trainers to come to our home and help us work out on the Cadillac of Pilates equipment. I know Oprah works hard and like everyone has to carve time into her day for stuff like that, but still . . .*

Between us chicks, for us, Oprah's Boot Camp looked so difficult that we didn't even make the attempt. Unless we had Oprah herself cracking her whip behind us, we just knew there was no way we were going to be able to stick to it. As diets go, this one is a little too strict for our taste. What ever happened to just using a little common sense and eating normal foods in reasonable portions? We think that this diet might be successful for chicks who don't have a lot of weight to lose, because they won't have to stick to it long. But if you're aiming for a thirty-, fifty-, or hundred-pound loss, we don't see how anybody could stay in Oprah's Boot Camp that long! Here are some thoughts, questions, and concerns from our chicks in Boot Camp who survived to tell the tale.

Q: I know I can't live on green vegetables; they all taste the same to me. Can I at least add tomatoes? What about dairy, such as yogurt? Isn't calcium supposed to be good for weight loss?

3FC: Although the plan does say just green vegetables, we did notice that official Boot Camp members, including Oprah's own staffers, are eating other nonstarchy vegetables. You can have tomatoes, bell peppers, summer squash, eggplant, and more. Once you increase your list of veggies, you can create a lot of really good meals. Most people are also eating some dairy, though they limit it to low-fat or nonfat types, and usually have no more than one cup daily. This seems to work better for the group. And you are right; studies have shown that the calcium in dairy products can help weight loss. However, it needs to be in a dairy product; the effect has not been the same with calcium supplements. We think you should grab your yogurt and not worry about it.

Q: How do I know which to choose? **Make the Connection, Total Body Makeover,** *or Oprah's Boot Camp?*

3FC: Begin by asking yourself what your goals are and how much effort you want to put into this process. If you want quick results and are willing to severely limit your food choices, Oprah's Boot Camp is the way to go. It's tough to follow, but you will see results. If you can't handle the limited food choices but are willing to work out, go for *Total Body Makeover.* You'll work hard, but you can eat what you want to eat, within reason, of course. A lot of women prefer a balanced diet, with a gentle push and easy-to-follow guidelines. *Make the Connection* is a great place to start, and it's a classic!

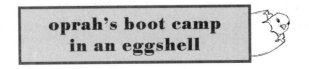

oprah's boot camp in an eggshell

Professional Counseling None.

Support System Message board on Oprah's Web site at www .oprah.com and the option of creating buddy groups on her Web site. No official interaction or guidance.

Fitness Factor *Lots!* Intensive workout, no slacking.

Family-Friendly Not very. Oprah's diet plan is very strict and, with its lack of grains and its other restrictions, particularly in the first four weeks, not balanced for the whole family. Be prepared to feed your family extra foods.

Pros If you can stick it out, it really works.

Cons It is rather extreme at first and may be difficult to stick to.

$$ Cheap! You should buy Bob's *Total Body Makeover* book, dumbbells, and ordinary healthy foods.

The Person This Diet Is Best For Someone who is seriously dedicated, understands the commitment, and is looking for quick initial results.

DR. PHIL'S ULTIMATE WEIGHT-LOSS SOLUTION

Have you ever given up on a diet because the weight loss was too slow? If you're anything like us, the answer to that question is probably *Duh! Of course!* We've all been hung up with instant gratification blues at some point in our lives. Dieting isn't usually a whole lot of fun, doesn't taste rich, sweet, or creamy, and generally doesn't give us overnight results. Going in, we know that, and we think we're prepared to stick with it, for better or worse, until fat do we part. As soon as the scale gives us a disappointing performance two weeks in a row, we're packing our bags and moving on to another diet that works better. It's not the diet that failed us, though; it's our unrealistic expectations.

Lucky for us, Oprah has delivered straight-talking Dr. Phil to set us back on the straight and narrow path to long-term success! Dr. Phil has heard every excuse, bad habit, and dirty diet secret in the fat chick arsenal, and he exposes them all in his book *The Ultimate Weight Solution.*

Diet and exercise are the bottom line of weight loss, but emotional, psychological, and philosophical hang-ups are the real obstacles that can stop us cold. Dr. Phil's book helps prepare us for the reality of the dieting experience. He strips away the fantasies and expectations and excuses and forces us to look the idea of long-term weight loss right in the face from the beginning, so that disappointment won't knock us off course later.

The information that Dr. Phil gives us is the same common sense that we all have but sometimes don't pay attention to because we can't always manage to see the forest for the treats! The sad fact is, as pointed out in his book, statistics show that diet programs have only a 5 percent success rate. Dr. Phil, however, claims an 80 percent success rate with his patients. What is his secret to success? In a word, self-control.

The predominant themes in Dr. Phil's Seven Keys to Weight Loss Freedom are all based on self-control and basic diet and exercise common sense. It sounds simple because it is. But if losing weight is this easy, why aren't we all at goal weight? Well, Dr. Phil says because the truth hurts! Dr. Phil reaffirms what we all know but are in denial about. This isn't going to be quick and easy, so put those flashy headlines out of your head. This book delivers the raw facts.

Dr. Phil teaches us realistic expectations. A healthy body is realistic, and a perfect body isn't. Realistic goals are a must. If you're five feet tall, don't reach for a six-foot model's physique. There is no diet that will turn Danny DeVito into Brad Pitt. We also shouldn't expect to lose five pounds a week. It's sad but true that we're inundated with hype about fast "fat" loss that is no more than water weight fluctuation.

So the good news is that you will reach your goals through Dr. Phil's Seven Keys to Weight Loss Freedom. As you learn the keys, you will become more focused and in control of your weight loss. The keys will teach you how to think proactively, gain control of emotional eating, prepare your environment, and eliminate its triggers, overcome impulse eating, make the best food choices, exercise effectively and *like* it, and develop a support network. Whew! We get exhausted just thinking about it, which is to say, this book isn't exactly light reading.

Of these seven keys, five of them involve personal steps that you will work toward on your own. The other two keys are the diet and exercise program, which we'll take a peek at now.

Dr. Phil's eating plan is called High-Response Cost, High-Yield Nutrition. It is compiled of foods that will help you lose weight and gain control of your eating habits. Dr. Phil points out that most diets today either cut out food groups entirely, or concoct special combinations of foods to bring about rapid water weight loss. While these diets work in the short term, they don't allow you to go back to your old eating habits without gaining the weight back. Dr. Phil's approach teaches you how to control your eating patterns instead. All foods are either "high-response cost, high-yield" or "low-response cost, low-yield." These aren't exactly catchy phrases, but once you understand the definitions, you can call them whatever you like!

The high-response cost, high-yield foods are, in general, foods that either take some time to eat or digest, or take awhile to prepare. They are also nutritious, such as the Shrimp Zucchini Salad on page 219. These are foods that you won't grab on the go and scarf down without thinking about it. Vegetables, fruits, meats, and whole grains are good examples. Low-response cost, low-yield foods are the processed, convenient foods that don't require much cooking or effort to prepare or digest. These are generally empty calories, or otherwise nonnutritious foods, such as candy bars, cheeseburgers, chips, etc. You can choke down these foods on impulse, and they can be in your belly before your tongue ever knows what hit it. You need to avoid these foods as much as possible.

The daily portions are mapped out for all food groups, such as three servings of protein, two servings of dairy, and four servings of vegetables. No groups are left out. If it's too difficult to keep up with the exact requirements, you can divide your plate into four equal sections. One fourth of your plate gets a protein, one fourth gets a starch, and the remaining half gets fruits or vegetables. You still need to learn portion control, though. No volcano stacks of rice on a fourth of an industrial-sized dinner platter!

Intentional exercise is another crucial key of Dr. Phil's weight-loss plan. We've heard it over and over, but here it is again. Exercise is a priority for anybody who wants to lose weight and successfully keep it off! As Dr. Phil so delicately puts it, "You must stop living like a lazy slug." The ratio of activity to eating has to be level in order to keep the weight off. The more you exercise, the stronger you will get, and the more control you will have over your body. Dr. Phil also contends that exercise will help reduce our urges to overeat.

Dr. Phil also tells us very clearly that we should make sure we get at least three to four hours a week of moderate exercise, which is pleasure walking, housecleaning, yard work, etc., and at least two to three hours of vigorous exercise per week. Vigorous exercise is aerobics, swimming, weight lifting, strenuous sports, etc. A lot of people don't want to hear that, but we can always count on Dr. Phil to give it to us straight!

Now, we know that Dr. Phil can rub some chicks the wrong way. And it's true, he is a little bit of a know-it-all, and he can sometimes make us feel like we're listening to a lecture from Dad. But regardless of what anybody thinks about Dr. Phil's personality, he really does have a lot going for him in the world of weight-loss motivation. Dr. Phil has his feet on the ground psychologically, and he's not afraid to tell us everything that we need to know but don't want to hear. He really will help you "get real" about weight loss and realistic expectations and goals. His program is helpful for anybody who has dieted and failed in the past, which is, like, 105 percent of us.

Lastly, his words stick. Compare with an infomercial: thirty minutes of inspirational talk and I'm ready to become a real estate magnate and live in Hawaii. The next morning, I've already lost the phone number. Dr. Phil digs in deeper and helps you approach weight loss logically. Here's some of what our Dr. Phil chicks had to say, when we asked them to get real about getting real.

Q: It sounds like Dr. Phil thinks that everybody has a problem with compulsive or emotional overeating. I don't have a problem with food, so can't I just follow the diet and skip the tongue-lashing?

3FC: If you can go straight through the diet without any issues, yeah, sure! Chances are, though, we all have *some* sort of issue or we wouldn't be overweight in the first place. The basic weight-loss plan can stand alone from the rest of the system, just as the keys to mental and emotional success can be worked with another diet and exercise plan. However, they truly are meant to work together. If you are only interested in the diet and exercise plan, do yourself a favor and spend a couple of extra hours reading *all* the keys, whether or not you take the quizzes, as they could mean a big payoff on your bottom line, no pun intended!

If you really don't want to work through all the keys, then don't. But if you have problems sticking to plan, or if you develop negative feelings while on this plan, you need to give in and review the keys. Unlike your bathroom scale, the Seven Keys to Weight Loss Freedom are very forgiving and you can always go back for a second helping.

Q: Are meal-replacement drinks okay? Dr. Phil considers them low-response because they are a convenience food, right?

3FC: A meal-replacement drink would fit the definition of low-response since you only have to pop the lid and kick it back. However, if it is a nutritious meal-replacement drink, then Dr. Phil says it is okay in moderation.

Moderation does not mean a drink for breakfast, a drink for lunch, and a sensible dinner. Drinks and bars are both okay if you're in a pinch and have no other choice. Look at it this way: if you are in a situation where you would normally grab fast food or a low-response, low-yield snack, go for the meal-replacement drink. Check your labels and make sure the calories are not too high, that you are getting a fair amount of protein and fiber, and that there is not an abundance of sugar.

Q: The diet allows one tablespoon of fat per day? How can I manage that? Get real, Dr. Phil!

3FC: That requirement is for added fat, like olive oil or nuts. You'll already have some fat in meats, eggs, fish, and low-fat dairy products, so you will have additional fat in the diet. Your extra fat for cooking or garnishing will be cut down.

dr. phil–approved low-fat lovelies

1. Grill or broil meat whenever you can to reduce the fat.
2. Poach or steam meat or vegetables in a broth.
3. Make a light cheese sauce with low-fat cheese and skim milk, with a pinch of flour.
4. Use fat-free marinades or high-flavor vinegars on meats and veggies, and sauté with nonfat cooking spray.
5. In the skillet, try using a teaspoon of olive oil per serving, and add fruit juice or a splash of wine to aid in flavor and moisture.
6. Top foods with salsa instead of higher-fat choices, like butter and cheeses.
7. Use a spritz of butter spray, or butter sprinkles on your plate.
8. Use a steamer for fish and vegetables.
9. Try mustards and fat-free dressings instead of mayonnaise.

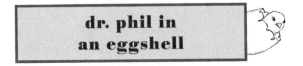

dr. phil in an eggshell

Professional Counseling None face-to-face, but you have the complete, in-depth program from the doctor himself.

Support System Dr. Phil has his own on-line community on his Web site at www.drphil.com, plus he outlines the importance of a support system in one of his seven keys.

Fitness Factor Intentional exercise is one of the seven keys and vital to the success of the program.

Family-Friendly Absolutely. There is nothing on this plan that you and your family cannot do for the rest of your natural life.

Pros This is a regular way of eating, so it will not require switching plans when you get to maintenance. There are no food groups dropped from the plan.

Cons The diet plan is based on foods that take longer to prepare. Cooking isn't always easy with a busy lifestyle. Convenience foods are to be avoided. The plan is heavy on the psychological aspect of weight loss, so it takes a while to absorb.

$$ While whole foods can be more expensive, this program poo-poos convenience and junk foods, which tend to be expensive, so you will probably save money.

The Person This Diet Is Best For Someone who has problems with emotional eating or who has a strong history of diet failure and is patient enough to take a long look at herself. Also good for people who like to cook.

recipes from the front lines

BOB GREENE MAKES THE CONNECTION

Breakfast doesn't have to be tedious, involve anything with "Grand Slam" in the title, or stick to your ribs all morning. Try something new that is quick and light.

tomato basil eggs

Serves 1

1 small slice tomato, or 1 sliced cherry tomato
1 fresh basil leaf, chopped
1 egg
Dash salt and black pepper to taste
¼ ounce Neufchâtel cheese (light cream cheese) cut into two
    cubes, ½ inch each

Preheat oven to 425°F. Spray a ramekin with cooking spray. Lay tomato slice in bottom of ramekin, and top with chopped basil. In a small bowl, lightly beat egg with salt and pepper. Pour egg over tomato and basil. Gently lay Neufchâtel cubes on top of egg. Bake in the oven for about 10 minutes, or until puffed and very lightly browned.

Per serving: 97 calories, 7 grams fat, 2 grams carbs, 0 fiber, 7 grams protein

DR. PHIL'S ULTIMATE WEIGHT-LOSS SOLUTION

Here's a recipe that is full of flavor and easy to make, and still fits the bill of high-response, high-yield fare. This salad is simple but packs a lot of flavor.

shrimp zucchini salad
. . . .

Serves 1

½ teaspoon minced garlic
2 teaspoons red bell pepper, finely minced
½ teaspoon lemon zest
2 tablespoons vegetable broth
4 ounces shrimp, peeled and deveined
1 tablespoon fresh lemon juice
1½ teaspoons canola oil
Dash salt
Dash black pepper
1 small baby zucchini, about 3 ounces, thinly sliced
1 cup mixed salad greens
½ ounce freshly shaved Parmesan cheese

Sauté garlic, red bell pepper, and lemon zest in vegetable broth for about 30 seconds. Add shrimp and continue to sauté until shrimp is done. If necessary, add another tablespoon of broth. Remove to small dish and set aside.

Combine lemon juice, canola oil, salt, and pepper in a small mixing bowl. Add sliced zucchini and toss well to coat. Place salad greens on a salad plate or bowl. Top with the zucchini

● *Continued on next page* ●

mixture and shrimp, and toss lightly. Sprinkle with shaved Parmesan cheese. Make sure you use a good quality cheese, for best flavor.

Per serving: 297 calories, 14 grams fat, 12 carbs, 3 grams fiber, 31 grams protein

Words to Live By

My idea of heaven is a great big baked potato and someone to share it with. —OPRAH WINFREY

We can't become what we need to be by remaining what we are.

—OPRAH WINFREY

mediterranean chicks don't get fat

the mediterranean diet

DESPITE OUR NATIONAL obsession with dieting, Americans are just getting fatter. In fact, Americans have the highest obesity rate in the world. France, on the other hand, has one of the lowest. The French people, along with others from Mediterranean countries, are thinner than us, even though they eat foods that we would consider taboo on many diets, such as croissants stuffed with Brie cheese, chocolate after every meal, or baklava for dessert. How do they eat all that good food and still stay thin?

This hot topic has been the subject of several recent books, the most notable being *French Women Don't Get Fat* by Mireille Guiliano. In her book, Guiliano describes the typical French lifestyle and the way the French manage food and daily activities to maintain their Parisian model physiques. Dr. Will Clower is the author of *The Fat Fallacy*, a guide to eating and living the French way to attain weight loss and better health. Here are the main principles of this eating philosophy that will help us stay Paris thin, even though we're eating dinner in Des Moines.

- **Breakfast.** Start your day off with a memorable breakfast. Take your time and enjoy it, and your breakfast experience will improve the rest of your day physically, psychologically, and emotionally.
- **Portion control.** Mediterraneans do not overload their plates with pasta, eat footlong overstuffed subs, or devour Grand Slam breakfasts. Their croissants are half the size of ours. An after-dinner chocolate is just one small, sinfully rich square.
- **Eat slowly.** Many people on the other side of the globe take the time to savor their foods; they turn their meals into memorable experiences. They don't gulp down their dinner so fast that they can't remember what they ate. By eating slowly, and consuming moderate amounts of fat, they give their bodies a chance to become full and satisfied on smaller portions.
- **Eat fresh foods.** Highly processed foods are not as popular in other countries as they are in America. Instead, fresh markets, filled with fruits and vegetables, are preferred over cans and boxes in supermarkets. If you do eat packaged foods, read the ingredient labels to make sure there's natural food inside, not a lot of chemicals. Dr. Clower says, "If it ain't food, don't eat it." This goes for artificial sweeteners, food colors, and any other additives.
- **Attitude.** In Mediterranean countries, mealtime is an experience to be appreciated. In America, our meals are typically treated as a necessity, with little thought given to the sensual properties of the food or the social joys of the company. Love your food at mealtimes, and the food will love you back!
- **Exercise.** It's impossible to get away from this requirement, no matter where you live. The French, and other Europeans, tend to walk much more than we do. They are constantly on the go, where we are usually stuck in traffic. Make a conscious effort to move more.

The "Mediterranean diet" is a regionally inspired plan that is more a style of eating than a structured diet. This diet can be confusing because it isn't all laid out with serving sizes or points, which we've become accustomed to when choosing diets. You're pretty much on your own when choosing foods and portions on the Mediterranean diet, but it's not really as scary as it sounds, and the food selections make it worth the extra effort to exercise moderation. If you spend a few weeks on the Mediterranean, you'll probably never want to go home again!

While the Mediterranean diet is not specifically a weight-loss plan, like Weight Watchers, you can easily lose weight on it. You'll eat a lot of fresh fruits, vegetables, and grains. You won't eat much meat or many processed foods. Some of us chicks are skeptical about eating anything that doesn't get served up with a basket of fries. Don't be afraid; it's not all hummus and eggplant. You're going to be able to eat pasta and even pizza, but don't expect to eat like you do at your local pizzeria. This diet takes its inspiration from the old, traditional Mediterranean foods, which do not include cheesy bread or hot wings.

Obviously, the Mediterranean diet is based on the foods of the countries that border the Mediterranean Sea, including Spain, France, Turkey, Greece, Italy, Egypt, Morocco, and others. There isn't just one diet that all of these countries follow, but they all do share some common characteristics. Each of these shared components should be included, because they all work together to provide maximum health benefits. Studies have shown that adopting just one or two of these characteristics did not always make a weight-loss difference, but including most or all of the changes did.

PRINCIPLES OF THE MEDITERRANEAN DIET

● This is mostly a plant-based diet. You will eat lots of fruits, vegetables, whole grains, and legumes.

- Fish and other seafood may be eaten a few times per week. Chicken is eaten less often, and beef and other meats are limited to just once a month. The preferred source of protein is legumes.
- Fruit is the preferred dessert and is usually eaten plain or just lightly sweetened. Lightly sweetened doesn't mean floating in a cobbler. You may have traditional sweets once or twice a week, so you are not completely giving up your treats.
- Chicks get to drink one glass of red wine every day. Men can have two glasses. A glass a day does not equal a bottle on the weekend. Moderation!
- You can have dairy every day, though it should be consumed in moderation to reduce the amounts of saturated fat in your diet. Think yogurt and cheese rather than milk.
- This is not a low-fat diet but allows moderate levels of mainly monounsaturated fats such as olive oil and nut oils. Saturated fats are very limited, and trans fats should always be avoided.
- The foods you will eat are generally fresh, whole, natural, and not heavily processed. You won't eat a lot of faux foods or high-sodium frozen dinners and condiments. Good-bye, Oscar Mayer. Hello, Jolly Green Giant.
- Regular exercise is just as important as the various food suggestions.

The White Stuff

It's hard to escape the warnings of the evils of the "white stuff"—warnings that have been dished out by everyone from Atkins to Oprah. White stuff includes refined flour products such as bread and pasta, as well as sugar and white rice. Whole-wheat products are definitely higher in nutrition and should be included whenever possible, especially since many Americans don't usually get whole grains from any other source. Yet when we think of real Italian pasta, we don't envision the brown pasta that graces our own supermarket shelves. In fact, the bulk of all pasta eaten in Mediterranean countries is white and has been for two thousand years. At one point, whole-wheat products were considered the food of the pauper, while white wheat was the food of the prince. Even couscous, a staple of countries including Morocco and Israel, is just a semolina pasta product. So Mediterranean people have managed to retain their good health while eating the white stuff. Even sugary sweets can be consumed once or twice a week, or on special occasions. Who couldn't resist the occasional serving of baklava? It's the next best thing to pecan pie! The lesson learned? Choose whole wheat when possible, limit portion sizes, but don't be too afraid of the white stuff.

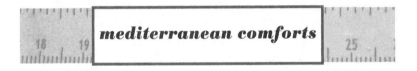

mediterranean comforts

One of the first hurdles of the Mediterranean diet is accepting the fact that we have to give up our traditional ideas about what comfort food is, down here in the Bible Belt. So for all of us who don't feel loving until there are cookies in the oven, here's a list of Mediterranean substitutions for the comforts of home.

The Mediterranean Diet	Versus	*The Bible Belt Diet*
pita bread		buttermilk biscuits
olive oil		Crisco
eggplant, roasted		baby back ribs
over a fire pit		catfish and hush puppies
shrimp scampi		Tater Tots
couscous		chicken nuggets
roasted chicken		corn dog
shish kebab		

Since this diet contains very few processed foods, which are usually calorie- and/or fat-laden, you will probably eat fewer calories overall, while eating higher quantities of food that keep you satisfied. Recent studies have shown that the moderate-fat Mediterranean diet is more successful than a standard low-fat diet for losing weight and keeping it off. Many believe that this is because the diet is easier to stick to long-term because the food is so good. What other diet encourages eating pizza, Greek salads, and honey-soaked figs? Chances are you probably won't need to count calories when you adopt this style of eating, since nearly everything you eat will be good for you and fairly low in calories. As always, you just need to watch your portion sizes. It would be diffi-cult to apply the Mediterranean diet to low-carb plans such as Atkins, because those plans are too restrictive and would not allow all of the components of the Mediterranean diet. However, you can apply the characteristics of the Mediterranean diet to many other diet plans, such as Weight Watchers or the South Beach diet.

Are you still confused? Or are you salivating and wondering how you can apply this philosophy to your own diet plan? If you want to know more, here are some well-tanned Mediterranean chicks to tell us how this diet helped them lose weight.

meet the mediterranean chicks

Shannon from Georgia

Our family's tight budget has often meant spaghetti dinners made from jarred spaghetti sauce and a huge platter of pasta. It was cheap, filling, and easy to overeat. Before I knew it, I weighed 236 pounds. When I heard about the Mediterranean diet, I thought that I'd be able to find a way to continue our spaghetti dinners but still lose weight. I don't know what I was expecting, maybe a fat-burning herb seasoning. I started ex-perimenting with recipes that I found on-line and was thrilled that they fit into our budget. I had to work to curb my pasta habit, but I learned more about portion control than I ever knew before. I've been eating more vegetables and less pasta, and have lost 60 pounds so far.

Karen from Tennessee

I discovered the Mediterranean diet by accident. My husband is Greek, and I was researching Greek cuisine so that I could cook some of his favorite childhood dishes, instead of our usual fish and chips or meatloaf and mashed potato dinners. We started eating more shellfish, grains, and vegetables such as eggplant. I really loved the food and it was fun to surprise my husband with what I was learning. He was first to notice that I was losing a little weight, and we knew it had to be the new food. I thought, "Hey, there must be something to this!" and after Googling Greek diets, I learned about the Mediterranean diet and how popular it was. I kept on cooking, and started exercising more, and went down three dress sizes!

Diane from Oregon

I'm a vegetarian, so it's been kind of hard to find a good diet plan that I could live with. Most of the diets are geared toward meat eaters. My doctor recommended the Mediterranean diet and said he'd been following it for years. I thought it was confusing at first, but after I got the hang of it, I liked it and saw results quickly. The foods were things I've eaten for years, but the guidelines put the plan into perspective for me, so I ended up eating less and making better choices. My doctor was so thrilled with my results that he put my picture on the bulletin board in his office to show other patients!

Q: I'm very happy counting points because it is the easiest way for me to lose weight. Can I do the Mediterranean diet while on Weight Watchers? There seems to be a lot of olive oil on this plan.

3FC: The Weight Watchers Flex plan is so flexible that it's easy to apply the Mediterranean concept to it. You just need to count the point values of the foods you choose. There is one stumbling block to watch out for. Weight Watchers members frequently substitute highly pro-cessed, nonfat foods to conserve points, such as fat-free sour cream or other dairy products. Frozen diet meals, such as Weight Watchers Smart Ones dinners, are also a popular choice of Weight Watchers members. Unfortunately, these products are so highly processed that they should be avoided on the Mediterranean diet. You'll want to eat freshly prepared meals using natural ingredients, such as the polenta recipe on page 234.

The Weight Watchers Core plan may seem ideal for the Mediter-ranean diet, until you consider what you have to avoid. The Core plan requires a lot of vegetables, whole grains, and lean meats, but it also prohibits many fruits, all sugars, red wine, and some of the carbs that the Mediterranean diet needs to be balanced. Plus, it encourages only fat-free dairy, such as nonfat cheeses and sour cream. You can't get all of the components of the Mediterranean diet into the Core plan.

Q: How do I do Phase 1 of the South Beach diet if I'm eating the Mediter-ranean diet with it? There are too many grains. Can I skip them?

3FC: Phases 2 and 3 of the South Beach diet are very similar to the Mediterranean diet, but Phase 1 is a challenge. On the Mediterranean diet you will eat lots of fresh fruit, whole grains, and a glass of wine each day, which we know are taboo on Phase 1 of South Beach. You can do Phase 1 as it is in the book, and then make the transition to Phase 2 by choosing Med-diet-friendly foods. The purpose of Phase 1 is to help kill your carb cravings and to get rid of a few pounds of wa-ter weight. If you don't need this assistance, more power to you! Just move directly to Phase 2.

There are a few things to keep in mind when blending the Mediterranean with South Beach. You may need to curb your string cheese or ricotta crème habit. The Med diet doesn't allow quite as much dairy as is allowed on South Beach. Another obstacle is the South Beach diet frozen dinners and sandwich wraps that have be-come popular. One glance at the half-page-long ingredient labels on these products is all it takes to realize that they are not the natural, unprocessed foods that you should be eating with your new lifestyle. However, you can eat very satisfying meals of grilled fish, lentil chili (page 235), pasta with tomato and vegetable sauce, and fresh fruits.

a typical south beach diet phase 2 day with mediterranean flair

Breakfast ¾ cup blueberries with ½ cup nonfat, sugar-free vanilla yogurt, sprinkled with a tablespoon of wheat germ

Lunch Roasted tomato soup, salad, and a bowl of fresh grapes for dessert

Snack Hummus and pita wedges

Dinner Spicy Lentil Chili, whole-wheat pita wedges for dipping; fruit salad for dessert; a glass of red wine with or after dinner

---

Q: I love Mexican food, but Mexico isn't exactly a Mediterranean country. Can I eat enchiladas and my other favorite spicy foods on this plan?

3FC: Absolutely! Many Mexican dishes rely on tomatoes, peppers, onions, black beans, and other vegetables. You'll probably want to choose vegetarian options most of the time and limit dishes with a lot of beef and saturated fats in them. But be realistic: you probably won't find many suitable choices at your local taco shack. Look for restaurants that offer authentic Mexican cuisine, and ask questions if you are not sure what's in the dishes. Remember the basic guidelines:

fresh food, portion control, and taking your time to enjoy. Many Mexican-style foods are already designed as individual portions, such as enchiladas or fajitas. Add a homemade salsa for flavor and freshness. You might even want to explore Spanish foods, such as paella. If you like spicy foods, you can zing up just about any Mediterranean dish with hot spices, such as our hummus recipe on page 236.

Q: I've been on the Web doing searches for Mediterranean diet and I can't find anything about weight loss. I've been on South Beach, but I miss my carbs. Can I really expect to lose weight if I eat this way?

3FC: The Mediterranean diet can be used for weight loss, or it can just be a lifestyle choice. We like that there are no forbidden foods except junk foods on a diet plan like this. You can have a mixture of whole and refined grains. You can eat fruits, potatoes, and other foods that some other diet plans don't permit. The key is portion control. The people who live in Mediterranean regions are much healthier because they eat more natural foods and fewer processed foods that contain chemicals and mystery products. They use good fats such as olive oil. They also practice portion control as a matter of course. Americans, in general, just eat too much! That is what we have to learn to get away from. For many people, weight is less about what we eat than how much we eat.

Most of the Web sites devoted to the Med diet focus on it not as a way to lose weight but as a way to regain health, and especially to protect our hearts. It's a healthier way to live. However, there is a book called *The Mediterranean Diet: Newly Revised and Updated* by Marissa Cloutier and Eve Adamson that does emphasize weight loss. It discusses various foods you should look for and even includes a few sample menus and recipes. Most of the books on the Mediterranean diet do not offer menus, so you need to base your choices around your own needs.

If you want to lose weight, decide how many calories you want to consume, then plan your Mediterranean menu to stay within your target count. It's the calories that count for weight loss in the end. And, as always, exercise is very important for weight loss. You are in complete control and can choose the foods you enjoy. It takes a little planning, but you learn more that way.

Q: I don't like wine and don't understand why it's required by this diet plan. Shouldn't we avoid alcohol when dieting?

3FC: Red wine is loaded with antioxidants and has been shown to help reduce the risk of heart disease when it is consumed regularly and in moderation. It is common to have a glass of red wine with dinner in Mediterranean countries. Do you have to drink it? No, it's not required, it's a personal choice. Plus it won't help you lose weight any faster. A lot of people don't like to drink alcohol, or they just don't like the flavor of wine. Purple grape juice also contains antioxidants, but you would have to drink more of it to get the same benefit, which would add up to more calories. Pomegranate juice may have even more antioxidants than red wine, and it tastes good!

Q: Since there isn't a menu or plan with this diet, how do I know how much to eat?

3FC: Now is a good time to learn what food portions should be. We've become so used to platters of pasta as served in restaurants that we don't know when to stop eating at home. Don't be afraid to use measuring cups until you familiarize yourself with correct portions. Then you can eyeball it. You don't need to count calories or carbs when you choose to eat like the French or other Mediterraneans, but you do need to get control of the amount of food you eat. Train yourself to eat until you are just satisfied and never stuffed. Don't take seconds, even if your grandma insists. Limit yourself to small amounts of rich foods, such as cream sauces or breads. If you are still hungry, help yourself to more vegetables, or have a fruit for dessert. It shouldn't take long before this way of eating comes naturally to you.

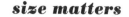

size matters

The French are known for love, romance, thin women, and rich foods, and they do it so well. They know something important that we Americans try to deny: size matters. Smaller really is better! Try our tips for portion control, so you too can savor the finer things in life, a little at a time.

- Fresh fruit is often portion-controlled by Mother Nature. Enjoy a fresh whole banana, apple, peach, or other fruit, instead of fruit salad, applesauce, or other processed fruit that arrives in a large tub.
- Put your large dinner plates in storage, and use the salad or luncheon plates instead. Since we tend to portion out foods by how much will fit on our plates, we usually eat less if using a smaller plate.
- Put a little less food on your plate than you think you will eat. Lay your fork down between bites, and chew slowly. You probably won't need to get another portion. If you do, make sure it's a healthy choice.
- When dining out, choose an appetizer as your main dish, or a child-sized entrée. You may even split a regular entrée with your companion. Just don't order a full-sized entrée for yourself if you think you may eat it all.

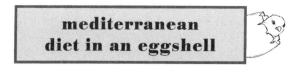

mediterranean diet in an eggshell

Professional Counseling None. You'll rely on your own sensibilities to get you through.

Support System Not really. You may find a few forums on-line that offer support for the Mediterranean diet, including 3FC. But there isn't anything official out there.

Fitness Factor Exercise is a main component of the Mediterranean diet, though you are on your own in making fitness choices.

Family-Friendly Very, since it is healthy and delicious for every member of the family.

$$ Very affordable because you'll eat little meat but a lot of vegetables and grains. You can also eat plenty of lentils and other legumes that can be purchased cheaply in bulk.

Pros Easier to stick to than most diets because the food is so good, and you can easily maintain it for life.

Cons You'll probably spend more time food shopping and in the kitchen since you will be preparing fresher foods from scratch, instead of depending on a lot of convenience foods.

The Person This Diet Is Best For Someone concerned about overall health and especially heart disease and cancer. Perfect for foodies who love this type of cuisine.

recipes from the front lines

This salad is low in Weight Watchers points but high in flavor. It is a perfect way to incorporate some of the Mediterranean diet into your Weight Watchers plan.

red pepper and goat cheese salad with polenta medallions

Serves 3

1 roasted red bell pepper, from a jar, cut in long strips
1 small tomato, chopped
½ cup fresh basil leaves, torn
½ small onion, sliced thin
2 tablespoons balsamic vinegar
1 tablespoon olive oil
Salt and pepper to taste
1 head bibb lettuce, or 1 bag of salad mix
1 ounce goat cheese
6 slices (¼-inch thick) purchased sun-dried tomato polenta

Combine red pepper strips, tomato, basil, onion, balsamic vinegar, and olive oil in a medium bowl. Add salt and pepper to taste. Cover and let sit at room temperature for about an hour. Or prepare in advance and chill until serving time. The tomatoes will release juices as they marinate, to create more liquid for the dressing.

Prepare polenta: Spray a nonstick skillet with cooking spray and heat over medium high heat. Add the polenta slices and carefully cook until lightly golden on each side.

To serve: Divide lettuce among 3 large plates. Top with pepper mixture. Sprinkle with goat cheese. Place polenta slices on the side of the plates and serve.

Per serving: 118 calories, 8 grams fat, 7 grams protein, 23 carbohydrates, 4 WW points

---

Enjoy the best of both worlds with this South Beach-Mediterranean blend. It's got everything you need—taste *and* nutrition—to help you lose weight and feel satisfied. This meal is so good, you won't remember that you're dieting.

spicy lentil chili

Serves 6

1 cup red lentils
Water
2 tablespoons olive oil
½ cup onion, diced
¼ cup celery, finely chopped
2 tablespoons garlic, chopped
1 medium tomato, cored and diced
2 cups canned vegetable broth
1 tablespoon Tabasco sauce
⅛ teaspoon turmeric
⅛ teaspoon cumin

● *Continued on next page* ●

⅛ teaspoon cayenne pepper
1 teaspoon sea salt
½ teaspoon black pepper
⅛ teaspoon chili powder

Bring lentils and 2 cups of water to a boil over high heat. Remove from heat. Place half the lentils and water in a blender or food processor and puree. Set aside.

Heat olive oil in a stockpot or Dutch oven over medium heat. Add onions and stir until they begin to soften. Add celery and garlic and continue to stir and cook for about 5 minutes. Add chopped tomatoes and cook an additional 5 minutes. Add vegetable broth, Tabasco sauce, and seasonings. Continue to heat until mixture begins to simmer. Stir in pureed lentils and reserved whole lentils and water mixture. Stir well and cook until lentils are tender, about 15 minutes. If chili is too thick, add additional water to thin.

Per serving: 226 calories, 6 grams fat, 12 grams protein, 34 grams carbs

Does the idea of hummus make you say *hmmmm?* Try our zesty recipe for a delicious and healthy hummus for snacks or entertaining. It also packs easily for a quick and healthy lunch at the office. Don't forget to pack the breath mints!

zesty red pepper hummus
. . . .

Makes about 2 cups

1 can (16 ounces) chickpeas, drained and rinsed
2 cloves garlic, peeled and coarsely chopped
¼ cup tahini

½ cup roasted red bell peppers
2 tablespoons fresh lemon juice
1 tablespoon olive oil
½ teaspoon cayenne pepper, or to taste

Combine all ingredients in the bowl of a food processor and pulse until mixture is smooth. Add a little water, if necessary, to thin the mixture to the right consistency. Transfer to a serving bowl and serve at room temperature with raw vegetables or pita chips.

Per ¼-cup serving: 127 calories, 6 grams fat, 4 grams protein, 15 grams carbs

Words to Live By

Everything you see I owe to spaghetti. —Sophia Loren

If I want a bite of chocolate cake, I will have it. I just won't eat the whole cake like I used to. —Judith Light

radical chicks
weight-loss surgery

LISTEN, BEFORE WE BEGIN to talk about an approach to weight loss as radical as surgery, we want to make sure that everybody understands surgery is *not* a quick fix. It's not as easy as it looks on some reality TV shows, where you go under the knife, spend a few days in funny-looking bandages, recover in no time thanks to the magic of time-lapse filming, and then emerge gorgeous and thin, looking trim and slim in a little black dress and perfect hair while everyone stands around and applauds your remarkable transformation. This is the real world, not TV, and when it comes to radical procedures like weight-loss surgery, you need to understand the difference.

Every chick needs to sit down and do a lot of soul-searching before considering a surgical procedure. And it's important when you're weighing your pros and cons to understand that this is not a simple, painless alternative to the struggle of saying no to cream pies and super-size. In fact, the decision to have weight-loss surgery runs far deeper than wondering if you can still eat your burgers deluxe.

Weight-loss surgery (WLS) changes you not only physically but emotionally and socially as well, and once you make the decision to pursue this course, you can never take a day off. Failure to stick to the diet plan that accompanies weight-loss surgery doesn't just result in a sugar and guilt hangover; it can result in severe illness or even death.

So why do some chicks choose weight-loss surgery? Well, because they have nowhere else to turn. These procedures are intended for heavy hens who have tried every other weight-loss option and failed. WLS is their last resort to lose weight and regain their lives, and for many, that last chance pays off.

Amy, of 3FC, had weight-loss surgery in 2003. She reached the point where she felt WLS was her last chance. She had dieted for many years, sometimes successfully, but was never able to keep it off. She would resume her old eating habits, usually because of stress, and always regained the weight. We watched her struggle not only with her weight but with the emotional pain she felt because she was not able to get it under control. We had mixed feelings about WLS and felt it should be reserved for extreme cases, and had a difficult time accepting Amy's choice. We were scared she would not survive the surgery. We were confused that she could not just lose the weight by dieting, because she'd done it before. But eventually, we accepted the reality of her pain and realized that this was truly Amy's last chance, so we chose to support her, and while she did hit some significant stumbling blocks along the way, her surgery has worked out well for her in the long run.

While there are risks involved with weight-loss surgery, there are many benefits, and often the risks of remaining obese outweigh the potential danger of surgery. According to the American Obesity Association, there are more than thirty obesity-related illnesses that can damage the quality of life and even cause death. It is up to you and your doctor to decide if surgery is a good choice for you.

According to Mark Lockett, MD and assistant professor of surgery at East Tennessee State University, the benefits of weight-loss surgery can be substantial. "Candidates for weight-loss surgery are morbidly obese and most studies suggest their life expectancies are significantly shorter than similar patients who are not obese, on the range of ten years or so. If a patient makes it through the surgery and recovery period, and ninety-eight percent do, then their life expectancy should increase."

Once you and your doctor have decided on weight-loss surgery, you will have to decide which type of procedure works best for you. There are several available. There is no best method, although there is great debate on this point in the WLS world, and not all surgeons perform all methods. If you study your options and feel strongly about a method not offered by your surgeon, you should get a second opinion. This is a permanent change and a very personal decision and you need to be sure you are making the right choice so you have no regrets.

You can elect to have restrictive surgery, which limits the amount of food that can be eaten by removing or closing a portion of the stomach. You eat less and feel full quicker. With restrictive surgery, the only thing that changes is the size of the stomach pouch, and the outlet size, which delays the emptying of food into the larger portion of the stomach. Now, that gives new meaning to the idea of food that sticks to your ribs!

You might also consider a combination of restrictive and malabsorption surgery. This procedure restricts the size of the pouch, plus it reduces the amount of nutrients and calories that can be absorbed by the body. In this process, the intestines are rerouted to alter the digestive system. As a result, you can only eat the foods that count, like proteins and nutrient-rich carbohydrates. Junk food and sugar are out; protein shakes, lean meat, and green veggies are in. You will also have to take vitamins and calcium supplements for the rest of your life.

Two of the most popular weight-loss surgeries are adjustable gastric banding and the Roux-en-Y gastric bypass.

Adjustable gastric banding (AGB), commonly known as the Lap-Band, is accomplished with the surgical insertion of a hollow silicone band around the upper portion of the stomach. The band divides the stomach into two sections, divided by a small opening. The first and smaller portion of the stomach, above the band, holds what you eat. This is also the section of your stomach that has all the nerves that scream "Feed me!" to your brain. When it is full, your brain is satisfied and won't know or care that you had only a two-ounce protein shake for dinner. Food is slowly passed through the banded entrance into the lower, larger section of stomach. Here your food will be digested normally. The band can be loosened or tightened by removing or adding a saline solution. This type of surgery does not involve moving or removing any of your organs, and it can be reversed.

Roux-en-Y gastric bypass (RGB) is the most commonly performed gastric bypass surgery in the United States. It reduces your stomach size, limiting the amount of food you can eat at one time. In addition, part of your intestines will be bypassed during the digestive process, reducing the amount of calories and, unfortunately, nutrients that can be absorbed. This two-pronged approach is one of the most effective methods of weight-loss surgery, but it cannot be reversed.

These procedures have one thing in common; after surgery, you must eat only quality foods. Postsurgical nip and tuckers will eat a very low-calorie diet. Since you will be eating less, every bite counts. You will eat very little sugar or fat. Failure to restrict your diet can interfere with your weight loss or make you ill.

To be approved for surgery, you generally need to be about a hundred pounds overweight. Specifically, your BMI, or body mass index, should be forty or more. A lower BMI may be acceptable if you experience an obesity-related illness such as diabetes, heart disease, or sleep apnea. You also will have to pass a psychological exam and attend support group meetings before the surgery. You also should have exhausted all efforts at losing weight through calorie reduction and exercise on your own. Getting approved for surgery, including undergoing the exams, is a long process. Don't be surprised if you have to wait six to twelve months from your first visit until the procedure. So much for the quick-fix idea!

Even if you meet the weight requirements, weight-loss surgery may not be for you. Here are some of the top reasons why people are excluded as weight-loss surgery candidates:

- You're addicted to drugs or alcohol.
- You have not exhausted your weight-loss options with diet and exercise.
- You have a stomach disorder.
- You're not willing to stick to a strict postsurgery diet.

- You think losing weight will solve other problems in your life.
- You don't have a family that will support your lifestyle change.
- You aren't willing to attend postsurgical therapy and follow-up visits.
- You have an eating disorder.
- You're a junk food junkie and can't give it up. (Although one indulgence may make you so sick, that could change!)
- You think of weight-loss surgery as a cure and not a tool.

Surgery is and will remain a controversial method of weight loss. This is a personal decision, and you should spend a lot of time reviewing your options before you make it. And it's important to work with your surgeon. She has your best interests at heart, and she will be sharing this experience with you, so don't be afraid to ask her about your concerns.

We asked our radical chicks to share some of their personal highs and lows with weight-loss surgery.

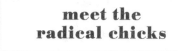

Amy 3FC from Tennessee

I had the Roux-en-Y weight-loss surgery in 2003. I'd reached a high of 285 pounds and was tired and frustrated with my inability to lose the weight. After careful consideration and discussions with my doctor, I decided to go with the surgery. Do I regret it? No, not anymore, but I do wish that I could have controlled my weight on my own.

I had a difficult time adjusting to the forced calorie control at first. Right after the surgery, I was convinced I'd made the wrong decision. I was depressed. I cried a lot, and I was angry with myself for going

● *Continued on next page* ●

through with the surgery. I realized that I had been influenced by celebrity success stories. I thought that if the stars had done so well with surgery, so could I. Once it was done, though, reality set in and I realized that I hadn't been prepared at all for what I had done.

In the end, it all worked out. I had a tough time for the first nine months, but I adjusted and I'm now very happy that I had the surgery. I've lost more than 130 pounds, I'm no longer diabetic, my sleep apnea is gone, and I feel very little pain from my arthritis. I also recently sealed my success with a tummy tuck!

Dawna from California

I know that somewhere down the line there could be health ramifications we did not know about at the time I had my surgery, and I took that into account when making my decision. I know, however, that I would probably have been dead or certainly disabled and unable to work within a few years, had I not had the surgery. If and when untoward effects happen down the road, I will have had many more happy, healthy, productive years than I would have had without the surgery. It is a chance we all take.

Terri from Maine

Food no longer controls me, and it is a wonderful feeling! Also, after ten years of being infertile due to morbid obesity, I just gave birth to my baby girl in December!

Deborah from Oklahoma

My first surgery was a gastric stapling. The staples came out when they did an MRI on my back, so I was back to over three hundred pounds. Having gained all the weight back and having bad reflux problems from the first surgery's having been halfway removed, I had Roux-en-Y. I out-ate that one and gained all but forty pounds back. It still made me feel better healthwise, and I have learned that now I have to change what I do instead of trying to out-eat every effort. I don't regret it at all because I needed it at those times in my life. For many people it is such a life-changing experience, and it was for me also. I wasn't successful because I didn't follow the rules after my surgery. I drank regular pop, soups, anything that would go down easy and lots of it. Very stupid of me, but I did it, so now I'm losing weight again the low-cal method. Surgery is a great tool to help people get on track, but you have to take care.

Becky from Colorado
I'm a much happier person when I feel like I'm in control of my life and have a hand in shaping my future. The out-of-control spiral that was my life has stopped since I had my surgery. Such a relief!

Q: If I go ahead and have weight-loss surgery, will I be able to eat normally again?

3FC: For the first few days after your surgery, you won't be able to eat at all. You'll suck on ice chips, and drink water, protein drinks, broth, or teas, about an ounce at a time. This will gradually lead to soft foods, like baby food, cottage cheese, yogurts, and pureed foods. You will have to introduce food into your system slowly and carefully. Remember, after surgery, your holding tank will only be about the size of an egg, and overeating could be damaging, or even fatal.

Food selection depends largely on the individual, although everything that you eat should be quality food that's nutrient-rich, because you don't have very much space to satisfy your nutritional needs. Many people experience discomfort after eating sugar or fatty foods, while others seem to tolerate them well. Amy has no problems with sugar, but greasy foods cause her to "dump." Dumping has various symptoms for different people, but Amy experiences chest cramps and nausea, followed by a deep, uncontrollable sleep. The pains can be intense and scary, because chest pain is also a symptom of heart disease. It can feel like you're having a heart attack, when it's only a cramp.

So hopefully, with the help of your doctor, you will redefine what eating normally is, and you won't go back to those extra helpings of the sweet potato soufflé. Regardless of which weight-loss option you choose, surgically or otherwise, if you want to lose weight and keep it off, you must change your perception of what eating normally is and make better choices for the rest of your life.

To Market, to Market

In the first few weeks following weight-loss surgery, you may feel some emotional turmoil or even find yourself in mourning for the foods you can no longer eat. Also, considering you are recovering from surgery, it isn't a bad idea to stock the refrigerator with foods you'll be eating until you are mentally and physically up to grocery shopping again. Here's a list from Maureen from New York City, who had RGB surgery in August 2004 and since then has lost more than 130 pounds. Maureen compiled this shopping list based on what she learned from her nutritionist. The items cover the first three phases (several weeks) of postsurgical eating. Your nutritionist should give you a similar list before you have your procedure, based on your needs and the type of surgery you've had.

- Protein powders
- Broth and teas
- Smooth soups (use a blender)
- Low-sugar/low-carb yogurts
- Baby food
- Crystal Light
- Unsweetened applesauce
- Instant oatmeal, plain—no sugar added
- Whipped cottage cheese or ricotta cheese

- Soft tofu
- Fat-free or 2 percent soft American cheese slices
- Sugar-free gelatin and sugar-free pudding
- Chewable vitamins and sublingual B-12 tablets
- TUMS and chewable calcium pills

Some equipment and supplies you may find handy are a blender, a food processor, one-ounce cups (you can find these at a restaurant or wholesale supply store), and an egg poacher.

Q: I want to get weight-loss surgery, but I've read stories about people being hungry and gaining their weight back. Can you gain all your weight back after surgery?

3FC: The answer is yes, you can gain the weight back, but you won't if you follow your doctor's orders. Most failures are caused by lack of support, or the patient's lack of knowledge about how to deal with her new lifestyle. So let us tell you again: *you must eat as prescribed.*

At first, when you're on liquids only, you will be drinking your meals for nutrition more than out of hunger; most patients don't feel hungry at all after surgery. As you progress, you will begin to eat more regular food, at more regular intervals. It is up to you to stick with the eating schedule exactly as prescribed for you, no matter how quickly you are losing weight. This rapid weight loss at the beginning, called "the honeymoon period" by many of our radical chicks, happens almost effortlessly. Soon after, though, you will be relying more on your own resources as your weight decreases and your body doesn't need as many calories to survive. If you start with exercising and meal plans from the beginning, you will find it easier to stick with when it counts—in the long run.

Some of our chicks found that they were more emotionally impacted by this surgery than they could have imagined. Amy felt this way. She was not prepared for the grief she would experience when she found that her old deep-fried and whip-creamed coping mechanisms had suddenly vanished. Stress eating was her only way to deal with life's problems, and surgery doesn't change that! Long-term support and therapy are vital to getting and keeping the weight off. The surgery is a tool, and you should become skilled in its use.

Q: Will I lose all of my excess weight? I was a size 6 when I got married, but now I'm a 24. Can I get back down to my 6s?

3FC: Anything is possible, but that doesn't mean it is likely. Your body is different now from when you got married, and you may never be that small again. You will probably carry the bulk of excess skin after you lose the excess fat. You should definitely exercise and focus on strength training as soon as your doctor gives you the go-ahead, so you will be as fit as possible when you reach your goal. Instead of reaching for a size-based goal, aim for a health-based goal, and proceed from there. Keep your concerns focused more on your inside than on your outside. Of course we all want to look good, feel confident, and be happy with ourselves, but a considerable amount of patience, as well as realism, is required.

We can't predict your dress size, but we can share with you what we learned from Dr. Lockett about what *not* to do after weight-loss surgery:

- Don't alter your post-op instructions and diet.
- Don't lie around the house. Get up, get dressed, and go do things even in the early post-op period. Those who get going the fastest do the best.
- Don't weigh yourself more than once a week. Scale watchers drive themselves crazy. The goal is not to lose weight so much as to improve the medical problems associated with the weight.
- Realistic expectations are a must. Don't expect to go from 350 pounds to 120 pounds. It doesn't work that way despite what many people think.
- Don't compare your weight loss with others'.

heavy hens give it up

We all have reasons why we want to lose weight, but when you've got a lot of weight to lose, there are some unique feelings that we heavy hens alone can relate to. The comments that follow were obtained through our survey, and they are very candid. These sometimes painful, sometimes joyful thoughts reflect the special problems women face when they have over a hundred pounds to lose; they touch on the deeply emotional aspects of obesity. If you also need to lose as much as we heavy hens did, perhaps these personal thoughts will remind you that you're not alone, and help get you started on your journey toward greater health and happiness.

What We Look Forward To

- No more friction bumps on our inner thighs from walking
- Buying underwear from Victoria's Secret
- Fitting into one size fits all
- Choosing hairstyles for reasons other than camouflaging our neck
- No more reliance upon clever camera angles
- Fitting in all of the amusement park rides without fear
- No more permanent red rings around our waist
- Smiling at the security television, instead of avoiding it
- Sex without fear of hurting our mate
- Wrapping a regular-sized towel around ourselves
- Knowing the paper gown at the gynecologist will actually fit
- Choosing our bathing suit, instead of the bathing suit choosing us

• *Continued on next page* •

- Washing dishes without getting our stomachs wet
- Not wondering why people are laughing
- No more fear of plastic chairs

What We Hate About Being Overweight

- Jeans with elastic waists
- Legs too fat for dainty sandals with heels
- Wearing a T-shirt over a bathing suit
- Not tucking in shirts
- Plus size signs over the clothing racks
- More expensive clothes
- "Queen size" pantyhose
- Granny panties

Q: Will I be able to eat in restaurants after weight-loss surgery? I travel a lot, and many of my meals are on the road. I don't really want to ask the servers for advice. It's rather embarrassing.

3FC: You will be able to eat in restaurants, but you'll have to make some adjustments. One of the most difficult problems is how to deal with the portion sizes. Restaurants serve large portions, and you'll only be eating a fraction of them. Expect questions from concerned servers or managers if you are only picking at your plate. Some people don't like to announce that they have had WLS, but in some cases, you might be more comfortable just telling them and getting it out of the way, rather than assuring everybody that yes, your dinner tastes fine.

Some patients get an identification card from their surgeon, explaining that they have had WLS, so they can get permission to order from the child's menu. Ask your doctor or nutritionist if she can make something similar for you to use. Restaurants are not obligated to accommodate you, but many will. Cafeterias are great choices for WLS patients, because you can look at everything in front of you and buy only what you can eat.

If you do order straight from the menu, you can pick something from the appetizer menu or choose a couple of side orders. Be careful with the appetizer menu: many of the choices are fried, sugary, or otherwise unsuitable. If all else fails, be sure to ask for a doggy bag, and you can have leftovers two or three times!

jiffypop's tips for successful weight loss through weight-loss surgery

Jane F. Perrotta, known as Jiffypop on 3FC, is the moderator of the Weight-Loss Surgery (WLS) forum. Once topping the scales at over five hundred pounds, and now maintaining a loss of almost three hundred pounds, she is the poster chick for successful weight-loss surgery. These are her best tips for having a successful weight loss, based on what she has learned through her own experience and through coaching others through the same process.

1. Research everything beforehand, learn all you can about the procedure, and join support groups to learn how it affects their lives.
2. Ask questions: of your primary care doctor, your surgeon, and other WLS patients. Go back and ask more questions. This is not the right choice for everyone, and no matter what you decide, someone will disagree. Once you've made your decision, ignore the naysayers.

● *Continued on next page* ●

3. Keep your eyes on the prize. Maintenance is even more important than losing. Put even more effort into maintenance than you put into navigating the presurgery evaluation and approval cycle.

4. Move yourself up in your list of priorities. The stakes are much higher after surgery than before, so make sure you have appropriate food, take your vitamins, get your blood checked regularly, and incorporate resistance training to help the calcium stay in your bones.

5. Any work you do to control your food demons *before* surgery will help you afterwards.

6. Find, and keep, a live support group, no matter how successful you feel after surgery. If your surgical group needs to make room for new patients, you may find yourself looking elsewhere to meet your needs. Look into a private group or Overeaters Anonymous, or seek a therapist who specializes in eating disorders. If you don't click with your therapist, find another one who "gets it."

7. Be prepared for changes in your relationships. Your life will change, and not everyone in your life may be willing or able to keep up.

8. Surgery won't change your emotional issues. It will help with the weight loss but not with whatever stresses or issues you may have. In fact, you will no longer be able to "eat your emotions," which can make coping more difficult until you learn new methods to handle stress.

9. Figure out how to deal with head hunger, and prepare for some degree of mourning. Get therapy or find alternate outlets to battle emotional or stress eating. (I knit!)

10. The first three months are hard. Expect a much more regimented life as you move through a staged diet, from protein shakes and liquids up to real food. It can be rocky, but it won't last. You can survive anything for three months.

11. Put your energy into figuring out how to live with the surgery rather than into trying to outsmart it. One group loses and maintains and the other group doesn't.

12. People lose at different rates, and some people, despite their best efforts, will not make their goal. Make sure you're following the rules and then stop obsessing.

13. Make the most of your honeymoon phase. Exercising and eating right will give you the best weight loss possible and will carry you throughout maintenance.

14. Your success is up to you and you alone. Including others in your plans is entirely your choice, but be aware that the fast, massive weight loss will make even the most well-meaning people wonder all kinds of bizarre things. You might have to say something if only to stop rumors that you've become a drug addict or you're dying of cancer.

15. Attitude is everything. If you go into this process thinking you're a failure or that this is a punishment for mistakes you've made in your life, you'll be miserable and have a very high risk of failure. If you embrace this as a second chance, you'll do much better.

16. Ask for help. It's out there. Even if you are bedridden or in a wheelchair, or have no cartilage in your knees, there *are* exercises you can do.

17. Realize that this is no quick fix and that you will still have to do the same hard work to get it all off and keep it off. You will need to exercise and watch what you eat for the rest of your life, just like everyone else does. Congratulations. You are normal.

Q: I am a stress eater. How will I do it with weight-loss surgery? Will I be "comforted" with smaller bites of food instead of the larger amounts I eat now?

3FC: If you are a stress eater, the first thing you must do is find another outlet for your stress. You cannot stress-eat after weight-loss surgery. It is imperative that you work on this before your procedure. You'll need to pick up a hobby, or maybe some alternate activity, like exercise or even meditation.

Amy was a classic stress eater. This was one reason we all worried about her when she had surgery. What would Amy do when things got stressful? What would she do when she was bored or lonely or anxious? We were afraid she would continue to eat, and die.

Amy has done well with portion control, and she has not suffered ill effects from stress eating, although she does still do it on occasion, but to a small degree. Amy did not realize how similar her emotional eating patterns would be after surgery. She knew her surgery would change her stomach, but it didn't occur to her that it wouldn't change her emotional response to life. Not only were life's problems and stresses still there, but she had new problems. She was afraid to swallow some foods. She was afraid of choking, or of dying. Not only was she unable to eat a lot, but she couldn't eat the same comfort foods she had in the past, like candy bars and chips. For years, food was everything for Amy. It is like that for many overweight people, so be sure that you get counseling before surgery to deal effectively with your demons.

What is the best preparation? "There may be no way to adequately prepare anyone," says Dr. Lockett. "Everyone is different and responds differently. The psychological exam that is required prior to surgery is of some value, but support groups pre- and post-op are the most important thing. All WLS patients should be in a support group, even if it is just on-line at Obesityhelp.com, for instance."

Support groups are vital for at least two years after surgery, but Amy and some other chicks at 3FC think they may prefer to stay in them for life.

The Real Skinny on Cosmetic Surgery

Tummy Tucks and Excess Skin

Excess skin is a common problem among women who have lost large amounts of weight. How much excess skin will you have? This can vary widely from one person to the next and can be affected by factors including heredity, skin tone, and time spent in the sun. Younger women will usually have less than older women, because they have more elasticity in their skin. The amount of weight you lose will also come into play, since an extra 250 pounds will have done more damage than an extra 100. How quickly you lose the weight is also important. If you lose 100 pounds fast, you stand to have more excess skin because your body didn't have time to adapt. Weight-loss surgery patients frequently face this dilemma, though it can happen to anyone. It's really impossible to know how much excess skin you will have until you get there. But carrying around the excess skin is still much better than being very overweight.

Can you prevent it? Remove it later? Our chicks have asked about this many times.

Meg Heinz, a personal trainer and one of our forum moderators, has become an expert on loose skin. After losing 120 pounds through diet and exercise, she had a considerable amount of excess skin. She researched the topic and chose to have her loose skin surgically removed. She has shared her knowledge and experience with the rest of us.

Q: Will exercise affect the way my skin looks when I reach my goal weight?

Meg: Exercise alone can't make your skin tighten up; however, building muscle as you lose weight and afterwards can help to fill up some of the loose skin.

Q: Are there any creams or lotions that I can rub on my skin that will make it tighten up?

Meg: No.

Q: *Are there any vitamins or supplements that I can take that will make my skin tighten up?*

Meg: No.

Q: *When will I be able to tell whether my skin will tighten up after weight loss?*

Meg: Try not to worry prematurely about potential skin problems before you reach your goal weight. Many body changes happen as you lose the last ten or twenty pounds. Most plastic surgeons tell you to wait at least six months after you reach your goal weight and stabilize there to see how your skin reacts to your weight loss. However, not much is likely to change after a year.

Q: *I've reached my goal weight and waited six months and still have a problem with excess skin. What can I do?*

Meg: At this point, it comes down to two choices: live with the skin or have it surgically removed. Excess skin problems can usually be camouflaged under clothing quite nicely. If you don't want to live with the skin, you can schedule a consultation with a plastic surgeon to discuss surgical options. You might want to consider talking to a doctor just to find out what all your options are, even if you don't think that you would consider surgery.

Q: *What kinds of plastic surgeries are done for excess skin?*

Meg: Here are the names of some of the various procedures:

- Arms: brachioplasty
- Thighs: thigh lift or lower body lift

- Face/neck: face lift
- Breasts: breast lift, mastopexy
- Butt: butt lift, lower body lift
- Entire lower body (abdomen, butt, thighs): lower bodylift, belt lipectomy

Many of the above can be combined with lipo to remove excess fat. Frequently multiple procedures are done together to save on expenses.

Q: Does plastic surgery leave scars?

Meg: Yes. Unfortunately it's a trade-off between scars and excess skin. Most scars can be camouflaged by clothing or a bathing suit or underwear, although those on the arms and knees and other exposed areas are more visible. Scars go through a maturation process as they heal, starting off as red and raised, and fading to thin white lines over the course of a year. Your doctor will suggest products and techniques (like massage) to minimize scarring. You need to avoid tanning and sun exposure on your scars for a year.

Q: How much does all this excess skin weigh? Will I lose weight if I get rid of the skin?

Meg: "Dry skin" (skin drained of all its fluids) doesn't weigh much at all. (They drain the fluids back into your body in the OR before they remove the skin.) Frequently, however, some fat is removed along with excess skin and that adds some weight to what's removed. The total weight can range from just a pound or two to twenty or more pounds, depending on the amount of excess skin and attached fat that you have. Everyone's experience will be different. A plastic surgeon who examines you can answer that question for you.

You can read our latest info on excess skin at www.3fatchicks.com/cosmeticsurgery.

Liposuction

If your problem is a stubborn fat deposit that you can't get rid of, liposuction might be for you. Some chicks have done all they can to master their thighs and crunch their abs, but they still have a couple of speed bumps on their curves. If this sounds like you, liposuction might be just what you need. In liposuction, a surgeon vacuums out your excess fat cells from under your skin. The surgeon will insert a hollow tube into the fatty area, basically plunge the fat loose, and suck it out. Common side effects are bruising and swelling, but as with any procedure, rare complications can occur, including death.

Lipo won't tighten up loose skin, and it won't get rid of cellulite. It will get rid of stubborn fat that just doesn't want to go away. This procedure is not intended as a method of weight loss. Even the most diligent dieter and strength trainer can be left with fat deposits that just won't budge. Lipo is, in fact, the only way you can spot-reduce. The procedure, which can be done under local anesthesia, is generally much more cost-effective than traditional cosmetic surgery. Ask your cosmetic surgeon or dermatologist if lipo can help you.

Words to Live By

All our dreams can come true, if we have the courage to pursue them.
—WALT DISNEY

In two decades I've lost a total of 789 pounds. I should be hanging from a charm bracelet. —ERMA BOMBECK

laying the golden egg

A S IS TRUE OF any great journey, on the road to better health and wellness, just when you think you've arrived, you realize that you are just beginning! The most important challenge in any commitment to a fitter and thinner lifestyle comes when you've already lost the weight. Keeping the weight off can take just as much effort as losing it in the first place. You can never go back to your old style of eating or eat like your thin friends, or you will regain the weight, and for good reason. You may be surprised to learn that your metabolism is slower now than it was when you were overweight or when you were originally thin. Now, perhaps more than ever, you have to really pay attention to what you are doing.

Learning how to maintain your commitment to a new lifestyle, not only during the initial weight-loss phase but for the rest of your life, is a process of getting to know yourself, emotionally and psychologically as well as physically. Many chicks gain weight through emotional eating to soothe other problems such as stress, loneliness, or troubled relationships. Maybe you were bored, or frustrated with a job that didn't challenge you. Whatever the reasons were behind your extra weight, keeping the weight off means facing those demons, and finding a better way to cope with your feelings, as well as your waistline.

We know that if you've gotten to this point, you feel much better than you did. You're more energetic, you look fabulous, and your health has improved tremendously. You have to keep this success in mind and remember what you're working for. If you back off, or let those nasty demons rear their ugly heads, it can all slip through your fingers like a greasy french fry.

We 3 fat chicks were once notorious yo-yo dieters. If our jeans were too tight, we'd follow a quick weight-loss scheme, then go back to our old eating habits. And of course, it should be no surprise that the weight came back on as quickly as it left us—and straight back onto our thighs—until we realized that we had to make a plan not just for next week or next month but also for the rest of our lives.

Losing the weight is the adventurous, exciting part of the journey. It's keeping the weight off that requires elbow grease. Our most inspirational weight loss role models have taught us a few lessons. The first lesson we learned about keeping the weight off was to actively invest in our weight maintenance on a daily basis. You can't just lose the weight and forget about it. We had already learned the little things that make a big difference in the long haul, and we couldn't forget them now. For example, we learned that if we start out the morning with exercise, we are less likely to give in to temptations later in the day. Likewise, if we take the time to measure ourselves with a tape and weigh regularly, it is easier to stay at goal, since we are aware of the slightest change in the wrong direction.

We began to understand what it meant to be fully accountable for our actions. If we screwed up, we had no one to blame but ourselves. For us, the most important difference between then and now is our commitment to ourselves, to each other, and to the support of the community of chicks that we connected with through our Web site.

The inspiration and determination to get started on the climb of your life is the first step in any successful dieting program. The next step is learning how to maintain your commitment to your new lifestyle, not only during the initial weight-loss phase but for the rest of your life. So for all of you who are trying to lay a golden egg, here are some tips from our high-maintenance chicks, to help you along on your new path, so that the next diet you go on will be your last.

The Six Golden Gateways to Successful Maintenance

1. Make Yourself a Priority

You're never going to achieve your goals as long as you're the last person on your list each day. You're going to have to give up a few things in exchange for other activities if you want to keep off this weight. You may think that your life is too busy to accommodate your new lifestyle, but it isn't. You simply can't keep putting yourself at the end of the schedule. Diet and exercise are a priority for health, just like practicing good hygiene or visiting a doctor when you're sick. You're not selfish for putting your health ahead of washing your husband's underwear! When you take care of your health, you benefit your whole family. Beverly learned this and, as a result, has lost 190 pounds. By making herself a priority in her own life, she has kept the weight off.

Beverly from Arkansas

I absolutely have to make taking care of myself a priority or I would never bother. I could come up with a hundred excuses for putting off exercise, like eating crap out of convenience and pretending the dryer is shrinking my clothes. But where would that get me? Oh yeah, I remember, my old life! We have to take care of ourselves in order to be the best possible wives, moms, and women we can be, period. Do I feel guilty sometimes? Absolutely! But I figure I can still take my daughter to the park an hour from now, after I exercise. The laundry will get done . . . eventually; the floor doesn't need to be vacuumed right this minute. It's a trade-off—learning how to balance all the most important things in life to achieve the best possible outcome. So, everybody is not completely happy all of the time? They will get over it. Plus—and you all know it's true—if momma ain't happy, ain't nobody happy!

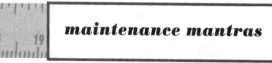

maintenance mantras

Many of our high-maintenance chicks have mantras that they describe as the little voice in their head that spurs them on when they feel like giving up. We asked them to share some of these inspirational "hooks" with us, so that you can try out a few for yourself. Repeat some of these maintenance mantras to yourself the next time you need a pep talk!

Falling down is not failure. Failure is staying down.
— MEL, PERSONAL TRAINER, MODERATOR OF 3FC

It gets easier over time . . . It gets easier over time . . .
—JENNIFER, NEW YORK

Never trade what you want at the moment for what you want the most.
— BEVERLY, ARKANSAS

You can quit this very second if you really want, but is that what you really want to do? —JAN, FLORIDA

Is——(fill in the blank with your favorite forbidden food) really worth sixty minutes of cardio? — MELANIE, MODERATOR OF 3FC

I don't do that anymore. — MEG, MODERATOR OF 3FC

Breathe: it can change the pattern of your thoughts. Learn to wait: once you can wait, you can do almost anything. And remember: it all counts. — ROBIN, CALIFORNIA

hazard signs on the hungry highway

One of the most difficult parts of maintaining weight loss is that we fat chicks, like most of the rest of the world, have an epic capacity for denial. We can feel like we're steering clear of temptation and never even notice that the road we're on is headed straight to the nearest burger stand. So for all of us queens of denial, who can wind up ten pounds heavier faster than you can say chocolate chip cheesecake, here's a few of the hazard signs and suggestions for how to steer out of your skid.

Danger Signs

- I forget to eat a snack and then I'm so hungry that I overeat at mealtime.
- I do not want to exercise, and I start making excuses to myself.
- I start picking leftovers off my kids' plates.
- I stop drinking water, which only makes things worse.
- I start picking and nibbling at high-calorie food—a slippery slope that leads right to a binge.
- I buy or make certain food for "others." Who am I kidding? It's really for me and I'm the one who ends up eating it.
- I don't have food planned or prepared in advance. And I sure don't make very good decisions when I'm hungry!

How to Steer Out of Your Skid

- I carry fruit and veggies for snacks everywhere I go.
- I try to exercise more.
- I stop buying treats "for the kids."
- I try to be accountable for what I eat.

• *Continued on next page* •

- I try to pay more attention to my positive inner voice, and I say my mantras a lot.
- I steer clear of trigger items.
- I pay more attention to water consumption.
- I plan ahead, so nothing is left to chance.
- I try to get more rest.

2. It's Okay to Slip Up a Little

A successful diet is not an all-or-nothing approach. That would be a miserable, not to mention impossible, way to diet! To err is human, so don't expect yourself to be perfect. Slipping up doesn't have to mean you'll gain the weight back, though. Just accept that you cheated a little, and then move on and try to stay on program the next time you're tempted. How many times have you said, "I've already blown my diet today, I may as well keep eating and start my diet again tomorrow"? The second you realize you've goofed up, just stop. Don't wait until tomorrow, because you're guaranteed to feel worse then. If you stop now, you can feel proud of yourself later, knowing that you realized what was happening and you took control.

One thing you do have to keep in mind, though, is that you can't have continual slip-ups. If you are constantly experiencing setbacks, then you should reevaluate your lifestyle, because you will put the weight back on if you keep it up. When you chose your weight-loss diet, we hope you picked a diet plan you could stick with, because you usually have to keep it up for the rest of your life. It becomes a lifestyle, not a diet. You eat just a little more than you did while losing weight. You keep up the exercise and continue to make good choices. You can have slipups or even planned treats, but you need to draw the line at what defines success and maintenance. Decide how far you can go without losing control, and whatever you do, don't cross that line.

Jamie found a realistic diet plan that she could live with for the rest of her life, and in her case, the right diet has made all the difference to her long-term weight-loss success.

Jamie from North Carolina

I can't count how many times I reached my goal weight and then gained the pounds right back. I never really ate bad foods, I just ate too much food. I was fooling myself to think I could go on a strict diet that I usually hated, one where I couldn't wait to get back to "normal" food, which I usually overate. Enough was enough. The last time I decided to lose weight, I wanted to eat my regular foods, since I knew I'd get back there eventually. So I counted every calorie that passed through my lips, and I exercised, since it was all about calories in versus calories out. I couldn't believe how much easier this was for me! When I reached goal, I kept on counting calories and just ate a little more. I still exercise, since it's also part of the big picture. I learned the hard way that I couldn't avoid paying attention, just because I was at goal. If you don't keep track of what you are eating and doing, the weight will slip back on before you know it. Good health should last forever, but it only happens if you make it happen.

3. Long-Term Success Isn't Automatic

Some things in life simply don't come without some hard work up front. We would much rather have the weight loss occur instantly and never have to worry about gaining it back, but it won't happen that way. Weight loss requires patience and hard, consistent work. In the world of weight-loss maintenance, there is no immediate gratification, and no buy-now, pay-later plans. You have to put your cash on the barrel every time you eat a meal. Here's how one of our most successful high-maintenance chicks explains it:

Barb from Ontario

I think that as a society, we are conditioned to live on credit. Buy a house, live in it now, and pay for the next twenty-five years. Buy a car, drive it now, and pay for it the next five years. Weight loss is not like that. You can't decide to lose weight and get fit and be a size 8 in good shape today and then pay later. You have to work now for results later, which is not something we're all used to doing anymore!

So why do some people start losing, keep losing, and then maintain their weight loss while others fail? I think it is mostly a mind-over-matter thing with a lot of determination thrown in. I recently realized that it was like a snowball rolling downhill. We only have to summon the determination to start the thing rolling in the first place, and then it will gain momentum on its own. Success causes more effort and effort causes more success. Then we just have to find it within ourselves to give it the occasional push when it starts to slow or stall. I think that's where most people fail. The momentum stops and they are resigned to let it.

4. Move It or Lose It

The chances are slim to none that you will achieve your weight-loss goal without exercise, and you have even less of a chance at keeping that weight off without it. Exercise is not only a calorie burner; it is essential to our system. Our hearts and lungs and bones need a solid cardio and strength-training program. The members of our Maintainers' Forum unanimously agree that exercise is part of a weight-loss maintenance success.

Anne from Arizona

Exercise is just fantastic! Possibly the best thing I've done for myself. I went from total couch potato to triathlete, and no, I didn't even have to get a perfect body to make that happen. I feel so much better, so much more relaxed, and so much more in control when I exercise. I'm still exercising now that I'm pregnant, but I've dropped the frequency, intensity, and duration quite a bit. Once you get started exercising, it is so tough to quit. Even when I broke my foot last year, I still managed to go swimming and pool running with a floaty belt. There is always a way, no matter what's going on in your life, to fit in a little healthy activity!

5. Forget the Head Games

Emotional eating can slow down or destroy our attempts at weight loss and maintenance. Eating is not always about the food; often it's about how food makes us feel. It can be comforting or distracting, or give us a sense of pleasure we don't always get elsewhere. Although this kind of emotional eating comforts us in the moment, we always feel lousy afterward. Guilt, shame, physical discomfort—these are just some of the aftereffects of emotional eating. And we *know* we're going to regret it later, but we still do it anyway. Now is the time to get over it. Learn some new habits. We lost our weight, not our problems, so it's important to deal with your issues and find a better solution than eating. Plan ahead, so you have some recourse the next time an emotional food craving hits.

Mette from Norway

I've always known that I overeat when I'm very hungry. I also overeat when I feel depressed, rejected, sad, and down. I do tend to take care of myself with sweets: eating cookies always makes me feel better!

The changes in my routine felt stressful because I didn't want to make them—like exchanging cookies for dumbbells! Feeling anxious and insecure didn't help either. I even managed to identify new high-risk situations for overeating: I noticed that I also overeat when I don't sleep enough, drink enough water, or rest when I'm tired. It's weird that I interpret every signal of discomfort from my body as a sign to eat, but I found a way to turn to exercise and real self-love—rather than just consuming mass quantities of empty calories—and that, in the long run, was truly a comfort!

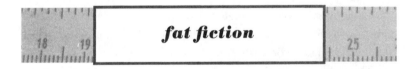

fat fiction

All chicks need a curvy heroine! Read a few of these books recommended by some of our chicks for another perspective

• *Continued on next page* •

on being overweight. From chubby girls to scorned women, you'll find stories to make you laugh and cry and hopefully become inspired in your own weight loss. You can see a current list of all of the favorites at www.3fatchicks.com/books.

Blubber, Judy Blume
Bridget Jones's Diary, Helen Fielding
Fat Chance, Deborah Blumenthal
Good in Bed, Jennifer Weiner
In Her Shoes, Jennifer Weiner
Lady Oracle, Margaret Atwood
Life in the Fat Lane, Cherie Bennett
Losing It, Lindsay Faith Rech
Night Swimming, Robin Schwarz
One Fat Summer, Robert Lipsyte
Slim Chance, Jackie Rose
Something's Wrong with Your Scale, Van Whitfield
What Are You Looking At? The First Fat Fiction Anthology, Donna
    Jarrell, Ira Sukrungruang

6. Lifelong Success Is Not Just Wishful Thinking

In a nation where everyone is dieting but obesity rates continue to rise, it seems like weight-loss success is just wishful thinking, but it's not. Lifelong success is completely within our reach, but you have to make a conscious effort to make it happen. We're not going to kid you; it will be hard work. You'll have to work at it for the rest of your life. The good news is that it does become a lot easier after a while, and you'll soon learn that you don't want to do it any differently.

Meg from Pennsylvania
Three years of living maintenance every day has given me the confidence of knowing that the only way that I'll gain the weight back is if I make a lot of

really bad choices. I now know—beyond the shadow of a doubt—that the power to keep the weight off is totally in my hands.

Regaining isn't going to happen to me passively; I would actively and consciously have to make bad decisions—ranging from not monitoring my weight to not exercising to eating the wrong foods—in order to put the weight back on. Knowing that keeping the weight off is completely under my control and in my hands makes maintenance a lot easier in my mind. I know what to do to keep the weight off and I fully intend to keep doing it every day of my life. This new body (and new life) is a gift beyond compare, and I'll never ever choose to give it up.

Last Words That We Hope Will Last a Lifetime

There are no quick fixes to lifelong problems, and dieting is no exception. When we make a decision to diet, we are making a decision to change our life, and everything we do from that point forward, no matter how small or how grand, will impact our success. Our hope is that you will take the knowledge and experience that we've offered you in these pages and put them to use for the rest of your life, because the diet never really ends, it just becomes a better lifestyle. And if you take nothing else away with you, we, and all of the chicks who have contributed to this book, hope you realize that no matter how tough the struggle may seem at times, you are not alone!

INVESTING SUCCESS

SUCCESS

How To Conquer **30** Costly Mistakes &
Multiply Your Wealth!

Advantage World Press is proud to publish the
Investing Success™ series of books. Look for these future titles:

- Investing Success For Women

- Investing Success For Couples

- Investing Success For African Americans

- Investing Success For Baby Boomers

- Investing Success For Retirees

- Investing Success For Christians

- Investing Success For Young Adults

- Investing Success For Small Business Owners

- Investing Success For Families

INVESTING SUCCESS

SUCCESS

How To Conquer 30 Costly Mistakes &
Multiply Your Wealth!

Lynnette Khalfani

ADVANTAGE WORLD PRESS

Published by Advantage World Press
(www.AdvantageWorldPress.com)
P.O. Box 452
South Orange, NJ 07079

Printed in Canada
First Edition: January 2004

Book Design by Pamela Terry, Opus 1 Design
Editor: Tawana Bivins Rosenbaum

This publication is designed to provide accurate and authoritative information in regard to the subject matter covered. It is sold with the understanding that the author and publisher are not engaged in rendering legal, financial or other professional advice. Laws and practices vary from state to state and if legal or other expert assistance is required, the services of a competent professional should be sought. The author and publisher specifically disclaim any responsibility for liability, loss or risk that is incurred as a consequence, direct or indirect, of the use and application of any of the contents of this book.

SPECIAL SALES
Advantage World Press books are available at special bulk purchase discounts to use for sales promotions, premiums, or educational purposes. Special editions, including personalized covers, excerpts of existing books, and corporate imprints, can be created in large quantities for special needs. For more information, write to Advantage World Press, Special Markets, P.O. Box 452, South Orange NJ 07079, Fax (973) 324-1951, or E-mail: specialmarkets@advantageworldpress.com.

Publisher's Cataloguing in Publication Data

Khalfani, Lynnette.

Investing success : how to conquer 30 costly mistakes & multiply your wealth! / Lynnette Khalfani. -- 1st ed. -- South Orange, NJ : Advantage World Press, 2004.

p. ; cm.

(Investing success series)

Includes index.
ISBN: 1-932450-50-5

1. Investments--Popular works. 2. Finance, Personal--Popular works. 3. Business--Popular works. I. Title.

HG4521 .K43 2004   0401
332.6--dc22

Attention readers: If you've ever made an investing mistake and learned a valuable lesson from it, share your story and help other people. Your investing experience could be featured in an upcoming book in the *Investing Success*™ series. To submit your story for inclusion in a future *Investing Success*™ book, please send it via E-mail to: *mystory@InvestingSuccess.net* or write to:

Investing Success™
c/o Advantage World Press
P.O. Box 452
South Orange, NJ 07079

Special note to financial advisors: Please help teach the public about how to avoid or fix investing mistakes. Send your insights to: *advisorshelp@InvestingSuccess.net*

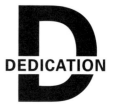

DEDICATION

This book is dedicated to my daughter, Aziza, and my son, Jakada. You both have given me more riches than I could ever count. Just looking at you each day is sheer joy.

I pray you will follow Mommy's example of finding your life's mission, pursuing it with passion, and creating your own wealth.

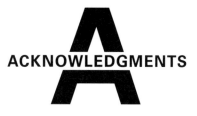

ACKNOWLEDGMENTS

I have so many people to thank for all their hard work, encouragement, and assistance in helping me bring this book to life.

To Akil, my husband: I know I tested your patience many times with my promises (rarely kept) that I only needed to work "five more minutes." I truly appreciate your input, support and understanding – not to mention the numerous meals you prepared and brought down to the basement office when I was glued to the computer. Thanks also for being a wonderful father to our kids, especially during those times I was so engrossed in my work.

To my sister, Deborah Darrell: I couldn't have asked for a better marketer, business partner, publicist and strategist. I love you and will forever remember how you took my passion for this project and selflessly made it your own. You've been a big blessing to me, and a positive influence throughout this endeavor. Is there any way I can bottle just half of your organizational skills and efficiency?

To Pamela Terry, of Opus 1 Design: what an amazingly talented person you are! You "got it" from Day 1. And up until the very end, you continually improved upon my vision for *Investing Success*, creating an awesome cover and beautiful interior design. I hired you for your outstanding creative skills. But you turned out to be far more valuable than I imagined. Thanks for serving as a good sounding board, and for the constant stream of information, resources and contacts you offered as I learned the ins and out of publishing.

To Earl Cox, of Earl Cox & Associates: I'm so lucky to have you on my team. I'm also so very impressed by your industry knowledge, and your sales and marketing savvy. Your consulting services and publishing expertise have benefited me immeasurably. Many thanks for those marathon brainstorming sessions, your intensity, and honesty.

To Tawana Bivins Rosenbaum: all I can say is thank God for editors like you! I'm still in awe of your eagle eyes and keen attention to detail. You made this book a much more readable, clean and inviting text. I look forward to learning more from you as I continue the *Investing Success*™ series.

To Tim Askin and Michael Shmarak: what a pleasure it has been working with you over the years. Each of you has been a tremendous resource for me as financial journalist and author. No matter how crazy my deadlines were, I always knew I could count on you to help me find fantastic sources of information and first-rate financial experts. I want you to know all your efforts were (and still are) very much appreciated.

To all the people who took the time to be interviewed by me, both market professionals and investors: you added so much to the body and scope of this work. I know your insights will be instructive to readers. Thank you for your expertise and your candor.

Finally, I must give heartfelt thanks to the many friends, family members, and colleagues who supported me or who poured over *Investing Success* and offered advice, feedback and constructive criticism. All of your comments were helpful. Special thanks, Mom, for suggesting the subtitle of the book. You're the best!

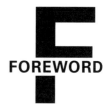

FOREWORD

As Lynnette Khalfani so wisely points out, all investors make mistakes from time to time. But the most successful investors are those who are able to learn from these blunders and make wiser decisions in the future.

As someone who has lived and breathed investing for more than 40 years, I can honestly say that many of our most serious mistakes come from our hearts, not our heads. The amazing bull market of the late 1990's created a euphoria that was hard to resist, and an atmosphere that caused a lot of people to ignore time-tested investing basics and throw discipline out the window. Now that we are hopefully witnessing a recovery from the worst bear market since the Depression, it is equally important that investors maintain a cool head and not allow their fears to interfere with thoughtful long-term decisions.

Therefore, I encourage you to take Lynnette's well-researched advice to heart. Set specific, measurable, and realistic goals. Create an asset allocation plan that suits your risk tolerance, time frame, and goals. Buy a diversified mix of investments, being careful not to over concentrate in any one asset class, sector, style, or industry. And perhaps most important of all, make a commitment to being a lifelong investor.

These basics are more important now than ever. They are our investing compass points, and I urge you to take them to heart. I strongly believe that the American stock market is still the best place for long-term investing, and that with a wise investing plan – combined with a cool head -- you can meet your financial goals. I wish you the best.

Charles R. Schwab
Founder and Chairman
The Charles Schwab Corporation
August, 2003

For individual investors there are two sides to the investing equation: first you must know the "right" things to do; second you must avoid doing the "wrong" things. There are hundreds of books that deal with the right way to invest and this topic is subject to a wide diversity of opinions. In this book, Lynnette Khalfani has, to our benefit, decided to concentrate on the second, and equally important, part of the investing equation. She has pointed out what to avoid. And no one is likely to dispute any of the points she so clearly makes on the pages that follow.

The investing world can be a very unfriendly place for the unprepared or under-informed investor. In fact, it can be a veritable minefield for individuals who don't pay attention to their investments or who completely put them under the control of a third party. One misstep can blow apart a lifetime of savings. What Lynnette has done in this book is literally placed large red flags on the investing landscape: showing us the areas to avoid, showing us where the wealth-threatening mines are buried, and marking a pathway through this minefield to the end goal of increased wealth.

As president of an organization devoted to creating investor education material and as a professor of investing studies at the college level, I have personally worked with hundreds of individual investors. In analyzing the activities of those who have performed poorly, it has become apparent that the same mistakes are made over and over again. And even the most savvy of investors makes them. These are the mistakes that are clearly described in this book. Once they are recognized, they can be avoided.

In a clear, concise and easy-to-read manner, Lynnette has detailed the mistakes that prevent investors from attaining the financial goals they really want and are capable of reaching. This is a book you will want to read thoroughly the first time and then scan again each time you review your portfolio of investments; perhaps quarterly, perhaps annually. Avoiding investing mistakes is key to increasing your wealth and therefore this book deserves a place in the library of every individual investor.

Leland B. Hevner
President,
National Association of Online Investors (NAOI)
July 15, 2003

TABLE OF CONTENTS

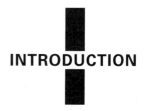

INTRODUCTION

Have you ever wondered what separates successful investors from marginal ones or from those who get clobbered by Wall Street? The best investors aren't always better stock pickers. Most of them don't boast Ivy-league degrees. Nor do they have access to "inside" information. In truth, the most successful investors – that is, the ones who consistently make money in up and down markets – are simply the people who make the fewest investing mistakes, and those who *quickly* fix the blunders they do make.

Too often, unsuccessful investors think: "If I could just pick the next Microsoft, I'd be rich," or "If only I had sold my stock at its peak, I'd have a fortune." Well, it certainly helps to identify industry-leading companies as potential investments. And "selling high" may bring you one step closer to fattening your bank account. However, the reality is that just buying good investments and selling them for a profit offers absolutely no assurance that you will be a successful investor. In fact, if you *only* master those two elements of buying and selling, you almost certainly will fail miserably as an investor.

THE "BUY LOW, SELL HIGH" MYTH

"Now wait a minute," you may be saying. "Isn't that the very definition of smart investing: knowing *what* to buy and *when* to sell? And what about that old adage: 'buy low and sell high?' Isn't that what this whole investing business is all about?" Actually, nothing could be further from the truth. Here's why:

All the buying and selling savvy in the world won't maximize your wealth if you make any number of costly investing missteps.

Consider, for example: What happens if you trade so much that commissions eat away at your profits? What happens if poor planning or impatience leads you to pay extra taxes to Uncle Sam? What happens if you trust an unscrupulous stockbroker, trustee or accountant, and he skims funds from your account? What happens if your investing strategy fails to take advantage of the benefits of compounded interest?

So sure, you might buy some "winners" for your portfolio — and even sell them at the right time. But what happens if that Wall Street darling you loaded up on nosedives inexplicably right after you purchase it? No bad news from the company. Nothing terrible about its management, product or the industry in which it operates. Just negative overall "market conditions." These are just a fraction of the possible dilemmas that await beginning and long-time investors alike.

MASTERING THE FIVE PHASES OF INVESTING

Despite conventional wisdom, shrewd investing clearly entails far more than buying and selling know-how. Successful investing involves mastering a multi-faceted process, and side stepping the dangers lurking at every turn. These dangers must be avoided to maximize investment performance and multiply your wealth.

By now, you may be asking: "If investing transcends buying and selling, what else is there?"

The investing process involves five distinct phases:

1) Strategizing to meet your personal goals;

2) Buying the right investments;

3) **Holding** and adequately monitoring the investments in your portfolio;

4) **Selling** investments in a judicious manner; and

5) **Dealing effectively** with investment intermediaries such as stockbrokers and financial planners.

Once you recognize the many traps that arise during these five stages, you can readily avoid these perils. And what if you've *already* erred and somehow stepped onto an investing landmine? Don't despair! (You're reading this book, so while you might have "lost your shirt," life and limb remain intact, right?) The key is to better navigate those ticking time bombs going forward.

Remember: you don't have to be perfect. The best investors just make the fewest mistakes, and they readily recover from the fumbles they do commit. The sooner you realize this basic yet powerful truth, the sooner you can begin to turn almost any perilous situation into a profitable one. That is a central message throughout *Investing Success*.

But if you don't remember anything else from *Investing Success*, I would hope that you would remember this most crucial point:

Unsuccessful investors focus on products. They're constantly asking: "What's the best stock to buy?" or "What's the hottest mutual fund?" And if they make poor choices, they are reluctant to properly remedy the situation. By contrast, successful investors focus on the process of investing. They ask: "What should I be doing to grow my portfolio?" or "What strategies will help me reach my goals?" If they err at some point, they are eager to fix their blunders, learn from those miscalculations, and minimize future missteps.

This is a big distinction between unprofitable investors and enormously profitable ones. So, if you find yourself worrying too much about products, you may have to change your mindset to become a successful investor. Also, if you fall into the trap of blaming others for your financial predicament, you may have to re-think things.

As a financial journalist, I realize that corporate scandals, accounting improprieties, and research conflicts of interest have cost the investing public trillions of dollars in recent years. While there is plenty of blame to go around, in the final analysis you are ultimately responsible for your own finances. After all, no one cares about your economic well being more than you do, right? Even if you've lost money on Wall Street in the past due to outside influences, as you read this book I want you to take an honest look in the mirror — and decide whether you also fell victim to your own investing mistakes. It's tough medicine, I know. But I honestly believe that only after you recognize your own mistakes can you remedy them, and start to build true wealth.

THE GENERAL CONCEPT BEHIND *INVESTING SUCCESS*

I hope you didn't pick this book up expecting to be berated for your investing shortcomings (or to give a copy to someone else to berate them for their mistakes!). That's not what this book is about. On the contrary, I want to make it clear that mistakes are a natural – indeed a healthy and very necessary – part of becoming a successful investor. To think that you will completely avoid all investing mistakes is wholly unrealistic. Did you learn to walk without falling down a few times? Of course you didn't. Just as you learned as a toddler to put one sure foot in front of the other, so too will you learn to stroll confidently down this exciting place called Wall Street. Besides, if you didn't make some bad decisions as an investor, I doubt you would really learn what does and does not work, how you should and should not conduct your financial affairs, nor why it's necessary to look at investing as a long-term process, as opposed to a one-shot event.

WHAT DOES A JOURNALIST KNOW ABOUT INVESTING ANYWAY?

I also think it's important to tell you how I came to write *Investing Success*. Some people may ask, and legitimately so, what qualifies me to write an investing book. After all, I'm a financial journalist – not a stockbroker, financial planner or money manager. Well, the truth of the matter is that it's precisely *because* I'm a personal finance journalist that I'm able to share the valuable information you are about to read.

The advice contained in this book isn't Lynnette Khalfani's wisdom (as much as I'd like to claim credit for it). To be sure, I have my opinions and I offer them candidly. But primarily, I've tapped the collective wisdom of hundreds of financial experts and investors just like you. Over the past decade, I've interviewed well over 1,000 financial professionals – from market strategists to hedge fund experts to chief investment officers and so on. When I talked to members of the financial planning community in particular, I noticed patterns in what they would say concerning their clients. Over and over again, people seemed to be making the same types of costly, and largely avoidable, investing errors.

I further saw investors' tendency toward financial mistakes when I began writing a personal finance column for Dow Jones Newswires in 1999. Readers frequently wrote me with investing questions and dilemmas. Later, when I did regular "Financial Fitness" segments on CNBC, the same thing happened. On a weekly basis, viewers would log onto CNBC.com and pose a variety of questions about whatever financial topic I reported on that week. Almost invariably, readers and viewers expressed a higher degree of comfort getting information from me than from their paid advisors. This initially surprised me. I later discovered, though, that these individuals appreciated the fact that I was a neutral third party. I had no investment products to sell, no commissions to earn, no vested interest in their finances.

The same thing is true today. So no, I don't work for a Wall Street brokerage house and I don't have a license to sell securities. Nor is that my intention. If I became such a professional, then I'd probably only give you one person's point of view (my own), or perhaps the bias of my firm. But as a journalist, I'm more than happy to be able to offer you my educated opinion, as well as a wide range of informed ideas from some of the top minds in finance.

HOW TO USE THIS BOOK

Because a winning investment program involves the five crucial areas described above – strategizing, buying, holding/monitoring, selling, and dealing with financial intermediaries – I've organized this book into five easy to understand parts according to those criteria. Furthermore, each chapter is devoted to one investing mistake.

If you are planning your debut plunge into the financial markets, ideally you should read *Investing Success* from cover to cover before spending a dime on any investment. Going through each chapter and each investing mistake sequentially will help you think about investing as a step-by-step process – as opposed to a haphazard series of events that mystify and overwhelm unwitting investors.

Realistically though, you probably won't get your hands on this book before you commit money to an investment. But it doesn't matter if you've just made your first investment or your 500th. What lies between these pages will help you become a more successful investor.

Even if you are a seasoned investor, you too will be best served by reading the text straight through because it will re-focus your thinking, and highlight mistakes you may be making or overlooking. Some highly experienced investors may know what their problem areas are – say, you have difficulty selling investments – and can flip right to those chapters.

There are also several handy symbols used throughout *Investing Success* to guide your reading:

 NOTE & REMEMBER: For statistics, facts, resources, and other straight-forward information.

 For action items. This is where I give you suggested things to do.

 For insights that I want you to think about or visualize, and counter-intuitive points that may cause you to re-consider certain beliefs.

Finally, at the end of each chapter, I offer a "**$ummary $uccess $trategy**." This is the place that succinctly highlights what you should do to avoid or fix the mistake covered in that chapter.

Don't beat yourself up if you find that you're guilty of committing some of the investing faux pas outlined in this book. Countless others – myself included - have made some of the same mistakes. In order to illustrate how widespread investing mistakes are, I have incorporated plenty of first-hand accounts and other information from individual investors with a range of investing know-how from all walks of life. Some of these investors, like famed billionaire Warren Buffett, are legendary and their names are immediately recognizable. One well-known investor is Charles Schwab, founder of Charles Schwab & Co., Inc. During an interview in 2003, he candidly told me "I've made enough investing mistakes to fill *three* books." But *Investing Success* doesn't just capture the know-how of celebrated market professionals.

Other people included in this book you've probably never heard of, but their stories will sound familiar, as they may mirror your own experiences or those of someone you know.

Because investing is such a dynamic process, I hope that even after you close the last pages of *Investing Success*, you will refer back to it whenever you contemplate how to make smarter investment decisions.

Best wishes in your investing endeavors! I know you'll be greatly enriched — and sleep better at night — if you conquer the following 30 investing mistakes.

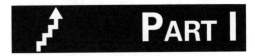

PART I

STRATEGIC SLIP-UPS

FAILING TO SET SPECIFIC, MEASURABLE, AND REALISTIC GOALS

Do you remember when you were a kid and some adult asked you what you planned to make of yourself in life? That initial conversation probably went something like this:

> **Adult:** Johnny, what do you want to be when you grow up?
>
> **Johnny:** I want to be a fireman.
>
> **Adult:** That's great, Johnny. Why do you want to become a fireman?
>
> **Johnny:** So I can help save people. And also because I want to drive down the street in a big, red fire truck with the sirens going 'Whirr!!! Whirr!!! Whirr!!!'

In the case of my son, who's in pre-kindergarten, his answer is more along the lines of: I want to be a fireman, *and* a baseball player, *and* a teacher, *and* a veterinarian, *and* a (fill-in-the-blank) …

You've got to love kids. They're super-ambitious, and so hopeful about the future. Many of them truly believe that they can achieve anything in life that they want. As adults, especially those of us who are parents, I think we all strive to nurture that natural optimism in children. For young people, having such carefree (translation: unfocused) dreams for the future is a good thing.

However, for adults, particularly those of us who invest, such unbridled optimism can be dangerous. Don't misunderstand me. I'm not saying that you can't have high hopes from a financial standpoint. What I am suggesting, though, is that we can't afford to completely mimic the carefree optimism of children. Youngsters have the luxury of giving little or no thought to the *specifics* of their goals, nor *how* and *when* those aims will be achieved.

WHAT ARE YOUR GOALS?

So many people simply say: "I would like to save more money," or "I want to invest for the future." Well, the first question you really need to answer is: For what *purpose* do you want to save or invest?

We all have personal goals. Some people would like to retire before they turn 60. Others want to build a dream house on the beach. Maybe your ambition is to be able to afford to send your kids to a private college. Or perhaps you're itching to quit your job and form your own company.

All of these personal goals are also financial goals, because it takes money to achieve them. For example, you certainly can't retire in comfort with an empty bank account. Neither can you launch a business without some start-up capital.

Take a few minutes to review the general goals listed below. Do any of them match your own? If so, think about whether each applicable goal is a short, medium, or long-range mission for you.

> **Short-Term goals:** can be achieved in 1-2 years maximum
> **Medium-Term goals**: require 2 -10 years to accomplish
> **Long-Term goals**: require saving/investing for 10+ years

- Pay off credit card debt
- Establish a cash cushion or emergency fund

- Buy a new automobile or a second car
- Retire comfortably
- Make large contribution(s) to church, synagogue, etc.
- Obtain a down payment on a first home
- Fund a family member's college education
- Start a business
- Pay for a wedding
- Pay off student loans
- Return to undergraduate or graduate school
- Take a cruise
- Buy a boat or yacht
- Create a non-profit organization
- Purchase a vacation home
- Travel around the world
- Fund a charitable trust
- Save for a new baby
- Acquire residential or commercial rental property

GOAL-SETTING IS THE FOUNDATION OF SUCCESSFUL INVESTING

Numerous studies show that people who engage in active goal setting – i.e. thinking about their goals *and then writing or typing them out* – overwhelmingly fare better than people who don't set written goals. This is true in investing, and throughout life in general.

There's some science behind this, as well as some common sense. When you write down your goals, and especially when you look at them everyday, they serve as a constant reminder of what you want to achieve. A written mission keeps you focused. It gives you motivation. And perhaps most interestingly, declaring your objectives in black-and-white kicks your subconscious mind into high gear. Without you even trying, your brain starts thinking and strategizing about ways in which you can meet those goals — even while you're sleeping.

 Investors who don't bother to define any personal goals lack focus. They buy investments indiscriminately, under the false assumption that simply "being in the market" is somehow beneficial. In reality, such misdirected actions are highly harmful. They frequently result in wasted time, money and energy.

Individuals with hazy or generic goals (like "I want to be rich") are unable to reach them due to an unrealistic or unknown assessment about what it takes to get there. Remember when I said earlier that a lot of people express a general desire to "invest for the future?" Financial planners say that a common refrain among investors is: "I want to have a comfortable retirement."

What exactly does that mean? As you might suspect, it is highly subjective and individualized. For some people, having a "comfortable retirement" may mean making sure their 30-year mortgage is paid off. Others might view free-and-clear ownership of a home as low on the list of priorities. Also, what kind of money are we talking about to achieve "comfort," or *your* preferred quality of life in retirement? Will you require $2,500 or $5,000 monthly, $10,000 or perhaps some other amount? Determining these quality of life preferences are what leads us to the importance of setting the right kinds of goals: so-called SMART goals.

READY, SET, GOAL!

So far, you've figured out *why* you're investing, or why you *want* to invest: It's for retirement, that new boat or the 4,000-square-foot house you want to custom build. Whatever they are, your goals remind you that investing *isn't* about building wealth simply for wealth's sake. Investing should always begin as a goal-oriented process, helping you meet real-life needs and aspirations. As you can tell, goals are personal and values-based.

Still, you'll miss the mark if you stop here. You're far from done in the goal-setting department. Now that you've lumped your goals into short, medium and long-term time tables, you'll want to really hone in on several key points. Namely, you must establish specific, measurable and realistic goals; also known as SMART goals. SMART is an acronym that describes goals that are:

- **S**pecific
- **M**easurable
- **A**ctionable
- **R**ealistic
- **T**ime-Bound

Here is an example of a well-crafted SMART goal:

"I want to save $25,000 for a down-payment on a $250,000 4-bedroom, 2 ½ bath colonial home with a pool that I will buy three years from now."

This goal is **specific** – in terms of the dollar amount required, the cost of the house, as well as the type of home desired. It's **measurable**, because you can readily figure out how much you would have to save each year (roughly $8,009 assuming a modest 4% annual return) to come up with the $25,000 down payment. It's **actionable** because no amount of dreaming, wishing, or thinking alone will generate the money. You'll have to *do* something. That could mean making automatic deductions from your paycheck, reducing frivolous spending, or working a second job to meet the goal. Depending on your income, expenses, debts, etc., this may be a stretch goal. But if you earn $50,000 a year or more, this goal is nevertheless realistic. (Even if you don't earn $50,000+, this goal is **realistic** if you are prepared to make financial sacrifices. For instance, do you really need to eat out twice a week for dinner or to get 150 premium-cable channels in your home?). Finally, this goal can keep you on course because it has a definite **time** frame: three years.

SO HOW MUCH WILL THESE GOALS COST?

Ultimately, you will also need to figure out how much money it will take to meet your personal/financial goals. For many short and medium term goals, you probably have a pretty good idea of the costs, so you can just plug in the appropriate numbers. For example, the new car you want retails for $25,000, or you have $10,000 in credit card debt you'd like to get rid of – and sooner rather than later. But what about those far-away goals, like your retirement in 20 years?

There are scores of retirement calculators on the Internet that will quickly tell you, based on a series of assumptions, one of two things:

> 1. *The amount of money you will have accumulated at retirement* if you make "X" amount of annual contributions;
>
> **or**
>
> 2. *The amount of money you need to save annually* in order to accumulate "X" amount of funds at retirement

To illustrate how these calculators work, let's assume you are 40 years old, you wish to retire at age 65, and that you've already stashed away $50,000 in an Individual Retirement Account or 401(k) plan.

Example 1. If you put away $500 a month for retirement, how much money will you have accumulated at retirement in 25 years? The answer depends on how much you plug in as an expected rate of return. Use a figure between 7% and 10%, depending on how much risk you think you'd be willing to assume. Don't make the mistake of having an impractical (and/or improbable) outlook about your expected investment returns. (In other words, don't assume you'll rack up 25% annual returns. That's an unrealistic projection).

Based on our hypothetical savings of $50,000, and annual contributions of $6,000 ($500 a month times 12 months in a year), you will save $781,059 by retirement. That assumes you will generate 8% returns annually.

Example 2. What if you already know how much you want or need during your golden years? Let's say it's $1,000,000. The next step then is to figure out how much annual savings is necessary to help you reach your $1,000,000 goal. Again, based on the same set of assumptions: you have 25 years to retirement, $50,000 in current savings and you expect your investments will return 8% each year.

In this scenario, to wind up with $1,000,000 upon retirement, you must contribute $8,995 annually (or $750 a month) to your nest egg. Here are a handful of web sites with retirement calculators and useful worksheets that are more comprehensive, yet easy to use:

- www.smartmoney.com
- www.quicken.com
- www.money.cnn.com
- www.kiplinger.com

There are literally tens of thousands of sites out there you can utilize. In early 2003, I did a search on Yahoo! using the key words "retirement calculator." I came up with whopping 206,000 hits!

Many web-based calculators will walk you the through the primary assumptions that a financial planner would in helping you to figure out your expected retirement savings. But be sure to recognize the shortcomings of many calculators and what they can't offer.

- They can't help you figure out how much you can realistically afford to set aside given all your current obligations (mortgage/rent, car payments, credit card debt, utility bills, not to mention basics like food and transportation).

- Also, while most calculators take inflation into account, others don't.

- Some web sites offer general guidance about how your expenses in retirement may rise (such as higher travel and medical expenses) or fall (no more commuting costs or buying suits for the office). But others make no mention of that.

- Moreover, some retirement calculators fail to consider at all the impact of other money you may have coming. Besides your savings, your post-retirement income can be derived from sources such as Social Security benefits, trusts, annuities, pensions or an expected inheritance.

HOW A FINANCIAL PLANNER CAN HELP

This is where having a good financial planner can be of value. He or she won't just calculate the specific dollar amounts it will take to fund each of your goals. Based on a careful, tailored assessment of your personal situation – your individual risk tolerance, your health, the amount of money you have already saved, the funds you can continue to save regularly, and any other relevant information – that advisor can offer feedback on everything from how feasible your goals are to how you can best prioritize them.

Furthermore, after reviewing your entire portfolio, and evaluating the securities in which you'll be investing, an advisor can use historical investment averages as a benchmark for setting your targeted investing returns. If you get good service and an advisor who will act as your "financial quarterback," the fees you pay will probably be well worth it, especially if you are a procrastinator and the advisor can get you going with a workable financial plan.

Let's assume for now, however, that you're flying solo. (At least, you are while you're reading this book). Here's where your work begins.

Based on what you've just learned, **write out your top five personal goals**.

If you're feeling especially ambitious, list 10 of them. Note whether they are short-term, medium or long-range targets. Also, be sure to make them SMART goals; nothing generic or pie-in-the-sky.

_____

_____

_____

_____

_____

_____

_____

_____

_____

At this stage, if you've actually taken the time to _write down_ your goals (and I hope that you have!) you're ahead of 90% of the pack. Many people _think about_ and _say_ they want this or that goal. But relatively few individuals take the time to commit their words and goals to paper. For investors, that's a big mistake.

You *must* have detailed, written goals in order to direct your plan of action. Otherwise, you're not investing wisely. You're really just dreaming of getting rich.

And again, there's nothing wrong with dreaming per se. It's just that you've got to ground those dreams in reality. After all, you're not a kid anymore. You're a grown-up, right?

$UMMARY $UCCESS $TRATEGY

TO CONQUER INVESTING MISTAKE #1:

Set specific, measurable and realistic goals. Write out your unique dreams, such as saving a certain amount for your child's college tuition or retirement by a certain age. Goals help you remember that investing is done for a purpose.

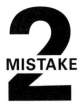

MISTAKE

INVESTING PREMATURELY

This chapter is probably going to "tick off" a lot of people in the brokerage industry. It may make a lot of you investors angry too – at least at first. Nevertheless, there is something that millions of investors need to know. And since your stockbroker probably won't tell you this, I will:

Many of you have absolutely no business being in the stock or bond markets right now.

That's right, I said you shouldn't be currently investing. Why on earth would I say that? Especially in a book that's telling you about investing. Simply put, a lot of you don't yet have your financial house in order. And investing at this stage is investing prematurely, probably to your long-term detriment.

Allow me to explain myself here.

As a financial journalist over the past decade, I've interviewed hundreds of people who have lost money in the financial markets. Some losses were relatively small. In other cases, the losses amounted to tens or hundreds of thousands of dollars. Needless to say, the financial hit these investors took hurt.

FINANCIAL WORRIES RUN DEEP

But there is another, less obvious – and often overlooked – cause behind these investors' dismay. A big reason investors have so much angst over their mistakes and losses in the financial markets is because they're also anxiety-ridden over their general lack of financial security.

Surveys consistently show that each New Year's holiday, one of the top resolutions for Americans (besides losing weight) is getting their personal finances in order. By and large, the average American's finances are in shambles – and most people know it, even if they don't quite know why they have financial problems.

To compound the situation, some investors (consciously or not) are mistakenly counting on their investments to "fix" a whole lot of things that have long been neglected in their lives: things like planning for their family's future and getting their debt under control. These investors erroneously think that as long as their portfolios keep growing, they'll somehow be financially prepared to handle any circumstance. So when that quarterly statement arrives in the mail, showing that they've lost money, these investors get panicky. Deep down they fear that their investments have gone awry – just like the rest of their financial lives.

While many of these individuals were busy reading the *Wall Street Journal*, analyzing stock charts, or pouring over mutual fund data, what they should've been doing is putting their energies into taking care of the basics of their personal finances.

I can sum up the financial basics in two words: Will DIED. Or maybe it's better put this way:

Will	Will and Testament
D	Debt
I	Insurance
E	Emergency Stash
D	Disability

GET A WILL WHILE YOU'VE GOT A LIFE

At some point, all of us will die. It's an obvious fact of life. But it's also a reality that most of us don't like to think about, much less *talk* about, or *act* on.

Remember September 11, 2001? Of course you do. Who can forget the attacks on the World Trade Center in New York, the Pentagon in Washington D.C. and the airplane passengers who overtook their hijackers before crashing in the mountains in Pennsylvania?

Of the thousands of people who died on Sept. 11th, many of them were young men and women in their 30s and 40s. Most left behind young children, spouses, or other loved ones. Unfortunately, what many of them *didn't* leave behind was a will: a simple legal document expressing their wishes and how they would like their personal and financial affairs to be handled upon their demise.

> Unfortunately, in today's world, people die prematurely from all kinds of dangers, accidents, diseases and other causes. That's one reason why having a will is critical.

HERE'S WHAT A WILL CAN DO:

- Provide for your loved ones by letting you determine when and what assets should go to various family members, friends or charities

- Allow you to designate a guardian to care for your minor children
- Avoid the time and expense of an unnecessarily lengthy probate. (A will must be probated, or proved valid by a court. With a well-prepared will, your estate can be settled much more quickly)
- Minimize the chances of family squabbling after your death, because you've clearly expressed your wishes
- Reduce the emotional turmoil your loved ones will experience, since at least there is a plan laid out

Despite these advantages, it's estimated that more than 70% of all Americans don't have a will. And yes, yes, yes, I know you're busy. Join the club. We've all got too much to do and not enough time to squeeze in everything. But answer this question: what is your priority? Is it handling your financial affairs or watching television? According to Nielsen Media Research, the average adult in the U.S. spends more than 4 hours a day watching television. Can you turn off the TV for just one week? No sports, news, soap operas or dramas. Spend that time instead thinking about and acting upon how to best leave your personal affairs.

When you do die, you'll be doing the people you leave behind a big favor if you've prepared your will. In the event of your death, they'll already have to deal with a big emotional blow. Don't compound their grief by burdening them with unnecessary worries over things like: Who would Sarah have wanted to take care of the kids? Or why didn't Dennis leave a will?

EXCESSIVE DEBT: THE ULTIMATE FINANCIAL DOOM

How much credit card debt are you carrying right now? Less than a thousand bucks? More than $3,000? Have you hit the $10,000 mark?

Take a look at the following statistics. They help explain why many people think Americans are in the midst of a credit-card frenzy.

The Debt Toll Rises ...

- The typical U.S. household has 13 cards, including bank, retail and debit cards
- The average credit card debt for those with a balance totals $8,940
- The average annual interest rate on credit cards issued nationwide is 14.7%

Source: Cardweb.com

Here are the two sides to this issue. On the one hand, critics say the credit card industry has kicked its marketing machine into massive overdrive when it comes to offering credit cards to consumers.

> According to the Consumer Federation of America (CFA), credit card issuers mail five billion solicitations annually. That works out to roughly 50 per U.S. household, which explains why you probably get at least one credit card offer each week.

"Credit card issuers are shamelessly escalating their marketing and available credit to stratospheric levels," says Travis Plunkett, CFA Legislative Director.

On the other hand, the credit card industry says it is simply making credit available to a public that desires to do everything from buying clothes, to renting automobiles and booking hotel rooms.

A WAY OUT OF DEBT

Here's my position: For better or worse, Americans have an unprecedented amount of debt. Only you know if your personal level of debt is a burden to you. If that is the case, then it's time you acted to do something about it.

If you're an investor carrying more debt than is comfortable, you may have wondered whether it is more prudent to invest first or pay off your credit card bills first. In most cases, the answer is a no-brainer: pay those credit card bills first.

A simple example illustrates why. Assume you have a $3,000 balance on your Visa card, which is costing you 14.7% in annual interest. And let's say you came into $3,000 – maybe a job bonus or a refund check from the IRS. Well, if you wanted to invest that money in the financial markets, you'd have to rack up a 14.7% return (after taxes) to match the effective return you could get from paying off your Visa credit card. Can you (or anyone else for that matter) *guarantee* a 14.7% return if you invest? Absolutely not. So if you're really serious about investing or wanting to invest (and I trust that you are since you've picked up this book), do yourself a favor and get that credit card debt in check first.

I know some of you are thinking one of two things:

1) If I wait until I pay off all my credit-card debt, it could take years!

or

2) I'm *already* investing, via my 401(k), IRA, or mutual funds, and there's NO WAY I'm going to stop investing until I pay off those blasted credit card bills!

In both cases, don't worry. In the second half of this chapter, I'm going to tell you how you can best handle your debt *in less than 30 days* – no matter what your situation. If you follow my advice, you'll be prepared to invest – and you won't make the mistake of investing prematurely.

INSURANCE

Let us revisit the issue of the Sept. 11th victims. Many of those killed worked on Wall Street. They were stockbrokers, traders, analysts, and so on. The irony is that these Wall Street professionals spent a huge amount of time and effort trying to make money – for others and themselves. Yet, lots of them neglected to make the one sure bet that would have brought financial security to their loved ones. By doing one simple thing, buying life insurance, in addition to playing the stock market, they could've provided far more long-term protection for their family members.

Learn a lesson from that tragedy: purchase life insurance coverage right away to provide for your family in the event of your death. Obtain a policy that would give your beneficiaries a payout that is at least five to seven times your annual salary. Depending on your personal situation, more may be advisable. (For example, if you have young children, you may want to make sure their college educations are paid for in the event of your death). Remember, life insurance isn't an investment per se. It's designed to replace your income and give financial stability to your family in your absence.

WHEN DOES $500 RESULT IN A $1,000,000 PAYOFF?

Before you say you can't afford to buy life insurance, realize this: for a healthy 40-year-old man who is a non-smoker, a 20-year term life insurance policy with a $1,000,000 benefit is well under $1,000, with policies in the $500 to $700 range being the most common. Isn't that kind of protection worth it? Therefore, take a fraction of the money you're committing to stocks or mutual funds and buy a good life insurance policy. Later on in this chapter, I'll tell you where you can find the right kind of life insurance policy at a cost you can afford.

EMERGENCY STASH

Did you know that in May 2003, some nine million people in the U.S. were unemployed? The national unemployment rate also rose to 6.1% - the highest jobless level since July 1994, according to the Labor Department. Anyone who has ever been downsized knows the stress and the financial challenges that a layoff can bring. If you've never been through a layoff, count yourself fortunate. But don't be fooled into thinking that it couldn't happen to you simply because your boss really likes you or your job performance has been excellent.

> Indulge me a moment here. Assume your boss came to you and said: "I'm sorry, but the economy is weak, our company's having hard times, and unfortunately, we're going to have to eliminate your position." What would you do? (I mean after you picked up your jaw).

How long would you be able to pay your mortgage or rent? Would you be able to keep up with those credit card payments … without having to use one card to pay off another? Think about all the luxuries you currently enjoy. How soon would you have to fire the gardener, eliminate trips to the hair or nail salon, forego restaurant dinners, or cut back on renting videos each weekend? If you've been investing, would you have to sell some of your investments to pay for your monthly living expenses? If so, that would lead to a nasty tax hit.

SET ASIDE THREE TO SIX MONTHS EXPENSES

To avoid cramping your current lifestyle and to minimize your stress in the event of a financial emergency, it's vitally important that you work towards building a three-to-six month cash cushion. This means that if your monthly expenses are $3,000, you should have an emergency stash of at least $9,000. A cushion of $18,000 is far better. Does saving three to six months of your expenses seem like a pipe dream that will take forever? If you continue reading the remainder of this chapter, I'll show you some smart ways you can very quickly get the emergency cushion you need – and prepare to invest wisely. Alternatively, you can make accumulating your cash cushion one of your short or medium range financial goals.

DISABILITY PROTECTION

I've already explained why you need life insurance – it's to provide for your family members after your death. But life insurance alone doesn't adequately protect your family. What if you somehow get injured? The fact is that your chances of being disabled during your working years is four to five times greater than your chances of dying during the same time period. In fact, in any given year, one out of 10 people will become seriously disabled.

Let's hope you're not one of those individuals whose badly injured in a car accident or some other such mishap and is unable to go to work. You don't want a disability to cost you your house, your lifestyle, or your savings and investments. The answer? Get a disability insurance policy as quickly as possible.

QUICK-FIX SOLUTIONS TO GET YOUR FINANCIAL HOUSE IN ORDER – AND PREPARE YOU TO INVEST

If you've been reading this chapter closely, you probably realize that I'm not saying you have to be 100% debt free, have a million dollar life insurance policy, purchase expensive disability coverage, etc. before you start to invest, or continue to invest your money. Instead, I'm simply saying take care of the basics. Get some kind of life insurance. Protect your income stream as best you can. Do a bit of financial planning before you venture into stocks, bonds, mutual funds and other investments.

Here's how anyone can quickly put their financial house in order – or at least patch it up sufficiently in order to invest with a much higher degree of financial security.

GET THE WILL TO DRAW UP A WILL

This is one area where you can't afford to procrastinate. To create a will, you basically have two options: retain a professional or do it on your own.

Option 1.

Call a lawyer, make an appointment to see him/her as soon as possible and get a will drafted immediately. Make that call today. Your family is depending on you.

Option 2.

If you're more of a do-it-yourselfer, or if you can't afford to hire an attorney, I recommend using a good software program that will walk you, step by step, through the process of creating your own will. These are a few helpful websites to aid you in this endeavor:

- www.nolo.com
- www.ezlegal.com
- www.standardlegalsoftware.com
- www.legalzoom.com

If you use a software program, I'd still recommend having an attorney who specializes in wills give your document a once-over. This review will be much cheaper than hiring the lawyer to actually create the will. But getting that feedback will give you peace of mind and the assurance that everything is done properly, as required by the laws in your particular state.

One caveat to all you procrastinators out there: Please don't do what I did. My husband and I prepared our wills– and then we took seven months to get the darned things notarized! The wills just sat up at our house, lacking witness signatures and a notary public's seal. Without these crucial final touches, our wills were invalid.

SLAY THE DEBT DRAGON

Here's how you can conquer your debt dilemma, and get ready to invest with the least amount of financial worry:

- If you've got the money, for goodness sakes go ahead and pay off at least some portion of your credit card debt. (I'm amazed at the number of financial planners who tell me that their clients have plenty of money sitting in the bank, but nevertheless have many thousands of dollars in high-interest credit card debt).

- What if you're cash poor but house rich? Then seriously consider taking out a home equity loan to convert your credit card and consumer debt into mortgage debt. (All that interest you're paying on charge cards, student loans, and/or automobiles is not tax deductible. But you can write off up to $100,000 annually in interest on mortgage debt, including a home equity loan).

- If you're short on cash, don't own a home or haven't got equity in your house, immediately call your credit card companies and ask for a lower interest rate. If you've been paying on time, you'd be surprised at how readily they will agree to a rate reduction. (They don't want to lose your business to the competition).

- If you find yourself able to only make minimum payments, cut up your credit cards or at least stop carrying them with you. Eliminate all future credit card spending for which you can't pay off the entire balance by the time the bill arrives.

- For those drowning in debt, and in need of expert help, consult a debt-counseling agency. Two reputable resources are *www.debtreliefclearinghouse.com* and *www.debtadvice.org.*

- Bottom line: Establish a realistic plan for aggressively paying off your debt. *As long as you stick with it*, **you won't be harming yourself by simultaneously investing and reducing your debt load.**

INVESTIGATE INSURANCE OPTIONS

- Find out if you have life insurance coverage from your employer. Verify the exact amount of your benefits. Companies that offer this perk typically give your heirs a lump sum payout based on your annual salary.

- Go see your human resources specialist or employee benefits administrator as soon as possible. Ask about whether you can increase your coverage on the job. Often, you can double your life insurance benefit amount – say, from 1 ½ times your salary to three times your salary – for a very modest deduction from your paycheck.

- Read up on the two kinds of life insurance: permanent and term. For most people, term is the best option and the most affordable. Go on the Internet to learn more about each. Then head to these web sites to comparison shop for the best available policies:

- www.insurance.com
- www.selectquote.com
- www.insure.com
- www.quickquote.com
- www.insweb.com

5 WAYS TO ESTABLISH AN EMERGENCY STASH

We've all heard it said that you should "save for a rainy day." Well, try telling that to someone who's barely able to pay all their *current* obligations, including utility bills, credit cards, car loans, housing, and so forth.

I know it can be a hardship to put money aside to prepare for the unexpected. For years, my husband and I struggled to do it. But now we save every month – automatically. And so can you. You can build your emergency stash little by little if you make your savings systematic, and if you truly commit to saving each and every month — no matter whether the roof starts leaking or the transmission goes out on your car.

Would you like to jump-start your plans to accumulate a cash cushion? Here are five easy ways:

1. **Sell stuff you don't need.** A yard sale featuring your unwanted electronics, clothing, furniture, household goods, computer equipment, art, etc. could net you a tidy sum to start your emergency fund.
2. **Cut out unnecessary spending.** Dispense with magazine subscriptions, cable television, daily lattes from Starbucks, etc. Divert the money you save into your emergency fund each month. **Shopaholics:** see my advice on page 40A.

3. **Slash your current monthly expenditures**. Most people pay more than they should for everything from long-distance telephone service to car leases simply because they don't take the time to shop around, according to Matt Coffin, CEO of Lowermybills.com. To see where you can cut your expenses, log onto *www.lowermybills.com*. Also log onto *www.capitaloneautofinance.com* to find out how to lower your monthly car payment by refinancing your auto loan.

4. **Get a second job** – even if only temporarily. Commit the extra funds solely to your emergency stash. Above all: make your savings automatic by having a fixed amount of funds transferred regularly from your paycheck(s) into your emergency fund. If you don't get the money in your hands, you're less likely to spend it. And chances are you won't miss it either.

5. **Secure a line of credit.** To develop an instant three to six month emergency reserve, obtain a personal line of credit. Rates vary from 6% to 14% depending on your credit history and the size of the credit line you establish. A better option for homeowners is to get a tax-deductible home equity line of credit. Most are currently under 6%. But caution: **Don't use the credit line for any reason other than a legitimate emergency.** The point is to have this credit line as your stand-by while you build up your personal savings. Having a credit line is also a good hedge against a job loss. If you ever get terminated, you already have the credit line at your disposal. But trying getting a credit line when you've lost your job, which is exactly when you'd need it, right? Well, be forewarned: Without a job, the bank loan officer will probably laugh you right out the door.

DISABILITY

Again, see the web sites listed above for insurance quotes. Additionally, look for these features in a disability policy:

- **Annual Inflation Rider** (Find a policy that pays additional benefits as the cost of living index rises)

- **Non-cancelability** (Get a policy that can't be canceled up to age 65, with the option to renew if you keep working)

- **Waiting period** (A one-to-six month period before your benefits begin is common. For the lowest priced coverage, pick the longest waiting period you think you could manage without financial aid, preferably 90 days or more for the best rates)

- **Definition of disability** (Select a policy that defines disability as an inability to work at your regular occupation)

If you are an individual who will diligently follow the advice in this chapter, congratulations. You're on the pathway to becoming a successful investor. You won't make the mistake that so many others do of investing before they're truly ready.

If you're a stockbroker or financial advisor, it may seem like heresy to turn away a client's money and tell that individual to first clean up his financial house. But think about it this way: When investment losses occur – and inevitably, they *will* occur – which client is more likely to phone your office completely stressed over the market, totally irate and practically demanding your head on a platter?

Client A: Whose investment portfolio just went down 10%, but she is debt-free, has a six-month cash cushion, adequate life insurance and disability coverage, as well as a carefully crafted will?

Or

Client B: Whose portfolio also went down 10%, but is struggling to make his credit card payments, has no savings to speak of, and lacks life insurance, disability protection and a written will?

You decide.

$UMMARY $UCCESS $TRATEGY

TO CONQUER INVESTING MISTAKE #2:

Handle some financial basics before investing. Pay down credit card debt, if you can. Draw up a will, get life and disability insurance coverage, and set aside a cash cushion of three to six months' expenses in case of an emergency.

THE SECRETS TO SHOPPING WELL AND LOOKING LIKE A MILLION BUCKS
(Without Spending A Small Fortune)

OK, so this part of the chapter is for all you serious shopaholics out there – gals and guys! But ladies, this information is particularly valuable to you if:

- You'd like to get your shopping habit under control; or
- You want to *look* like a million bucks – without having to actually *spend* that much.

For most of you, I'm guessing that you have plenty of bills to pay, not enough cash to go around, and you've made countless broken New Year's resolutions about managing your money more wisely. If this sounds like you, then *now is the perfect time* to get your act together! To save yourself big bucks, remember my Top 10 Rules for Money-Wise Shoppers. These are strategies that every true fashion aficionado knows (but will never tell):

1. NEVER PAY FULL RETAIL PRICE. EVER.

I'm not suggesting that you walk into Barneys, or even your local department store, and start haggling over prices. But any savvy fashion editor or stylist will tell you that nobody (in the know) pays the full asking price for anything these days.

Here are a few pointers:

- For starters, you can *wait until the item goes on sale* (trust me, it will!)
- *Shop sample sales* in major cities and get designer duds for a fraction of the retail price. These to-die-for sales usually happen after Fashion Week in New York, Los Angeles, London, Milan and Paris.
- *Buy classic styles off-season*. Great pieces look good season to season.
- *Hop online*. All of the following web sites sell designer merchandise both in and off-season: decadestwo.com (for vintage chic); yoox.com (for Italian designers); bluefly.com;

ebay.com (yes, ebay! It offers high-end designer clothes, including some that hit the Net before they're available nationally); overstock.com; and starwares.com (for celebrity duds).

- **Think Outlets, Outlets, Outlets.** The book *Buying Retail Is Stupid! The National Discount Guide to Buying Everything at up to 80% Off Retail*, written by Trisha King and Deborah Newmark, offers state-by-state listings of factory outlets. Last time I checked, this comprehensive, 396-page guide, could be bought on Amazon.com for just $2.55.

- Finally, *you can actually negotiate* in many boutiques and specialty stores. Don't be obnoxious about it. But when you find something you want, just sort of wrinkle your nose up a bit and, while holding the price tag, ever-so-nicely ask the sales person: "$75? Is that the best price you can offer me?"

2. DON'T SHOP ANOTHER DAY UNTIL YOU *ORGANIZE YOUR CLOSET FIRST.*

In your head, you may think you *need* another black skirt. But you probably just *want* one, because if you carefully go through your closet (that's right, sort out all those folded piles and even the stuff in bags and tucked away in the corners), you'll probably find that you have at least two or three – and likely even more – perfectly fine black skirts. So it's hard to justify buying yet another black skirt under these circumstances. By organizing your closet, you'll also be far less prone to making impulse purchases of other things you mistakenly believe you "need."

3. THINK LIKE A CELEBRITY.

When you see Halle Berry or Jennifer Lopez donning a gorgeous dress, wearing Harry Winston jewels, or even sporting a sexy pair of Jimmy Choo shoes, *realize that they rarely ever pay for clothes and accessories.* In fact, designers shower them with goods knowing that having these A-list celebrities wear their clothes will be good publicity and thus boost sales. The celebs themselves more often than not will wear the item once (if the designer is lucky).

But then that item gets donated to charity or tossed in the back of what I'm sure is the world's largest walk-in closet. In any event, consider this: Since multi-millionaire "superstars" aren't even paying to look like stars, why should you? If you keep in mind that a $1,000 dress you're pining away for is probably only realistically going to be worn by you just once (like the stars do), chances are you may be willing to forego splurging on that item if you can't really afford it.

Manolos And Mutual Funds

I'm not suggesting that you can't ever splurge. It's just that you have to be wise about it, and willing to exercise *some* restraint. So while you're *thinking* like your favorite celebrity, don't feel that you can't sometimes *dress* the part as well. After all, most of us would love to have a closet full of shoes like "Sex in the City's" Carrie Bradshaw, right? Well, you really don't have to choose between Manolos and mutual funds. Smart women can – and often do – have both. I know some of you may be thinking: "A pair of Manolo Blahnik shoes can cost upwards of $500. I don't have that kind of cash. But I really want them, so I'll just charge them." But please don't fall into the "debt trap." To get the red carpet looks that Hollywood actresses and New York models flaunt, find the best consignment store in the ritziest neighborhood you know. Go there and "recycle" your wares for cash. Use the money for mutual funds or, if you simply can't resist, those killer Manolos. With a little creative thinking and a willingness to splurge only occasionally, it is possible to keep that New Year's resolution about getting your finances together – without having to say goodbye to fashion.

4. TAKE A FRIEND SHOPPING.

And I don't mean your girlfriend whose Visa bill is constantly more than her rent. I'm talking about your level headed friend; the one who doesn't call you every other week to borrow money because her paycheck has run out. One suggestion though: don't drag along a pal (however well-intentioned) who simply can't have fun on your shopping quest. Instead, bring along your "I-know-how-to-enjoy-myself-too-but-I'm-not-going-to-squander my-rent-payment-to-do-it" buddy. What's the point of all this? A friend with a good head on her shoulders will keep you from making outlandish purchases and wasting your money. She'll make you accountable for your spending actions. And accountability counts.

5. ESTABLISH A PRE-SET LIMIT BEFORE YOU GO SHOPPING.

Just come up with a ballpark figure (say $500) and let that serve as your cap. Now here's where you get to *really* enjoy yourself – and not feel deprived. Mentally allow yourself the option of going 10% over your pre-set limit. So if you absolutely can't do without $50 worth of lingerie, but you've already reached your $500 limit, you can go ahead and make the purchase, and do so guilt-free. Any spending beyond that, though, and you're asking for trouble. This way, if you stick to your pre-set limit, you'll be patting yourself on the back. If you go as high as your spending-cap-plus-10%-limit, at least you've still stayed within the guidelines, without breaking the bank. Bonus: if you actually spend 10% under your limit, celebrate! One caveat: don't spend the 10% you saved (and then some) on an expensive dinner or some other one-time event. Instead, sock that money away into a "hands-off" savings account.

6. GO WHERE THE REAL BARGAINS ARE.

Serious fashionistas who can swing it go to London or Milan for fashion bargains. The cost of the airplane ticket can be well worth it if you pick up, say, Italian boots for $100 that you'd spend $450 for in the U.S. You'd obviously only use this strategy when you're planning to buy multiple items for which the savings alone would pay for the cost of your travel.

7. FREQUENT DISCOUNT RETAILERS.

Pick up the trendiest looks at stores like Target and H&M. Don't worry that the clothes didn't come from a so-called upscale retailer. Most times, no one will know the difference.

8. MAKE MENTAL COMPARISONS.

When you are tempted to plop down a big chunk of money for, say, a cashmere sweater (and yes, I know it's a beautiful one), ask yourself: is this *really* worth a full day's pay? For more expensive items, think: is this truly worth a week (or whatever time) of my labor?

9. DO SOMETHING RADICAL.

If you find yourself at the mall every week (or even every day), plan to make a radical change – if only temporarily. Make a vow to do ABSOLUTELY NO SHOPPING whatsoever for an entire month, or for whatever period of time you think you can stand it. You'd be surprised how much strength you can muster up if you put your mind to it. And while you're saving gobs of money in the process, you'll find other creative uses of your time – and cash.

10. GIVE AWAY SOMETHING.

Emulate your favorite celebrity and make a donation to a worthwhile cause. Surely you have something in the back of your closet, or packed away in the attic or basement, that you've not worn in a month of Sundays. Give it to a charity or a woman's shelter. There's truth in the saying: "What goes around, comes around." You give something to someone else in need, and your generosity will come back to you in some way. In other words: to get a blessing, first *be* a blessing!

INVESTING SUCCESS

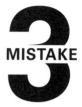

MISTAKE 3

OPERATING WITHOUT A PRUDENT ASSET ALLOCATION STRATEGY

If you set about to take a cross-country driving trip, chances are you would consider a map a "must have" item. Well, just as you'd no sooner drive from New Mexico to Maine without a roadmap, you also shouldn't put your investing program into high gear without the benefit of having an exact set of directions as to where you're going. Nevertheless, that's exactly what millions of investors do everyday when they invest without a clearly defined asset allocation strategy.

Recall briefly the investment goals I discussed in Chapter 1 of this book. Reflect especially on your own written goals. Those goals represent your final destination – or where you want to go. Your asset allocation strategy is the roadmap that guides you there.

After you take into consideration your current age, investment time-horizon, your ability to stomach risk, and your goals, you need to get down to the business of dividing fixed percentages of your money to stocks, bonds, and cash (and possibly other investments). That's what asset-allocation is. The idea is to build a portfolio where you establish target percentages (or percentage ranges) and invest money accordingly in differing asset classes. One big benefit to doing this is that you systematically diversify your investment holdings.

Over the past several decades, numerous hypothetical investment models have suggested the following recommended allocations, based on a person's age, risk appetite, and so on:

- Very aggressive portfolio: 100% stock funds
- Moderately aggressive portfolio: 70% stocks; 20% bonds; and 10% cash
- Moderate portfolio: 50% stocks; 35% bonds; 15% cash
- Conservative portfolio: 30% stocks; 50% bonds; 20% cash

But you should know that any formal statistical model is only as good as the specific assumptions that underlie it. Essentially, the makers of the models, and users of it, are assuming that certain investment trends will continue. The thinking goes something like this: "Well, historically, we know that stocks have returned roughly 10% over a 10-year cycle, fixed income investments have returned 6%, and so on."

Of course, statistical models are derived based on what happened in the past. No one can predict the future — so don't waste your time and money calling a psychic hotline to ask where the Dow will be next January! Still, asset allocation helps anchor your investing program. It's the right way – indeed it's the only sane way - to guide you through the investing process. Most accomplished investors will tell you in a heartbeat that it's impossible to pick winners and avoid losers year and year out. If you too want to become a savvy investor, take some time to craft an asset allocation plan.

Imagine that you are lost in a dark tunnel. Your only way out is with a flashlight. And in the midst of hearing bats, rats, and who knows what around you, you're thankful that your flashlight's batteries are working well. That flashlight is illuminating just enough of the tunnel ahead for you to walk through fairly confidently. Just as you have an end goal in sight for which you are investing (retirement, perhaps?), so too you have an objective here. Your goal is to make it safely to the tunnel's exit point. As you carefully make your way through the tunnel, you won't see every little jagged rock on the ground or every red ant crawling about that could potentially bite you. And truth be told, you don't need to see all those dangers. By and large, though, you will be able to make out the huge boulders to dodge, the big puddles of water you should walk around, and the walls that you must avoid running into. That flashlight will be critical to getting you to the light of day. As an investor, so will your asset allocation plan.

Having a well-prescribed asset allocation plan is crucial for several reasons. For starters, with a proper asset allocation plan, you will be less inclined to buy and sell based on emotions. An asset allocation plan also imposes discipline and consistency to your investing efforts. Additionally, an asset allocation plan reduces risk, since no investment category performs well all the time. And with a proper asset allocation strategy, when one category is faring poorly (say small cap growth stocks are out of favor), chances are another category you've also invested in (like large cap value stocks) are performing well.

This brings me to perhaps the single biggest argument in favor of asset allocation. Research shows that 90% of portfolio performance is determined by asset allocation. Take a minute and think about what that statement means.

It really boils down to this: In the final analysis, your ability to multiply your wealth by investing is not based on what individual stocks or bonds you buy. It's not governed by whether or not you have a high-priced fund manager. It's not dictated by whether you pour money into one sector versus another. Making money investing is chiefly determined by how well you divide up your money into different types of assets.

ASSET ALLOCATION GONE AWRY

Denis Walsh, president of Money Concepts, says one of the biggest mistakes he sees is people "buying investments that are far riskier than they realize." Walsh recalls, for instance, the height of the mania during the dot-com era. "I remember when we did asset allocation strategy for clients and they got angry because we didn't have enough in technology," he says, adding that some really irate clients left the firm.

No doubt those same clients were kicking themselves later when the tech meltdown occurred beginning in March 2000. Clearly, the absence of an asset allocation strategy leads to investors buying inappropriate investments, having portfolios that are improperly diversified, and under-performing the broader market.

DON'T FORGET REAL ESTATE

As you contemplate the best asset allocation for your individual needs, don't just think stocks, bonds and cash. If you have substantial assets to invest (roughly $250,000 to $500,000 or more), you'd be wise to also consider "alternative investments" such as gold, energy or other commodities. Even with far less money, many investors would be well served by diversifying with real estate. For those who want broad exposure to the real estate market, REITS, or real estate investment trusts are the best way to go.

Housing prices have skyrocketed in recent years and historically low interest rates have led millions of people to purchase their first homes or trade up to bigger ones. New home construction also remained strong in 2003, all of which led economists, Wall Street pundits, and others to debate whether or not a "bubble" existed in the housing market. If so, that "bubble" did little to dampen the performance of REITS, many of which continued to yield anywhere from 5% to 9%, thanks mostly to the hefty dividends they pay.

Perhaps best of all, REITS let you enjoy the benefits of owning residential or commercial property "without the hassles of being a landlord" says Leo Wells, head of the Wells Real Estate Investment Trust in Atlanta, and one of the best known and most widely-respected experts in the industry.

SOME SIMPLE RULES DON'T WORK

If you're unsure as to whether your portfolio should be aggressive, moderate or conservative (or some variation thereof), it will be money well spent to have a consultation with an investment advisor who can walk you through the process of determining what's right for you. You can also visit the plethora of investing web sites that allow you to take "money personality" tests and so on. These sites often also feature specific areas designed to assess your risk tolerance and asset allocation needs. That will give you some big-picture guidance.

What you shouldn't make the mistake of doing is using someone else's asset allocation strategy. What's best for your sister-in-law or your Uncle Tony isn't likely to be most appropriate for you.

You also shouldn't take this important strategic step and boil it down to an over-simplified method. Yet, that's what many investors have been told to do for years. They were advised to use the "Rule of 100."

For a multitude of reasons, I think you'd be smart to largely disregard the "Rule of 100." This outmoded rule asserts that people should subtract their age from 100 and use the final number as the percentage of assets to invest in stocks. Thus, a 40-year-old man using the Rule of 100 would invest 60% of his assets in stocks. The remaining 40% would be allocated to bonds and cash.

Here's why the rule of 100 doesn't make sense anymore (if it ever did). People are living longer than ever. Advances in healthcare and medicine, and improvements in technology mean that a person who is now age 65 can probably count on seeing age 85. Moreover, the 80-plus crowd is the fastest growing segment of the U.S. population.

Because of these factors, many financial planners say they won't even take on a client unless the person agrees to let the planner put together an investment strategy that goes out until the person reaches age 90 or even age 100.

In the past, people retired at age 65 and then lived maybe another seven to 17 years. But given modern demographic trends, the wise planner doesn't want his or her clients running out of money at age 82. (Besides, can you imagine the *guilt* those phone calls would trigger? Client: "You *promised* me I wouldn't run out of money, and here I am penniless, healthy as a horse, and *only* 89 years old!" Advisor: "Oh my goodness ... I'm so sorry! I didn't think you'd live *so long*!")

The wise planner wants his or her client to be gone long before the money runs out.

Interestingly, though, when financial planners talk to their clients about planning well into the future, many investors respond with all sorts of reasons about why they don't need to plan *too* far ahead.

Kathy Boyle, a veteran Certified Financial Planner™ practitioner in New York, and the head of Chapin Hill Advisors, has heard it all. She's had clients tell her everything from: "Oh, nobody in my family lives to age 100!" to "Cancer runs in my family."

It's as if forward-thinking advisors like Boyle are betting that their clients will live long and prosperous lives, yet some investors are betting that they'll die!

Take the smart odds: bet that you'll live to be very, very old and gray. And do yourself a favor by creating an investing strategy that assumes you'll be around for decades to come.

$UMMARY $UCCESS $TRATEGY
TO CONQUER INVESTING MISTAKE #3:

Create a prudent asset allocation strategy. Studies reveal that asset allocation determines 90% of portfolio performance. Assess what mix of stocks, bonds, cash or other investments such as real estate are most appropriate for you in light of your goals, time horizon, and risk tolerance.

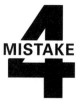

NOT INVESTING ON A CONSISTENT BASIS

Throughout this book, you'll read many accounts of investing moves gone awry. You'll also find a few stories that have nothing to do with investing per se. They do, however, offer practical guidance about how to conquer investing mistakes.

The first such story is a personal tale. It's about me.

IS THAT HOW I REALLY LOOK?!?

In early 2002, when I was a *Wall Street Journal* reporter for CNBC, I remember getting off the set after a long day's work, going into an editing booth, looking at a tape of myself and thinking: "I don't like the way I look. I look fat."

Sure, I'd heard that television adds 10 pounds to you. Still, I thought, I don't want to look *that* big on air! Seeing myself that way – through the unforgiving gaze of a television camera – was a big time eye-opener. At that point, I immediately resolved to lose weight – something that I'd never even given a thought to before.

For most of my life, I've known women who have battled obesity. I've also known waif-like women who dieted religiously and exercised like crazy. But I didn't fit in either camp. I wasn't fat and I wasn't skinny.

As a child, even though I was a bookworm, I'd been super active. I took ballet, tap and swimming lessons during grade school; I participated in sports and gym classes in junior high; and I was on the varsity track team in high school. As a college undergraduate at the University of California, Irvine, I played tennis only recreationally, but often enough to stay fit.

By the time I finished graduate school at the University of Southern California, however, my regular exercise was pretty much limited to walking up and down the steps to my Los Angeles apartment when I left and returned home each day.

WELCOME TO THE REAL WORLD OF DEADLINES

After graduate school, I entered "the real world," and started working as a journalist. After doing a stint as a reporter for the fast-paced Associated Press in L.A. – our motto there was "a deadline a minute" — I moved with my husband to Philadelphia. Though I maintained an impossibly hectic schedule – working at the *Philadelphia Inquirer* by day and at FOX-TV by night – large chunks of my days were spent sitting at a desk: on the telephone, doing interviews and writing news stories on a computer.

To make a long story short, my sedentary patterns started catching up with me. And my weight started mushrooming. I later had my first child, my daughter, just before I turned 30. And two-and-a-half years later, I gave birth to my son.

I reveal all this to explain that by the time I sat in that CNBC editing booth viewing myself on tape, truth be told, I *was* overweight. I just hadn't been paying attention.

But I was wearing a size 14 or 16 (depending on the clothing designer). I had not exercised in years. I rarely drank water, let alone the eight daily glasses recommended by doctors. And I was practically living on candy bars and vending machine food – despite the fact that I'm a vegetarian.

So what happened?

Simply put, I made a decision. At age 33, I resolved to lose weight to look better on television. (Yes, I admit that vanity was the driving force for my decision! But my secondary motives were to have more energy to play with my kids, and to not feel so sluggish and drained all the time).

Here's what I did.

I went to see a nutritionist. I read about seven or eight books on diet and exercise. I constructed a written plan. Then, starting in mid-April 2002, I got busy. And I mean ridiculously busy.

I worked out every day. I lifted weights. I cross-trained. I ran relentlessly on a treadmill in my house. (Sometimes, my husband actually had to tell me to give it a rest and let my body recuperate, because I'd want to work out in the morning and at night!)

All the while, I kept copious notes and charts of my progress. I also watched every thing that went into my mouth. I cut back drastically on carbohydrates, and (most excruciatingly!), I swore off sweets. For four months straight I did not eat any "treats." Not a single chip or even one bite of cake.

Can you guess what happened?

It probably won't surprise you to learn that I did indeed lose weight … 28 pounds to be exact. (My goal was 30 pounds. Truthfully, though, I don't know if I ever hit that target because when my perfectly adorable daughter – who was then four years old – started asking if she could weigh herself, I put the scale away; and haven't been back on one since).

I got down to a size 8 and was thrilled.

A year later, by the time I did my last report on CNBC in March 2003, I'm proud to say, I was still a size 8.

Friends, colleagues and viewers all noticed the change. Many people asked: how did you do it? I told them the key was just *deciding* to lose the weight, and then being *consistent* in executing my weight-loss strategy.

But can you imagine what would've happened if I'd worked out only sporadically? Or just quit exercising altogether after the first month? I can guarantee you that I wouldn't have had such drastic results in such a short period of time.

You know without a doubt that it would be foolish for someone to exercise once or twice a year in hopes of losing 20 or 30 pounds. Consistent, regular exercise is what would be required, among other things.

The same principle holds true for getting optimal investing results. Just like I couldn't get the body of my dreams without regular workouts, you can't realistically expect the portfolio of your dreams if you're investing only sporadically.

Nevertheless, scores of investors don't invest on a regular basis. They make the mistake of investing only when they have "extra" money. Some people falsely believe they need to have big sums of cash to invest, so they never get around to investing at all. Other individuals invest only sizeable figures on a yearly basis – using annual bonuses received from their employer or tax refunds they get from Uncle Sam. (By the way, I'm not suggesting that you shouldn't invest that IRS refund check or your year-end bonus. I'm merely pointing out that to invest with better results, it shouldn't be a once-a-year event. While we're on the subject, though, if you do get a big cash windfall, research shows that you're probably better off committing that money to the markets bit by bit, instead of in one lump sum).

There's another way that people exercise poor judgment in investing. Some investors flock to stocks or bonds only when they hear or read that the market is (or already has) moved upward. They want "confirmation" that the market or the overall economy is "strong" before they're willing to risk their money. Do any of these scenarios describe you – or anyone you know?

The problem with this approach is that when people fail to invest on a regular basis, they develop a haphazard approach to investing. They are inconsistent in their buying patterns and use a hodgepodge of criteria to determine "the best time to buy." They also become complacent about using proper investment strategies and they lack discipline. And finally, individuals who invest on a sporadic basis don't get the full benefits of compounded interest working in their favor.

I can't emphasize enough the financial harm that you do yourself long term by waiting to invest and not taking advantage of the power of compounded interest. To illustrate this point, assume you are 25 years old and plan to retire at age 65. If you socked away $3,000 a year for 10 years and earned 8% on your money, by the time you retired, you would have $510,090. Bottom line: your total investment of $30,000 gets multiplied 17 times. Pretty good, right?

Take a look though at what would happen if you waited 10 years to invest. In this scenario, you would start putting away $3,000 a year at age 35. And like most people who come late to the investing arena, you'd probably feel like you had to "catch up," correct? So let's assume that instead of investing $3,000 a year for just 10 years, as was the case in the first example, now you're going to invest $3,000 *every* year until you retire. The result is that you put away a total of $93,000 over the course of 31 years.

So how large does your pot of money grow? You wind up with $399,641 upon retirement. That's just over four times your total investment. Not terrible. But it's nowhere near as healthy a nest egg as you'd have if you simply started saving and investing earlier.

In the first instance, you end up with roughly $110,000 more at retirement. You also make annual contributions for only 10 years, as opposed to three decades. So you don't have to work as hard. On the contrary, your money is working hard for you.

When you invest regularly and consistently (now — as opposed to later!) it's like being in a 26-mile marathon, except you get to start at mile 10. That's

> the power of compounded interest. It gives you a
> huge head start so you can finish the race strong,
> even though you're not working as hard at the end.

As the saying goes: "successful investing is about time invested in the market, and not timing the market."

To remedy the error of investing on an inconsistent basis, or to avoid it if you're new to investing, plan to invest every month — or at the very least invest quarterly. Set up investment accounts that are linked to your employer's payroll system or to your bank accounts. Make investing automatic so that you don't fall into the trap of halting your investment regimen amid periods of heightened market volatility.

A systematic investment program also keeps you investing during those months where you could use some extra cash and might be tempted to forego putting money aside. (Admit it: If you don't have an automatic savings/investment plan, it's awfully easy to say something like: "Gee, I really need a new camera for our vacation; I'll just buy one using the money I was going to invest.")

And take some comfort from people who have long had money automatically withdrawn from their checking or savings accounts: most of them say they no longer even miss the money.

In a rising market, another benefit to investing with regularity is that you get to "dollar cost average." In dollar cost averaging, you commit a specific amount of money at fixed intervals – regardless of what the market is doing. In a bull market, dollar cost averaging works to your benefit because it allows you to buy more shares at a lower average price over time. This is accomplished because you are "buying on the dips," or when prices fall, as well as when prices rise.

In a bear market, though, where a persistent downturn is occurring, some stock market experts liken dollar cost averaging to throwing good money after bad.

And should you think about selling during such a downturn, be prepared for your financial advisors to try to talk you out of doing so.

In his book "Crash Profits," best-selling author Martin Weiss, who also heads Weiss Ratings Inc. in Palm Beach Gardens, Fla., suggests that stockbrokers will give you a slew of reasons as to why you shouldn't sell in a falling market. These brokers' advice ranges from "tough it out" and "hang in there" to "Don't be a fool and sell at the bottom," according to Weiss.

> All of this raises the question: should you invest regularly even in a down market? The answer is unequivocally yes. Here's why; later I'll tell you how. When you continue to invest through all market cycles you develop discipline. In fact, discipline gets imposed on your investing program even if your emotions start to creep to the surface.
>
> Also, you don't want to get in the bad habit of halting your investment activities every time the market hits a rough patch. If you do that, you're really just trying to time the market ... and how clear is your crystal ball?

Moreover, just because the broader market averages may be headed south, that doesn't mean your portfolio also has to go down. You can invest in ultra safe instruments, such as Treasury bills and other government securities. Weiss also recommends that you consider reverse index funds. They do the exact opposite of what the index they're benchmarking is doing. So if the S&P 500 Index falls 10%, an S&P 500-linked reverse index fund will rise by 10%.

You can also lighten-up on stocks and put more money in the cash markets. Better to remain a saver, and eke out even a modest return on your money, than to not put aside any money at all.

And in case you find this last bit of advice less than appealing, just remember that you're not alone if you are cautious about the equity markets, but continue to invest elsewhere. Even billionaire Warren Buffett, in his letter to shareholders released in 2003, said he was steering clear of stocks for a while because he saw limited upside potential. In discussing his recent performance, Buffett admitted that during "the last few years...my investment record was dismal." Buffett also said: "We love owning common stocks – if they can be purchased at attractive prices. In my 61 years of investing, 50 or so years have offered that kind of opportunity. There will be years like that again. Unless, however, we see a very high probability of at least 10% pre-tax returns (which translate to 6 ½-7% after corporate tax), we will sit on the sidelines. With short-term money returning less than 1% after-tax, sitting it out is no fun. But occasionally successful investing requires inactivity."

I doubt if many people would suggest that Buffett, who is clearly one of the world's greatest investors, is trying to "time the market." Rather, he's being savvy about where he puts capital – and in his case, it's very sizeable capital - at risk.

LABEL YOUR MOVING BOXES

To further increase your investing efficiency, earmark the funds you set aside as you invest regularly. So if you're saving an aggregate of $600 a month, that total shouldn't be thrown into one account and simply thought of as "investments."

Instead, you should clearly separate and label each account. If $100 is for your 10-year-old son's college education fund, have that money distinguished from your $300 a month retirement fund and your $200 a month account for the vacation you're planning two years from now.

Doesn't that make sense? After all, you label other things – from moving boxes to the seasonings in your kitchen spice rack.

Speaking of boxes, suppose you were about to move into a

nice big home. You'd spend a week or two packing up boxes with all kinds of stuff you've accumulated over the years – furniture, books, clothing, and so on. Now picture this scenario: the movers have come to haul away all those boxes, when suddenly you look down and realize that none of the moving boxes have been labeled. Yikes! You don't know which boxes are holding what. Is the china set in this box or that one? Where are your toothbrush, soap and other toiletries?

> Well, just as identifying your moving boxes allows you to readily visualize your household goods, "labeling" your financial accounts allows you to clearly "see" your investment goods. When you earmark funds – say, by specifying $250 a month for a new car in three years – you can also quickly and accurately measure your investment progress and determine whether or not you've met your designated goals.

There's another benefit to this strategy. If you or your movers came across a box labeled "spoons and forks," it would be obvious that the box should go into the kitchen, right? Similarly, labeling your investment accounts tells you where to put those funds.

And don't think it doesn't matter where you put your money, as long as it's invested somewhere. Nothing could be further from the truth. Financial planners say many investors who lump all their investments together frequently put the "right" securities into the "wrong" investment vehicle.

What do I mean by this? A perfect example of this is putting municipal bonds into Individual Retirement Accounts and 401(k) plans. IRAs and 401(k) plans are already tax-advantaged accounts. So if you place tax-exempt municipal bonds into those retirement accounts, you're not reaping the tax benefit of owning these tax-free bonds. In fact, you're converting tax-free income into taxable income because you'll later have to pay taxes on withdrawals from those retirement accounts.

Again, you might have the right investment – but be certain not to put it into the wrong account. It's kind of like having mislabeled the moving boxes, to take the previous analogy one step further. Wouldn't it be difficult (and frustrating) unpacking if you were in the kitchen surrounded by boxes that said "spoons and forks" and "pots and pans," but inside all the boxes there were really books for your home office and linens for the bathroom?

A PLAN BASED ON YOUR NEEDS

Raymond Lucia, a CFP® practitioner in San Diego California, has devised a unique method for having his clients "label" their money. His strategy is called "Buckets of Money™." Lucia, who wrote the book *Buckets of Money: How To Retire In Comfort And Safety*, suggests that you simply match your assets to your liabilities – creating "Buckets of Money™" to meet various needs.

"Buckets of Money doesn't involve some high-wire act like futures trading, currency arbitrage, penny stocks, or dealing in distressed real estate," Lucia writes. "You don't have to predict the future and you won't need to raise chinchillas, plant jojobas or be atop the crest of some so-called technological wave of the future. All you need to do is know your financial goals, divvy up your money accordingly, and then invest intelligently."

With the "Buckets of Money™" system, you purchase short-term assets, such as CDs and Treasury Bills and put them in "Bucket No. 1." That way you generate income for today.

Lucia recommends that you buy bonds and certain kinds of annuities to hold in "Bucket No. 2" if you desire inflation-indexed income "tomorrow."

Finally, he suggests that you acquire stocks and real estate in "Bucket No. 3" in order to achieve growth over the long-term.

Lucia reports that some 2,000 clients of his are now "bucketeers" – people who have "bucketized" their investments and reduced their portfolio risk as well.

$UMMARY $UCCESS $TRATEGY
TO CONQUER INVESTING MISTAKE #4:
Invest regularly with an automatic savings plan. Don't try to time market highs and lows. Commit to investing a fixed sum of money each and every month. Also, "label" your investment accounts to track your progress and know which funds should go where.

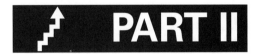

PART II

BUYING BLUNDERS

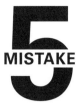

MISTAKE

PURCHASING INVESTMENTS WITHOUT HAVING PRE-SET BUYING CRITERIA

In the first section of this book, I walked you through some costly strategizing mistakes that ensnare investors. The next several chapters will discuss the buying goofs that all of us have made.

So let's start with a question: how do you currently decide which stocks, bonds or mutual funds are most appropriate for you?

Do you leave that to your spouse to decide?

Do you let your broker or financial advisor make the selections? Or maybe you actually research an industry extensively, and then pick what you think are the best companies in that sector?

Whatever investment-selection method you're using, I can guarantee you this: if you don't have established buying criteria, your investment strategy is off kilter.

Even if you've been successful at picking good investments in the past, invariably, at some point, not having specific buying criteria will come back to haunt you — for any number of reasons.

> Investors who fail to establish buying criteria inevitably end up purchasing the wrong investments. They are often unduly influenced by what others do or say. They're also more likely to duplicate their

investments, have an incorrect asset allocation mix, and suffer financial losses. Finally, investors who don't know why they should (or shouldn't) purchase a given investment have a much harder time later determining when to sell that investment.

Purchasing investments without some established buying criteria is akin to going shopping without a grocery list. If you didn't check the refrigerator and the pantry before you left the house, how do you know what you really need? Chances are you'll buy whatever looks good, or whatever you think is running low.

So there you are, pushing your cart down the aisle, and shopping without a grocery list. You see some item – maybe it's bread, eggs, or ketchup. Suddenly, you think: "Hmmm. Do we need more ketchup? Did we run out?" You go ahead and buy a bottle "just to be on the safe side." But then when you get home you find that you did, in fact, already have a container of ketchup – a full bottle no less.

The same type of foul up can happen with your investments. Without buying criteria, you can inadvertently duplicate your investments. You load up on things – such as small cap stocks – because you haven't checked your portfolio and you don't realize that you already own plenty of small-cap securities.

To avoid or fix this misstep, you must first know what you need – which begins with your asset allocation strategy. Remember the guidelines offered in Chapter 3 – with regards to selecting the right mix of stocks, bonds, cash and other securities? Once you have your overall investment roadmap set, you can drill down to the particulars: Namely you want to set criteria for buying stocks, bonds, mutual funds or other assets. In other words, what minimum set of hurdles must a company overcome to be considered worthy of your investing dollars? The idea is to establish some basic pre-requisites to weed out companies that don't fit your investing needs.

GENERAL STOCK-PICKING GUIDELINES

For starters, if you're evaluating individual stocks, start by analyzing the company's track record, history of generating revenues and profits, as well as its management expertise. For equities, also take into consideration a stock's price-to-earnings ratio and the health of the industry in which it operates. You should also be clear about the firm's competitive position. Is it the dominant force in the industry? Or is a small player going up against a number of much bigger rivals? All these factors, and more, will be important in helping you select investments that are in keeping with your overall asset allocation strategy.

And by the way, if some of these concepts are foreign to you, you're not alone. Nobody teaches you this stuff in school. In fact, Denis Walsh, of Money Concepts, says the lack of financial education in the U.S. is stunning. "It's shocking to me that you can get a degree, an advanced degree, and not know the first thing about how to manage money, let alone the difference between a small cap fund and a large cap fund."

To help investors, the National Association of Investors Corp. advocates the use of its Stock Selection Guide. The NAIC is an association of investment clubs. Its membership tops 600,000 investors who care – rightfully so – about investment education. NAIC members are encouraged to utilize research from Value Line in concert with the Stock Selection Guide. Even if you don't belong to an investment club, Value Line's independent research is highly valuable. (See more information on the topic of independent research in Chapter 25).

FIXED-INCOME INTELLIGENCE

If you are buying a company's bonds, or fixed-income securities, make sure you know the firm's credit rating as measured by Moody's, Standard & Poors, Fitch, or Weiss Ratings. What do these ratings agencies say about how reliable the company has been in paying interest to bondholders? Has it skipped any interest payments? Although bonds are generally less risky than common stocks, realize that bonds still have credit, interest rate and inflation risk. To educate yourself about various classes of fixed-income securities, visit the Bond Market Association at *www.bondmarkets.com.*

MUTUAL FUND BASICS

In evaluating which mutual funds to buy, you need to assess the fund's long-term track record. I would generally stay away from any fund that hasn't been around for at least five years; a 10-year history offers even better insights. You also should examine the fund's management. Who's running the fund you're considering? How long has that person been there and what's his or her philosophy? Additionally, how does the fund company go about selecting the companies in which it invests? Are securities selected by a single manager or does the fund use a "team" approach?

"I like seasoned managers," says stock-market expert Dan Strachman, the founder of Answers & Company. "Also, I don't care whether they pick Coke versus Pepsi. But I do care about the decision-making process they used to pick one or the other."

For mutual fund investments, you also need to think seriously about fees. Lipper Analytical Services is one company that tracks fund expense ratios. I'll discuss fees at length in Chapter 11. But for now, your primary consideration should be whether or not the fees the fund charges are reasonable or excessive. A good site for information is the Mutual Fund Education Alliance. Visit their web site at *www.mfea.com.*

QUANTITATIVE VS. QUALITATIVE RESEARCH

As you set your buying criteria, one decision you'll have to make is whether you want to rely on quantitative or qualitative analysis, or both. Quantitative, or technical analysis, refers to focusing on hard core numbers like sales, revenues, key barometers like price-to-earnings ratios, factors such as trend lines, and so forth.

For example, in 2003, the average S&P 500 stock traded at 32 times earnings – more than double the historical price/earnings multiple for stocks. If you are considering buying an S&P 500 stock and it's trading at only 14 times earnings, this data may give you insights into whether the company is reasonably valued.

Some say, though, that if you are a long-term investor you should rely not on quantitative measures, but on qualitative analysis. This simply means looking at the big picture. For instance, you might not know all the details about McDonald's market share, its average revenue per restaurant, and so on. But you may know, from a qualitative standpoint, that McDonald's is a fast food chain and that its brand name is recognized globally.

In this regard, qualitative analysis is more subjective. It's often easier to understand than quantitative inquiry. So if you aren't particularly technical, or if you don't have a lot of time, qualitative analysis may appeal to you.

$UMMARY $UCCESS $TRATEGY

TO CONQUER INVESTING MISTAKE #5:

Establish pre-set buying criteria before you purchase an investment. Pass on those investment ideas that don't fit your criteria. This will help limit unsuitable investments and guide you toward better-performing assets.

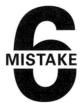

MISTAKE

RELYING ON TIPS AND "INSIDE" INFORMATION

Barbara Eng Nitzberg can still recall the first investment she ever made. It was back in 1989, and at her brother's urging she opened a Fidelity mutual fund account.

"I remember the check I wrote was the biggest I'd ever written," says Nitzberg, adding: "My hands were shaking."

By the mid-1990s, though "I'd become more knowledgeable and more comfortable with buying stock on my own," she says. But that also turned out to be the time she bought some of her biggest losers.

According to Nitzberg, who lives in New York, a big part of the problem was that she was getting – and acting on – bad advice. "I listened to people I knew, even if they didn't know what they were talking about."

Those friends and associates, however, were so gung-ho about various stocks that their enthusiasm was contagious.

"I tend to think it starts with a little dribble. Then all of a sudden everyone's talking about how wonderful this or that company is," Nitzberg says. "You get kind of caught up in that."

Nitzberg isn't alone.

Come on now. If we were forced to 'fess up, practically every investor would probably admit to having bought an investment – or at least having seriously contemplated doing so – just because a friend or someone we knew suggested it.

But this is almost always a bad idea.

> People who rely on "hot tips," pure instincts or so-called inside information often end up buying poor investments, and securities that don't meet their particular needs. Many times, these investments are also more speculative, volatile, and risky purchases. Thus, they more likely to cause investors to lose money.

It took Nitzberg awhile to realize that. But now she's glad she does her homework, and properly researches her investments.

"In the beginning, what I would consider looking at a company, was gathering company information. But I didn't know how to read a balance sheet. And I was too embarrassed to ask someone to teach me," she admits.

So instead she turned to companies' annual reports. But even there, she acknowledges, she didn't do a thorough job. "I'd read the nice part – the good glitzy part," of those fancy, colors reports. "Then I would go to two or three media sources and monitor" an investment before deciding whether to buy it.

These days, Nitzberg has a much better way of approaching investment opportunities. As a member of the New York chapter of the National Association of Investors Corp., she uses the NAIC Stock Selection Guide. "The Stock Selection Guide has given me a nice, standard, consistent way of evaluating whether something is a good prospect. Now I have a system," Nitzberg says. "It makes me feel more confident."

Among other things, the NAIC Stock Selection Guide lets you figure "the buy range" or the point at which you should consider purchasing a given stock. The Guide also aids you in determining whether a company is well managed. Finally, it helps you project sales growth and earnings per share for investments you are evaluating.

Nitzberg's story offers a valuable insight.

To put it bluntly: don't trust friends, relatives, colleagues, etc. to be your financial advisors. If they're not qualified experts, or if they haven't seriously investigated an investment, why should you seriously take their recommendations?

Taking a stock tip from a friend – even if it is a friend that you've known 20 years – is like trusting your barber when he says he can also install that new roof you need. What does he know about your roof – or any roof for that matter? You wouldn't want an inexperienced person fiddling around up there, because chances are you'd wind up with shoddy work. You'd want someone skilled and experienced to patch up that leaky roof.

The reality is that some things are best left to the experts. And I don't mean just financial services professionals. You too can be an expert – as long as you do your homework first.

Here's the best thing you can do when you get unsolicited advice from someone you think really doesn't know any more about an investment than you do. Nod your head politely, smile and let the information go in one ear and out the other. Now, if you think the person has good information, and presents you with some decent *facts* about why an investment might be a good opportunity, and you're interested, then take the time to do some research. There's no rule that says you have to buy today. Or that you have to run to the telephone phone and tell your stockbroker that you found a great new idea.

Take a breather. Evaluate the tip. And then see whether or not it's worth acting on.

And just like you shouldn't be so quick to follow a chum's recommendations, neither should you act on tips from strangers. And that's exactly what millions of people out in cyberspace are to you – strangers. Still, plenty of investors go into web site chat rooms and start to take advice from other participants. It's foolish because you have no way of knowing who is offering that advice. And even if they are qualified and credible, in how many cases will their mass-market prescriptions fit your individual needs?

THE RIGHT WAY TO USE THE 'NET

Having said all that, I'm not naïve enough to think that many of you won't turn to the Internet anyway. And, when done properly, that's actually a smart thing because the 'net is chock full of good information and educational tools for investors. In fact, Forrester Research predicts that by the year 2005, some 16 million U.S. households will get their first professional investment advice via automated online analysis. Another seven million households who use financial advisors will supplement that advice with advice from an online service, Forrester projects.

If you want to get online for information or advice, turn to a reputable site that specializes in this area. For instance, Financial Engines (*www.financialengines.com*) and mPower (*www.mPower.com*) are two well-known and trusted sources of retirement planning information.

Whatever you do, don't trust chat-room rumors, "inside" information from your broker or hearsay from your cousin Joe. Nothing other than smart, careful research should be enough to make you turn over your hard-earned money. You have to be willing to do the research yourself – or pay a professional to do it. When advisors suggest investments, make sure those recommendations are consistent with your overall strategy, risk tolerance and asset allocation plans.

When you research a company yourself, there are plenty of places where you can unearth information about a company's business prospects. A sampling of those resources: quarterly reports and other mandatory regulatory filings made with the SEC, annual reports and letters to shareholders, independent research and Wall Street research reports, and press releases from services such as PR Newswire and BusinessWire.

Another great resource to use is the Schwab Center for Investment Research. It consistently offers insights and information not found elsewhere. An example of these interesting tidbits: the Center found that for the two-month period from April until the end of May 2003, the S&P 500 gained nearly 14%. Schwab research suggested that similar returns were registered during a two-month period only 25 times since 1926, perhaps signaling a buying opportunity for investors.

Moreover, Charles Schwab & Co., Inc. gives some 3,000 publicly traded companies A, B, C, D, and F ratings. These grades give you an indication of what Schwab thinks of the companies based on four criteria: fundamentals, valuation, momentum, and risk.

Yet another online site worth examining is 3DstockCharts.com, which provides real-time charts of stock market buy and sell orders. The idea is to give investors a clear sense of what's happening in the market at any given time.

"Transparency and full disclosure are more important than ever," says John McNamara, CEO of 3DstockCharts.com

And again, while I don't suggest you spend your days glued to a computer screen, there is some valuable information to be gleaned here as well. For example, you can get real-time instant quotes. You can also see how many buy and sell orders are stacked up in a queue for a given stock. Perhaps chief among the highlights of

3DstockCharts.com's web site is that it has integrated data from all the major electronic communications networks, or ECNs: Island, Instinet, Archipelago, Redibook, Brut and the Bloomberg Tradebook. So you can instantly get from all the ECNs pre-market, regular, and after-market price changes.

INSIDER TRADING CRACKDOWN

What about getting tips from insiders who work at a company? Don't even think about it. First of all, if someone purports to know "inside" information about a company, what are the chances that you're the only person he's telling?

Besides, you don't really want engage in illegal insider trading anyway, do you? Federal securities regulators aren't taking such activities lightly, as evidenced by the prosecution of former ImClone Systems Inc. chairman and chief executive Samuel Waksal.

In June 2003, after being convicted of insider-trading, obstructing justice and dodging taxes, a U.S. District judge sentenced Waksal to seven years and three months in prison – the harshest penalty possible under federal guidelines. Waksal was also ordered to pay a $3 million fine, on top of an $800,000 settlement he'd made with the SEC to settle a civil lawsuit.

Not a fate worth risking, is it?

$UMMARY $UCCESS $TRATEGY
TO CONQUER INVESTING MISTAKE #6:

Thoroughly research an investment. Don't rely on other people's tips, idle recommendations, and so-called "inside" information.

CHASING THE LATEST HOT PERFORMERS

Going after the most recent investment "stars" causes investors to pay way too much money for what frequently turns out to be bad investments. In addition to risking market under-performance, investors who chase hot performers have difficulty selling if the investment turns sour because they're too concerned with "breaking even."

I can sum up this chapter in the following three paragraphs. But I'll go into more detail for those of you who really need convincing!

Here's the cliff notes version of this chapter: Don't flock to last year or last quarter's best-performing stock, bond, mutual fund or market index. Chances are, tons of other investors are too. Historically, investments on last year's "best performing" list wind up on this year's "worst performing" list. The Nasdaq Composite Index is a case in point. The technology-heavy Nasdaq rose roughly 86% in 1999. But in 2000, the index fell 39%.

Think about all the investors in Qualcomm Inc. who bought the stock near its peak. Many got caught up in the buying frenzy and investor excitement over this San Diego, Calif.-based maker of computer chips for mobile telephones. After watching Qualcomm zoom to $200 a share in early 2000, these investors spent small fortunes on the stock. Unfortunately, many also suffered losses of more than 50% when Qualcomm later came crashing back to earth.

Of course, Qualcomm wasn't the only such stock. Plenty of other companies watched their share prices travel the same upward trajectory – only to ultimately land at more realistic levels. In most cases, the stocks lost more than half their value.

But this is only really part of the story. Read on for more insights about the dangers of chasing returns – and how you can reverse this common investing faux pas.

DON'T GET TOO STARRY EYED

If you want to know about practically any one of the thousands of mutual funds out there, chances are Morningstar Inc. has detailed data on that fund – including its performance history, fees, the size of the fund, its investment objective and more.

But what Morningstar is best known for is its five-star rating system. In a nutshell, Morningstar assigns each fund it follows a rating of one to five stars. The rating is based on how well each fund performs compared to other mutual funds in the same category. Returns obviously matter, but so do fees and the level of risk associated with each fund, because Morningstar's rating system adjusts for both of those factors.

Having a top-rated fund from Morningstar gives a fund company or an investment firm major bragging rights. And when fund managers do climb into the top echelons of the Morningstar rankings, some companies spare no expense to let you know it. They take out full-page newspaper ads, they play up this information in quarterly mailings to shareholders, and they highlight their rankings in annual reports and prospectuses. Of course, they're very careful to include the disclaimer that "past performance is no predictor of future returns." Ironically, after all this blatant hooplah — which demonstrates the extent to which the Morningstar rankings are widely followed and highly coveted –- most Wall Street experts will turn around and tell you not to pay much attention to such rankings.

I'm going to give you exactly the opposite advice, with several caveats:

Do pay attention to the Morningstar rankings, but don't be a slave to them.

You should never use one fact – a Morningstar rating or any other single piece of information – as the entire basis for making a decision as to whether or not you invest, or stop investing, in a fund or stock. If investing is a puzzle (and indeed, it can sometimes be quite mystifying), then consider the Morningstar ratings one piece of the complex jigsaw you're working on. Also, don't invest in anything unless it meets your established buying criteria and you have properly researched the investment. So what if a fund has a five-star rating? If you already have a similar type fund and are achieving comparable returns, it's of little value to you.

Realize how the rankings affect *other* investors – and benefit from that.

The truth of the matter is that even though investors are warned over and over again not to chase performance, many people go out and do it anyway. Invariably what happens is that top-rated Morningstar funds will see big inflows of money because starry-eyed investors were wowed by a fund's five-star status.

What many of these investors don't realize – or are forgetting or betting against – is that historically, last year's star fund becomes this year's laggard. So by jumping into a fund after it's achieved five-star notoriety, you're coming late to the party.

Dan Strachman, the Answers & Company founder, bristles when clients are eager to jump into a given fund just because they saw that it just won a five-star rating from Morningstar. "I say: What do you care what it did last year? You didn't invest in it."

Strachman, who also wrote the book *Essential Stock-Picking Strategies*, adds that "the problem with a five-star mutual fund is that all the data show that a four-star fund manager performs better" right after the rankings are released. The reason? According to Strachman, these four-star managers are hungrier and more performance-oriented because they now want to rise a notch and achieve five-star status.

Since Wall Street pros are vying to be in those top fund spots and touting that information when they do make it there, I think it's unrealistic (and disingenuous by some) to simply tell investors: don't pay attention to fund rankings. Which leads me to another observation about this subject.

Here's one big reason why the Morningstar rankings are so influential. In a world of more than 20,000 stocks and funds, investors want and need a way to cut through the clutter. Otherwise, many people might not have any clue about where to begin in the face of so many investment options. For their part, top-performing funds and fund managers also need a way to stand out from the pack. To attract and keep investment dollars, they must show how they are better or different from the next offering. So, in effect, the Morningstar ratings serve as a universally accepted short-hand; a quick and easy way to segment funds into tiers. And we can all generally agree on what a five-star rating means, just like we all know what an "A" grade symbolizes in school.

Both are simple, easy-to-understand ways to classify and categorize – explicitly singling out the star performers – at least by one given set of criteria.

FINALLY, LOOK AT RETURNS IN A DIFFERENT WAY

One way to put a fund's performance statistics in proper perspective is to view any given fund as part of your overall portfolio. Moreover, you'll want to start focusing on absolute returns, instead of relative returns. This means you want to generate positive overall returns in your portfolio regardless of the relative yields among different asset classes.

Adopting a strategy that focuses on absolute returns isn't very common. Most mutual fund managers, instead of trying to make you money year in and year out, simply try to beat a given index. So say that manager is benchmarking his performance against the Wilshire 5000 Index. If the Wilshire drops by 8% in a given year, but the portfolio manager steers the fund to only a 4% loss, you can be sure that the typical fund company, rather than decry the loss of funds, will position the 4% downturn as a victory in a tough market.

If you're going to start looking at absolute returns, you have to accept the fact that you will sometimes have down investments. Remember, if you've diversified properly you didn't pick investments that would all move in tandem. In fact, they should not be highly correlated at all. That way, when your bonds are faring poorly, you can probably count on your stocks doing well, and vice versa. With this method, you won't worry about the latest, best fund; nor will you participate in every stock fund or sector run-up. But you will achieve greater overall returns than you would've by trying to pick a single stock in a universe of thousands and "hit a home-run" with that one stock.

I'd venture to say that many investors in stocks such as PMC Sierra and Nvidia weren't thinking about absolute returns when they bought into these companies in 2003. These investors were likely chasing returns. By mid-year, both stocks were up more than 100% — a surge some saw as a sign of pure speculation.

I know it seems counter-intuitive, but many successful investors say that it's precisely the time that others are fearful of being in the markets that savvy investors will find buying opportunities. Conversely, when most investors are in a feeding frenzy, smart investors take that as their cue to sit on the sidelines and be very selective about their investments.

Here's some advice from one investor who learned the hard way about chasing returns.

IN THEIR OWN WORDS:
INVESTORS SHARE LESSONS LEARNED

In younger years, I was a single gal earning a good six-figure income, working on Wall Street, living on top of the world, but clueless about investing. I devoured all of the investment advice that was available on the newsstands. I also didn't really understand why I was buying the stocks, bonds and mutual funds that my stockbroker was recommending, but obediently did what he instructed.

I thought that if I just bought the mutual fund that was at the head of the list that month, I couldn't lose. I would own this fund for several months or so when I realized it was nearer the bottom of the performers and another of the same mutual fund company's stock fund was now on top! Somehow, I always bought the wrong one at the wrong time.

What I know now is that I was buying a value fund *after* it had become a top performer and just before it was to become a bottom performer. Simultaneously, I was selling the growth fund to buy the value fund, as you now know, just before it went up! I was making one of the most common mistakes any novice makes.

The solution would have been to split my investment between the two funds and watch them slowly grow at different rates. Two steps forward, one back. Two steps forward, one back...

The biggest mistake was giving up on both funds, which are both still performing more than 10 years later. If I had known and kept both of them, this $10,000 would have been worth a lot more than the gold I invested it in! The funds would have been worth over $20,000 now and the gold is still worth less than $10,000.

I also know now that a good financial planner would have taken the time to explain all of this to me intelligently and I would have been better off for it. It's a mistake that I try to keep my own clients from making with their finances.

Mary-Jo P. Iacovino, AXA Financial Advisor
New York, NY

BEWARE OF PROMISES OF BLOCKBUSTER RETURNS

Sometimes, it's not just investors chasing returns of stocks and mutual funds that get them into trouble. Often times, investors seek out unrealistic returns elsewhere – only to get burned. Such was the case when a group of high net worth individuals handed over $900,000 to Eduardo McIntosh, a Boston area man later convicted of running an investment fraud scheme that cheated investors from all across the country.

In February 2003, McIntosh was sentenced to three years and one month in prison for taking investors' money, and promising them

40% returns on their money within one year, or five times their principal back within 10 days. Now what legitimate investment could "guarantee" such extraordinary returns? I certainly don't want to blame the victims here. But my point is that sometimes our desire to stretch for yield outweighs our common sense.

To test how much you know about investment scams, take the NASAA-CSA Investment Fraud Awareness Quiz at the end of this book.

$UMMARY $UCCESS $TRATEGY
TO CONQUER INVESTING MISTAKE #7:
Don't chase the latest hot performers. Last year's top funds are frequently this year's laggards. Better to look for investments with solid long-term track records.

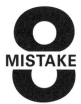

OVER-EXTENDING YOURSELF
WITH MARGIN

Have you ever been in a retail store and wanted a new suit, a dining room set, or anything else you couldn't afford right then and there? For many of you, chances are that didn't stop you. You probably whipped out a credit card and paid with plastic, correct? In this case, what you really did was borrow money – maybe at 14% or so - in order to take immediate possession of whatever you wanted.

Well, in the investment world, the same thing is possible. You can borrow money in order to buy stock. It's called buying on margin.

Here's how it works.

Normally, when you buy stock you pay for that investment in full. But let's say you establish a margin account, and now you want to buy $10,000 worth of stock. Instead of having to come up with the entire $10,000, you could maybe raise $5,000 of your own cash, and borrow $5,000 from the firm where you created a margin account.

Investment banks and brokerages are willing to lend you the money to buy stock because they have collateral: the stock you purchase on margin, other assets in your margin account, and other funds you have on deposit with the firm.

Bingo! You're able to buy more and different investments without having to fork over as much cash. Sounds fine, so far, right?

The problem is that some investors unwisely "over-extend" themselves through the excessive use of "margin."

Investors that are highly leveraged, due to too much margin, face a potentially crippling fate. If their investments or the overall market suffers a downturn, they could receive a "margin call" in which their broker sells securities in their portfolio or demands that they put additional cash into their accounts.

Unfortunately, many investors open margin accounts without fully understanding all the terms, ramifications and possible dangers involved.

Broadly speaking, here are some things you should know about margin accounts.

- **You can lose more funds than you deposit in the account.** If the value of the securities you purchase on margin fall below certain levels, your broker can ask you to provide additional funds to avoid the sale of your securities.

- **Your broker can sell securities without contacting you**. Don't believe, as some investors erroneously do, that your broker has to first telephone, mail or otherwise notify you about a margin call. The truth is that no such notification is required for a margin call to be valid. Now in practice, most firms will indeed try to contact you before they sell stock in your portfolio, but they don't have to. Besides, even if the broker does contact you, and you agree to meet a margin call by a certain date, the broker can still do whatever he deems fit to protect the firm's financial position, including selling your securities without notice to you.

- **You don't have the right to pick which securities in your account(s) should be sold in the event of a margin call.** Since those securities are collateral for the margin loan, your brokerage firm can legally decide which security to sell in order to safeguard its interests. This can be devastating if your broker sells some stock that you absolutely did not want sold, because of tax reasons or anything else.

Given these realities, here are some ways you can use margin wisely.

First, if possible, don't use margin at all. Again, think of the credit card analogy. If you're in a store and you have the cash, isn't it better to pay that way, than to incur interest and finance charges?

Second, know the rules that govern your margin account. In addition to certain requirements imposed by NASD Regulation, all brokerage houses have their own particular stipulations about their margin accounts.

Third, don't get over-leveraged. Do a "worst case scenario" calculation and determine a pre-set amount for maximum borrowing. Stick to this limit no matter how enticing the next investment opportunity appears.

In the best of all cases, you would never use margin if you didn't have the cash to buy stock. Does this seem contrary to the earlier advice I gave? Actually, it's not. What I mean here is that ideally, you'd only use margin if you have the money, but would prefer to deploy it elsewhere – to reap higher investment returns.

MARGIN MAYHEM THIS MILENNIUM

After the technology sell-off in 2000 and early 2001, investors nationwide suffered margin calls. Some who were especially hard hit had to sell stock from other accounts – thereby triggering unwanted taxes–in order to meet brokerage demands for payment.

Some of these investors were really just borrowing money to pay for stocks they couldn't afford – overvalued dot-coms priced at upwards of $100 a share.

And plenty of these investors found out another fact they didn't know about margin: that you are not entitled to an extension of time on a margin call. Sure, under certain circumstances, your broker may give you time to come up with the money to meet a margin call. But he's not obligated to do so.

To be as conservative as possible, remember to think about margin as kind of the equivalent of using your credit card to buy stocks. After all, credit is merely borrowed money. So you'd better use it wisely. And anyone who's dealt with credit card debt knows that it's all-too-easy to view that plastic almost as free money – at least until that shocker of a bill comes.

While some people might object, it's really not a stretch to compare margin to credit card usage. In fact, at some brokerage firms, if your account has a credit card or checks, you may also *create* a margin debit if your withdrawals (from checks, pre-authorized debits, or credit cards) exceed the sum of any available free credit balances plus your cash deposits on hand.

Another reason you should avoid excessive use of margin is that it may not just cost you money, it'll also cost you time. When you buy stocks on margin, you frequently have to spend a heck of a lot more time following your positions, monitoring your portfolio, and checking out the ups and downs of the stocks you own. Do you really want to spend your time that way?

$UMMARY $UCCESS $TRATEGY

TO CONQUER INVESTING MISTAKE #8:

Use margin wisely. Don't borrow money to buy stocks or other investments without carefully understanding the risks involved. And don't over-extend yourself by investing more money than you can realistically afford.

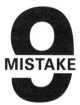

HAVING CONCENTRATED WEALTH

Do you know what investments are in your retirement plan at work?

If you're like most people, you may own a big chunk of your company's stock in your 401(k) plan. You may not realize it, but you may also have created what's known in the financial services industry as "concentrated wealth."

Concentrated wealth refers to a scenario where an investor has far too much of his or her assets tied up in a single investment. The ill effects of having concentrated wealth are many: a lack of diversification, heightened portfolio risk, and market under-performance. Even after the high-profile blow-ups at Enron and WorldCom, where employee-investors lost billions of dollars, people still tie up too much of their money in one stock.

Workers at WorldCom saw the value of the company stock in their 401(k) plans dwindle to a mere $18 million in July 2002 from $1.1 billion in April 1999. Employees at Enron also lost a fortune. At Enron, 58% of plan assets were in company stock. That was like betting the house at the racetracks – far too risky for any prudent investor.

Of course, not everyone develops concentrated wealth simply by buying a truckload of stock in one company. If you have much of your net worth tied up in a single business, it could be that you inherited stock, you may have founded a business, or perhaps you amassed or were granted stock from your employer over time. However it happened, if you have a great deal of money invested in one company, you should remedy the situation immediately.

 How much is "too much" invested in any one security? Most financial planners say putting 10% or more of your assets in a single company is courting danger. Others use a 25% threshold.

This single-stock phenomenon is apparently quite common. The Employee Benefits Research Institute says that company stock represents anywhere from 22% to 33% of the average holdings for people with 401(k) plans. Those numbers jibe with what other researchers have found. The Institute of Management and Administration's latest study of stock plans found that 27.9% of 401(k) plan stocks are invested in employer stock. And according to Boston Research Group, about 30% of 401(k) assets are in employer stock, and about 50% of those interviewed said they considered that stock riskier than money market funds.

Thus, even though investors know that pouring so much money into a single stock is risky busy, they nevertheless have not changed their behavior. And the consequences of this behavior – whether based on habit, denial, optimism or whatever – could be severe. "One of the biggest problems I have is to try and get people to understand and mitigate risk," says Ivan Gefen, a senior vice president with vFinance in Boca Raton, FL.

Professor Lisa Meulbroke, of the Harvard Business School, found that holding an individual stock is four to five times riskier than owning the Standard & Poors 500 Index. Her research also suggested that in order to compensate investors for the increased risk, company stock would have to be purchased 40% to 50% below its market price. That's a far cry from the typical 10% to 15% discount that some big employers offer their workers who want to buy company stock.

Various researchers over the years have demonstrated how owning a big chunk of a single stock can cause you to under-perform the broader market. A few samples:

- A November 1995 article published in *Trusts & Estates* magazine estimated that in a down market, a well-diversified portfolio might fall 9% or so. But the average single stock was likely to tumble 18%; and a risky stock was apt to suffer a 30% decline.

- A study in the November 1999 *CPA Journal* concluded that a $1 million investment in the S&P 500 from January 1970 through the end of 1998 outperformed a similar investment in the average single S&P stock by a whopping $18 million.

HOW TO HANDLE A SINGLE STOCK POSITION

One strategy to deal with a single stock position – and it's probably the one that will make you wince – is to sell some of that stock and pay the requisite taxes. While at first blush this may seem like the least attractive option, many experts say this is the best course of action when properly executed.

At Salomon Smith Barney, for example, specialists there who counsel high net worth individuals often devise what they call a "liquidation strategy" for their clients.

For some clients, they plan to liquidate 15% annually. And if the company's earnings grow 15% a year, in theory, the value of the investor's holding should gradually be replaced even while the client is simultaneously reducing his or her exposure to that one stock.

When you sell stocks in this manner, advisors often recommend that you re-invest the proceeds in a basket of diversified securities. You should also make sure you carefully weigh the tax consequences. This is an area for which you really want some professional advice.

CHARITABLE REMAINDER TRUSTS

You can also establish a Charitable Remainder Trust to liquidate big equity positions, diversify your holdings, and generate income. Such a trust works like this: Say you have $1 million in General Electric stock. And assume your basis in the stock is zero. If you sell your shares, you'll be required to pay 20% capital gains tax and you'd have $800,000 left over to re-invest.

On the contrary, with a Charitable Remainder Trust, you get to invest the entire $1 million in a tax-free environment. The way you do this is by donating the $1 million in stock to the trust. The trust, in turn, sells the GE stock. And because the trust is a tax-exempt entity, it pays zero taxes on the proceeds. You also get a tax deduction the year you fund the trust.

EXCHANGE FUNDS

Exchange funds represent another possible solution to the problem of concentrated wealth, though these vehicles aren't as popular as they once were. With exchange funds, you contribute your stock to a partnership, called an exchange fund. Other people do the same thing. Picture each investor as an owner of your own mini-mutual fund that you all have created. Every investor owns a bit of each company's shares.

The exchange fund then borrows money against the stock contributed and goes out and invests the money into an even more broadly diversified portfolio.

There is, however, a major downside to exchange funds. You have to stay in them for seven years. If you bail out early, you get dinged with a stiff sales load (commission). Another drawback: the partnership's holdings must contain at least 20% in any non-marketable assets, such as commercial real estate. Despite these disadvantages, for some people exchange funds may make sense to explore.

HEDGING STRATEGIES

What other alternatives are available to you to deal with your single-stock holdings?

For big stock positions, many say the best course of action is to hedge your position, and guard against a decline in the value of your shares. A detailed discussion of different hedging strategies is beyond the scope of this book. However, here is a quick summary of one popular way you can reduce the risk of having a concentrated equity position.

If you have $1 million or more tied up in one stock, consider whether it's worth it to cash out – without selling – by using so-called equity collars. A collar involves buying a put and a call at the same time, so you limit your upside potential, but at the same time you also limit your potential losses. (A put is an option that gives you the right to sell stock at a given price; a call is an option that gives you the right to buy a security at a certain price. Call options rise in value when prices in the underlying market go up. Puts gain value as underlying market prices decline).

Using an equity collar lets you lock in some of your profits and take a little cash out to boot, if you need to borrow money. However, these hedging transactions are subject to complicated "tax straddle" rules. Also, since many companies ban collars, you'd need to check with your firm to see if they would allow it.

Still, you should seek to reduce the dangers of having too much of your assets or net worth tied up in one stock, a situation that may set you up for a one-two knockout punch. If your company hits hard times, you risk your investment going down the toilet – and possibly losing your job.

> **$UMMARY $UCCESS $TRATEGY**
>
> **TO CONQUER INVESTING MISTAKE #9:**
>
> Put no more than 10% of your money into any one stock, bond, or fund. Avoid "concentrated" wealth, where too much of your money is tied to one investment.

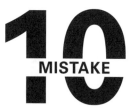

MISTAKE

LACKING TRUE DIVERSIFICATION

So much has been written about the benefits of diversification, that I think investors have a tendency to take it for granted. Please don't skip this chapter, thinking "yeah, yeah, yeah: I know I have to be diversified. I've heard that before." Trust me, you'll learn something new.

You've also undoubtedly heard the advice: "Don't put all your eggs in one basket." But to successfully navigate the buying phase of the investing process, you need more guidance than that.

You need more than just a basic definition of diversification. You really need to have a solid understanding of what diversification means, how it works, and how you can apply the concept to your portfolio.

To put it another way: Sure, you already know not to put all your eggs in one basket. What you may not know, however, is exactly where you *should* put those eggs – and how to handle your basket so that nothing gets broken.

This chapter will give you some key information in that regard.

HIGH TECH OR BUST

Back in the late 1990s, diversification to some investors meant having 10 or 20 stocks – and they all had to be in technology or have a dot-com behind the company name.

Nick Hodges knew plenty of those investors. Hodges, a CFP® practitioner who also has a CPA practice in Fullerton, CA, remembers a schoolteacher client planning for retirement.

The client's sister was also a CPA, and in 1999 "her sister was screaming at me for not investing her more aggressively," Hodges says.

The client, however, decided to follow Hodges' advice, and still invests $500 a month for retirement in a well-diversified portfolio.

"She stayed with me," Hodges says, "and she has an appreciation that her accounts didn't tumble like the rest of the market did."

Not every client followed his advice though.

Hodges also recalls a client with an $800,000 portfolio at the height of the Internet bubble. "He was very bright. And I tried to convince him that it was risky, and that he needed to be diversified," says Hodges.

But the client wouldn't budge. Instead, he took his money elsewhere.

"I talked to him months later, and his portfolio was at $400,000. Then another six months later, it was down to $200,000," says Hodges.

> Of all the ominous threats that investors face, a lack of diversification ranks high on the list. When people don't diversify their holdings, they duplicate investments unnecessarily, have riskier portfolios, experience greater volatility and are more apt to under perform the broader market – especially during periods of economic uncertainty.

Are you too looking to "strike it rich" and make a big splash in the investing world? Be careful, lest you belly-flop, as this investor did, and likewise squander hundreds of thousands of dollars.

Fortunately, there's a better way. And for many of you – especially those who are new to investing – you get to learn valuable lessons about diversification in the best way possible: painlessly and free of charge. How so? You learn from someone else's mistake.

> If the stock-market meltdown that began in early 2000, the Enron scandal that cost many employees practically their entire life savings, and a slew of other costly investing fiascos have taught us nothing else, it is this: real diversification is more than not being too heavily invested in one stock, bond or industry. It also involves expanding your investment portfolio across geographic boundaries, market capitalization ranges, asset classes, and investment styles, such as value versus growth.

Let's look at each of these features in a little more detail.

IT'S GOOD TO GO GLOBAL

If you want a well-diversified portfolio, you need to think globally. Too many people stick close to home when it comes to buying investments. But getting exposure to foreign markets can provide a big boost to your portfolio.

"As an investor, you want to have as many ponds to fish in as possible," says David Winters, chairman and chief investment officer at Short Hills, NJ-based Mutual Series Funds.

Of its six funds, the firm has two international offerings: Mutual Discovery, a global stock fund, and Mutual European, a sector fund. "What we're trying to do is make sure that we find opportunities no matter where they are," Winters says.

Experts say that to be properly diversified, anywhere from 10% to 20% of your portfolio should be in international investments.

And some feel that buying international stocks also gives you the chance to buy investments at bargain basement prices. "We're very picky about what we buy, and furthermore, we're very fussy about what we pay for it," says Amit Wadhwaney, portfolio manager of the Third Avenue International Value Fund in New York. He's constantly on the prowl for solid companies that are based overseas, where Wadhwaney believes you can get much better values.

"Why would you want to pay two to three times more buying a U.S. company," he asks, "when you can buy essentially the same thing or something better abroad?"

WHY SIZE MATTERS

Beyond geographic diversification, you also need to make sure you buy investments in different market capitalization ranges. Don't fall into the trap of only buying one type of security: such as small cap stocks. Make sure you mix it up with mid- and large cap offerings as well.

Having various asset classes almost goes without saying. But it's worth noting because some investors can get themselves in trouble by sticking to one or maybe two asset types. For example, ultra conservative investors may stick to only bonds or perhaps bonds and cash. With this type of strategy, you risk inflation (and taxes) eroding the dollar value of your holdings. Conversely, some super-aggressive investors err by continuing to invest 100% in equities. If you're 25 years old, don't have any kids and are putting away the money for a long-term goal, such as retirement, you can afford to ride out short-term fluctuations in the stock market. So an all-stock portfolio may be fine. But for most people, with less tolerance for risk, or shorter time horizons, you'll want to have a decent dose of bonds, cash, and/or real estate as well.

Finally, make sure you're not wed to one particular investment style. Often times, when growth-oriented investing strategies are in favor, value stock-picking strategies are out of favor; and vice versa. So to make sure you minimize your risk – and still capture some potential appreciation – cover your bases by picking investments that use both investment styles.

If you tackle all these areas, then your portfolio will be truly diversified. And again, a tremendous plus to having a truly diversified portfolio is that a balance of investments will help you weather economic downturns.

THE LINK BETWEEN ASSET ALLOCATION AND DIVERSIFICATION

Vern Hayden, a CERTIFIED FINANCIAL PLANNER™ practitioner in West-port, Conn. says people sometimes confuse asset allocation with diversification. But he explains it this way:

"Asset allocation is a discipline," he says, where you divide up your portfolio into stocks, bonds, cash, etc. Hayden says then you drill down a bit and figure out investment style. In other words, determine what percentage of large cap growth funds is prudent, and so on. Then you go about "matching great managers of great funds to those allocations," Hayden says. "The result of all of that is diversification. And it has a strategy ring to it."

$UMMARY $UCCESS $TRATEGY

TO CONQUER INVESTING MISTAKE #10:

Get truly diversified to reduce your investment risk. Proper diversification involves spreading your investments among various asset classes (stocks, bonds, etc.) throughout multiple industries (energy, healthcare, banking, etc.), over market capitalization ranges (small, mid-, and large-cap), across investment styles (growth and value), and geographically (domestic and foreign investments).

IGNORING FEES AND COMMISSIONS

Investors who disregard fees and commissions pay for that omission in diminished portfolio performance. Others simply pay too much for services that should be free or much less than they are getting charged. Small charges here and there may not seem like a lot in the course of one year. But over time, the numbers add up. The longer investors pay high fees, the more of a drag those fees are on investment returns.

UNDERSTAND THE BASICS

Before you can address the dilemma of high fees, you need to understand a few key things. First, you may have heard of an "expense ratio," but perhaps you didn't really know what it meant. An expense ratio is the fund's expenses expressed as a percentage of its assets. As a result, the higher a fund's expense ratio is, the higher its fees are.

You also need some big picture sense of where fees have been heading. According to industry data, fees rose steadily for the five-year period from 1997 to 2002. In 2002, management fees for large cap growth funds averaged 0.72% while large-cap value funds averaged 0.64%.

Additionally, you need a working knowledge of how mutual fund fees are imposed. By way of summary, here's a quick explanation of fees, delineated by share classes:

- With front-end loaded funds, or class A shares you pay an upfront sales fee that is deducted from your investment. The sales charge isn't included in the fund's expense ratio.

- With back-end loads, or class B shares, you pay no upfront fee. But if you sell before six years, you get hit with a redemption fee. Most B shares convert to A shares after six to 10 years.

- With level loads, or Class C shares, you don't pay a front or a back-end sales fee. Instead you pay a higher annual fee.

- With no load funds, you pay no sales charge at all. (But don't confuse that and think that there are no fees associated with your ownership of a no-load mutual fund). There are, indeed, other fees.

MONEY MARKETS ESPECIALLY VULNERABLE

If you're investing in money market funds with high annual operating expenses, you should really watch out. The reason? You might think you're getting a paltry 1% or so return on your money, but in reality, you could be yielding returns that are close to zero. Here's how: As of this writing – July 2003 – the Federal Reserve has the federal funds rate at 1.00%. (The fed funds rate is simply the interest rate that banks charge one another for overnight loans). And by raising or lowering the fed funds rate, the Fed is able to influence the money market arena – precisely the area that many individual investors (especially retirees) have money invested in taxable money market funds. Whenever the fed funds rate drops, so do yields on commercial paper, Treasury bills, and other short-term instruments.

Back in the late 1990s, the fed funds rate was a robust 5.5%. In 2000, it reached 6.5% - only to be slashed to 1.00% in 2003 as the Fed battled the economic recession. Nowadays, money market funds with yields of 1.2%, and a 1% expense ratio, are yielding a measly 0.2%. And if you take into account the fact that inflation is running at 3% annually, what you're really left with are negative returns, on an inflation-adjusted basis.

This issue is affecting millions of investors, given the massive amounts of cash sitting in money market accounts. As of June 2003, there was $2.1 trillion in money market assets, according to the Money Fund Report newsletter published by iMoneyNet Inc.

CRITICS ASSAIL HIGH FEES

In 2003, John Bogle, founder and retired chairman of the Vanguard mutual fund company, testified about this serious issue before Congress. "While the importance of cost applies to all types of mutual funds, it is most obvious in money market funds," he told the Capital Markets Subcommittee of the House Financial Services Committee. "Money fund performance comes down almost entirely to relative costs," he said.

In his testimony, Bogle related how 94% of the 263 taxable money funds for which he had data had gross annual returns for the years 1998 through 2002 of 4.6% to 4.9%.

Nevertheless, these same funds varied drastically in their fees, with annual expense ratios starting as low as 0.19% and climbing as high as 1.96%. Thus, the average net returns were drastically different: ranging from 2.6% to 4.58%.

Another telling statistic from Bogle: In 1978, mutual funds held $56 billion of assets and carried an average expense ratio of 0.91%. Today, the mutual fund industry boasts more than $6 trillion in assets, and the typical fund carries a 1.36% expense ratio. With a much larger asset base, one would think that fund companies could spread their fees over a wider pool of investors, thereby lowering mutual fund fees. Unfortunately, that hasn't been the case.

FEES UNDER SCRUTINY

But even before Bogle testified before federal lawmakers, mutual fund fees had drawn particular scrutiny. And the securities industry, under pressure to ensure fairness to investors, had begun to act.

In February 2002, the NASD announced the formation of a 22-person task force to recommend ways the mutual fund and brokerage industries could assure that investors are not overcharged when they buy mutual funds with front-end loads.

Usually, mutual fund companies reduce the sales load you pay as the dollar value of the shares that you or your family members own reaches specific levels, called "breakpoints."

For instance, take a look at the following breakpoint schedule, an example given by the NASD as guidance to investors:

Sample Breakpoint Schedule
Class A Shares (Front-End Sales Load)

Investment Amount	Sales Load
Less than $25,000	5%
$25,000 but less than $50,000	4.25%
$50,000 but less than $100,000	3.75%
$100,000 but less than $250,000	3.25%
$250,000 but less than $500,000	2.75%
$500,000 but less than $1,000,000	2.0%
$1 million or more	0.0%

Unfortunately, routine examinations by NASD revealed that investors weren't always getting the discounts due them. As a result, the SEC asked the NASD, along with the Securities Industry Association (SIA) and the Investment Company Institute (ICI), to take the lead in forming the task force. (The SIA is Wall Street's trade group, and the ICI represents the mutual fund industry).

Upon announcing the creation of the task force, NASD chairman and CEO Robert Glauber said the industry was "committed to helping investors receive restitution for missed breakpoints and ensuring going forward that they receive the discounts they are entitled to." He also said that "solving this problem is critical to investor protection."

To be sure, the issue of investors getting the discounts to which they are entitled is no small matter. As you can see from the chart above, if you were entitled to a 3.75% commission and you got charged 5% that was a sizeable hit.

Each mutual fund and family of funds set their own breakpoints and the conditions through which discounts are available. These terms and conditions differ from one fund to another, and they can also change. You can find out more information on breakpoints in the mutual fund prospectuses or Statements of Additional Information, and on many mutual fund company web sites.

To get a handle on this dilemma, the NASD required its member firms to do a self-assessment to determine how well these firms were complying with breakpoint reductions that should have been given to investors. As of this writing, the NASD was reviewing those self-assessments and determining how to best proceed.

WHAT CAN YOU DO?

Until the industry works this issue out, here's what I recommend.

- **Don't depend on your broker to give you the proper price breaks**. This is an area where you have to be proactive in seeking out and demanding the discounts you deserve.

- **Start by understanding how breakpoints work in general.** The NASD's web site, *www.NASD.com* is a good place for comprehensive information on this subject. Then look into how breakpoints are calculated and granted at your specific mutual fund(s).

- **Exercise your "rights of accumulation."**

  Did you know that you have something called "rights of accumulation" as an investor?

  A right of accumulation usually lets you receive discounted fees on a current mutual fund purchase based on a combination of that current transaction and previous fund transactions. The idea is that if your two (or more) transactions reach your fund's dollar breakpoint, you should be given a discount. For example, if you are investing $5,000 in a fund today, but previously had invested $20,000, those two amounts can be combined to reach a $25,000 breakpoint, which will entitle you to a lower sales load on your $5,000 purchase.

- **Write a Letter of Intent**

  It's very possible that you won't be able to immediately invest the minimum amount required to trigger a breakpoint discount. If that's the case, think about your investing plans for the next year or so. If you plan to make additional investments over the coming months (and remember the advice in Chapter 4 about investing on a consistent basis?), you might be able to get your fund company or investment firm to reduce your sales charges through a Letter of Intent (LOI).

  An LOI is a signed statement that you give your investment firm or fund company. This statement expresses your intent to invest an amount over the breakpoint within a given period of time specified by the fund. In effect, you're saying: "Look, I don't have a big lump sum to invest in order to get a price break, but I believe I should qualify for a breakpoint given the amount of money I will collectively invest" over the next year or so. Additionally, there's more good news concerning breakpoints. Often times, fund companies will let you include purchases you made within 90 days *before* the LOI is signed and within 13 months *after* the LOI is signed in order to help you qualify for a required breakpoint threshold.

A warning, though: If you fail to invest the amount stated in your Letter of Intent, and you don't hit the minimum dollar value for a breakpoint, the fund can retroactively collect higher fees from you.

• **Use Your Family Discounts**

The power and value of using your "rights of accumulation" or a Letter of Intent extends far beyond any one fund in which you might invest. These important tools can also be handily leveraged beyond what you, as one individual, can invest. When you exercise your rights of accumulation or initiate a Letter of Intent, you usually also get to count mutual fund transactions in other related accounts, in different mutual fund classes, or in different mutual funds that are part of the same fund family, toward your discounts. For example, your mutual fund company may give you a breakpoint discount by combining your fund purchases with those of your spouse or children. Also ask whether you can get credit for mutual fund transactions in retirement accounts, educational savings accounts, and even accounts at other fund companies or brokerage firms.

REGULATORS RESPOND TO THE FEES ISSUE

Because of "breakpoints" and other issues, it came as no surprise in June 2003, when the Securities and Exchange Commission released a 120-page report calling for better disclosure in the $6.4 trillion mutual fund industry. The same week, Rep. Richard Baker (R-La.), who is chairman of the House Financial Services Committee's Capital Markets subcommittee, introduced a bill that would require the SEC to adopt new rules on mutual fund disclosure. A key provision of the legislation would force fund companies to give investors more information about fees and fund manager salaries. For instance, under the proposal, fund companies would need to give you an estimate of your share of operating expenses, in dollar terms. Rep. Baker's bill also calls for fund companies to show portfolio transaction costs in a manner that would let you compare one fund to another.

While the bill wouldn't mandate that fund companies reveal salaries for fund managers, it would make fund companies describe how compensation is determined.

Regardless of what happens with the Baker proposal, or any related measures that are put forth, one thing is clear, this is an issue you must stay on top of.

WHAT ELSE TO DO ABOUT HIGH FEES

 For starters, assess how much your broker is charging you per trade and what the true cost is of your mutual funds. Look out for 12b-1, or marketing fees, imposed by mutual funds. Also analyze what up-front sales charges (commissions) are being assessed, as well as any back-end sales load. To find some of this information, check the fee table in your prospectus or in the most recent shareholder report.

Be prepared to switch funds if necessary. Unlike switches among stock, bond and hybrid funds, if you bail out of a money market fund that's not a taxable event. As the price per share of money funds is always a $1 per share, you generate no taxable capital gains.

Look for opportunities to cut brokerage and administrative costs you may be getting charged. Enroll in Dividend Reinvestment Programs. Ask for discounts when your assets reach certain minimums (most often $50,000 or $100,000). Remember that fees eat away at your portfolio's overall return.

Be aware of things like inactivity fees, which are imposed on less frequent investors. These charges typically range from $25 to $50 a year.

Ask for a breakdown of fees: you'll probably be surprised to see the slew of fees you're paying. Often times, there are account set-up fees, especially at online financial institutions. Of course, you'll be charged per transaction fees, or commissions to trade. Then there are other occasional fees, like the annual custodial fee you pay for your IRA.

CONSIDER INDEX FUNDS

Outside of the money market universe, index funds are typically the least expensive of all funds when it comes to fees, since no active management is required. International funds are usually the most expensive of all funds. They require more work and due diligence – in the form of research, travel, overseas phone calls, etc. – on the part of the investment firm or mutual fund company.

Occasionally, you'll hear about a mutual fund company that is waiving its fees in order to attract new customers or to entice existing clients to invest a certain minimum amount of money. Take advantage of these opportunities when you can.

But also recognize them for what they are: inducements to get you to invest money – kind of like credit card companies offering teaser rates. In this case, of course, you're not taking on debt. But by making the comparison to credit card offers, I mean that the reduced rates and fees only last for a certain period of time. After that, the normal fees will be charged. So be sure you know how long your "no fee" deal at a brokerage or mutual fund company will last. And find out in advance of investing what the new fees will be once the "no fee" offer expires. You don't want to accept what seems like a good deal in the short run, if that deal ultimately is going to cost you more money in the long run.

Also realize that the size of a fund, the asset class involved, the portfolio manager's trading habits, investor turnover, and the fund's geographic focus all impact a fund's annual expense ratio.

According to Morningstar, for the five-year period from 1998 to 2002, here are the breakdowns for the average growth stock funds:

> Large-Cap U.S. equity fund: Expense ratio = 1.18%
> Mid-Cap U.S. equity fund: Expense ratio = 1.27%
> Small-Cap U.S. equity fund: Expense ratio = 1.39%

Expenses are slightly less for value funds:

> Large-Cap U.S. equity fund: Expense ratio = 1.04%
> Mid-Cap U.S. equity fund: Expense ratio = 1.22%
> Small-Cap U.S. equity fund: Expense ratio = 1.20%

Now go grab your most recent prospectuses. Go ahead – do it right now so you can check your funds. How do the fees you're being charged stack up to the norm? If they're excessive, or if they're unclear, don't waste time and money: Set aside an hour or so to talk to your fund company or to employ some of the strategies I've suggested above.

FEES AND YOUR 401(K) PLAN

And what about fees in your 401(k) plan? According to data from the Barra RogersCasey/IOMA 2000 Annual Defined Contribution Survey, 64% of employers cover all the costs related to a 401(k) plans' administration and record keeping. That means about one-third of employers aren't doing so. And only 21% of employers with plans that have $1 billion or more in assets pay all administrative costs. Translation: the employees of these companies are also paying those administrative fees. Yet, 401(k) plans also don't typically reveal their fees on your quarterly or annual statements.

But here's where some research and sleuthing can add some perspective. A study by Hewitt Associates, the consulting firm that specializes in pension information, found that typical 401(k) administrative fees ranged from $75 to $150 a year per employee. Meanwhile, the 401(k) investment management fees ranged from having average expense ratios of 1.04% (for U.S. small-cap stock funds) to as little as 0.49% (for money market accounts), IOMA data show. Compare that to institutional investors, whose fund expense ratios can be as slim as 0.1% after three years, and you'll see why you need to take charge in demanding lower fees. Granted, institutional investors wield much greater clout because they have far more assets than you do. Nevertheless, as your 401(k) continues to grow, you should continue to request fee reductions.

By way of additional guidance, the 401(k) Association says that all your 401(k) fees combined should not be more than 1% of annual assets. You can ask your Human Resources department to disclose your 401(k) fees. But don't be surprised if H.R. simply hands you a bunch of legal documents. Another way to find out precisely what expenses are being paid for, and by whom, is to log onto the Labor Department's web site. There you can download a copy of an informative paper called "Study of 401(k) Plan Fees and Expenses."

$UMMARY $UCCESS $TRATEGY

TO CONQUER INVESTING MISTAKE #11:

Pay close attention to fees and commissions. Excessive fees and high commissions can eat away at your overall investment returns – especially in a down market.

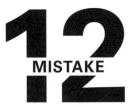

MISTAKE 12

BECOMING OVERCONFIDENT

I love to watch sports – and not just professional athletes in action. Sometimes, I get a kick out of watching teenagers on a basketball court.

Ever notice how when some 16-year-old kid strolls on the court with a new pair of Nike shoes, all of a sudden he thinks he's the greatest thing since Michael Jordan? He'll say something like: "Watch me slam, man! I'll dunk all *over* you!"

That kind of bravado reminds me of what happens to some investors. When a bull market gets in full swing, they start readying themselves for the slam-dunk. They're not satisfied to invest consistently and methodically, to diversify their holdings, and to let compounded interest and time work in their favor.

No, that would be too boring.

This investor is always thinking that if only he had the right trading tools, if only he had certain key information, or if only he could make his own stock picks, he could outsmart the market. He's kind of like the amateur golfer who thinks that with the perfect set of golf clubs, he could beat Tiger Woods. And what are the chances of that happening?

What makes investors feel so invincible?

Terrance Odean, a University of California professor who specializes in behavioral finance, has done some fascinating research in this area. His findings are very telling.

Individuals who get overconfident about their investing prowess can have that surge of self-assurance backfire on them. Overconfidence leads to poor decision-making, excessive buying and selling, diminished portfolio performance, and sometimes, financial losses.

To combat this investing faux pas, don't make assumptions about an investment. And please, don't be a know-it-all. Nobody can know everything about every stock or industry. Get help when needed, which is anytime you're even the slightest bit unsure about something or you don't have the time or the desire to learn about a prospective investment.

Interestingly, studies show that male investors express far more "confidence" about the investing process than do women. But very often women, research shows, tend to fare better in the investing environment. This chapter and chapter 22 will examine the role that overconfidence plays in portfolio performance.

Odean's research shows that people sell their winning investments more than their losing ones by a factor of about 1.5 to 1. Overconfidence plays a role in that, as do limited attention spans. Another contributing factor to overconfidence is the proliferation of all the information available to investors these days relative to previous decades.

Now there are financial news television programs, daily and weekly business newspapers, financial magazines, business talk radio shows, tons of Internet web sites devoted to investing, and the like. Armed with massive amounts of information from these varied sources is certainly enough to send your confidence into overdrive! But don't let your financial alter-ego – let's call it "Captain Crush-The-Market" — overtake all your good sense.

Yes, you may really be incredibly informed and knowledgeable. But it's foolhardy when you get so over-confident that if an investment doesn't pan out, you insist on being right – and declaring that the rest of the market is wrong. Your thinking is that somehow, some way, everybody else will come around to your frame of mind and your way of thinking. Well, if there were a herd of raging bulls heading in your direction, which would be easier to turn around: you or that entire stampede? It's so easy to get trampled by the market if you make the mistake of being over-confident. Try your best to be reasonable in your expectations and to keep your feelings of invincibility in check.

$UMMARY $UCCESS $TRATEGY
FOR CONQUERING INVESTING MISTAKE #12:

Guard against becoming over-confident. If an investment doesn't pan out, don't fool yourself into thinking that you're right and the rest of the market is wrong. The market is always right.

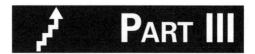

PART III

HOLDING/MONITORING MISHAPS

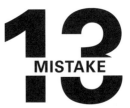

MISTAKE 13

MONITORING YOUR PORTFOLIO HAPHAZARDLY

Are you a person who likes to hold quarterly or annual yard sales? Or once a year, do you make a point to have a big spring cleaning – to get rid of the old clothes and stuff you don't really need? If you do, that's the same type of approach you should take to your investments. If you monitor your portfolio regularly you'll be able to see what you need, as well as what you don't.

On the contrary, not evaluating your portfolio on a regular basis can lead you to stockpile a lot of things you may not need – kind of like people who keep buying a new pair of black wool pants each winter, because they haven't been looking in the back of their closet, where there are seven other pairs of black wool pants.

I'll admit, I'm certainly a person who grapples with this one: the mistake of not monitoring my portfolio regularly enough.

If you're in the same boat, it's time for a life jacket.

When investors fail to adequately monitor their portfolios, they lose track of what they own, they forget why they even hold certain investments, and they maintain investments that are no longer appropriate.

There's another danger to haphazardly monitoring your investments. Most brokerages and investment banks require you to dispute any transactions within 30 days of receiving an investment statement. So, if your broker (or someone else) initiates a transaction that you didn't authorize, how would you know about it if you don't review your statements?

Checking those statements carefully when you get them will allow you to unearth any possible errors.

That's what happened to Margaret Bongiorno. One day she got a statement in the mail indicating that her broker sold $2 million worth of Sarah Lee stock that was in Bongiorno's account. At the time Bongiorno was an 84-year-old housewife from Long Island, N.Y. She denied giving her broker permission to sell the stock and the two sides wound up in arbitration. Thanks to her daughter, who was reviewing her mother's mail, Bongiorno knew about the transaction. But if she hadn't checked her statement she wouldn't have discovered the sale. So clearly, reviewing investment statements is especially important to check for mistakes and to make sure brokers aren't doing anything contrary to your wishes.

Here's another account from an investor who was wronged by a broker – but didn't find out about it until it was too late.

LESSONS LEARNED

IN THEIR OWN WORDS:
INVESTORS SHARE LESSONS LEARNED

> After much persistence from a financial advisor with (a Wall Street brokerage), I rolled over my IRA and opened a Money Market Account. Initially my account was handled with care and I had consistent contact with my advisor. My portfolio grew and I was happy. I trusted my advisor and the company she represented. Suddenly, she moved to New Jersey and was having personal problems. Unfortunately, I was not aware that she had made my portfolio very heavy in technology. Well, as we all know the market took a sudden turn and I lost many, many $$$$. (I had signed documentation to state I only wanted

medium risk). I should not have been placed in a high-risk situation.

I made many attempts to contact my advisor and my calls were not returned. I contacted the company and advised them that I felt my account was being mishandled. I was bounced from office to office. At this time I also noticed that my Money Market account had dwindled. Why, I asked myself? I had never withdrawn a dime. Finally, I am contacted by my advisor, who now surfaced in California. I confront her with my anger and anguish over the tremendous loss in my portfolio and the absence of $21,000 in my Money Market account. I checked over statements that had arrived and found the word "MARGIN" connected with my account. I was totally perplexed, as I honestly didn't have a clue what this meant. After investigating and searching on the Internet I found that she had purchased tech stock on margin. I never signed any paperwork that authorized her or the company to do such transactions. The CA office assured me that these funds would be returned. Well, I waited and nothing happened. My account was returned to NY for handling and a high-ranking individual at the company advised me that I should acquire a lawyer immediately. I acquired a lawyer and after much back and forth was given a settlement. It was not to my liking but it was better than nothing.

The lawyer does not give me the proper information on how this settlement should be handled and I end up paying the lawyer a third, IRS a third and me a third. It was one nightmare after another. I lost approximately $175,000.00, three years of mental anguish and lack of sleep. I learned to NEVER trust anyone, especially the big corporations. I felt that the company should have been held more accountable for their lack of supervision on the handling of my accounts. The lawyer should have been held accountable for misinforming me and causing me further monetary loss and sleepless nights.

Unfortunately, during the time that this was all happening I had severe illnesses in the family, which ended in death, and I did not give my portfolio my undivided attention. I stupidly felt that the company and the lawyer had my best interests at heart! These were very bitter lessons that I learned: not to trust anyone but yourself! I was made a fool of two times, but rest assured it won't happen a third.

V.B. , Ridgewood, NY

I know that in down markets in particular, the temptation is to file those statements away without even opening them. I once interviewed a woman in her 50s who was a long-time employee of a telephone company. In 2002, she stopped looking at her quarterly statements because every time she got one, it showed her retirement money had fallen by another $10,000 or $20,000. (She ultimately moved into annuities and says she feels less stressed about her investing).

But what she did – in terms of not looking at those statements — was actually very common.

So common, in fact, that Charles Schwab & Co., Inc. implemented a "Fresh Start" program in early 2003. The company found that scores of investors were simply stashing those statements in their drawers and not opening them. "Many people were just frightened and confused," company founder Charles Schwab told me during an interview. He said the goal of the program – where new clients could sign up for a free portfolio evaluation – was to get people to intelligently review their portfolio status, and to make changes if necessary. Simply ignoring a declining portfolio, he noted, would be a "big mistake."

So don't just stick your monthly or quarterly statements into a file (or worse yet, the trash) and never look at them.

- Open those statements.

- Check out your portfolio at least every six months, preferably quarterly to monitor performance and look at the underlying fundamentals of your investments.

- Also establish a system for regularly reviewing your investments. It could be a beginning of the year, mid-year or end of year assessment.

- Make a point to systematically check out everything in your portfolio.

- Ask yourself if the reason you bought an investment remains valid.

  None of this is to suggest that you should obsess over the quarterly fluctuations in your portfolio. After all, it's senseless to get bent out of shape based on a three-month time period in your 20 or 30 year investing plan. But if you stay on top of your investment portfolio with annual check-ups, you'll be more relaxed about your overall investing experience. And you'll find that there's no need to obsess over either the daily volatility in the stock market or quarterly blips.

$UMMARY $UCCESS $TRATEGY

TO CONQUER INVESTING MISTAKE #13:

Monitor your portfolio on a regular basis. Open your statements and review them. Check for errors. Make sure you've authorized any transactions that occurred. Don't just throw your monthly, quarterly or annual statements into a drawer or in the trash can.

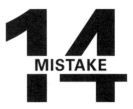

MISTAKE

14

HAVING YOUR ASSETS SPREAD OUT OVER TOO MANY ACCOUNTS

When scores of investors lost money in their 401(k) plans for the first time in 2001, some blamed employers who didn't offer enough variety in their retirement offerings to shield employees from the struggling economy. For example, out of every five 401(k) plans, only two had a small-stock fund option.

But sometimes, having too many accounts can also hurt your investing strategy.

> Having too many investment accounts makes it far too easy for investors to lose track of what they've bought, duplicate their investments, pay too much in fees, and thwart their asset allocation goals. All of this can lead to generating poor investment returns. A multitude of accounts creates extra headaches during tax season. There's an emotional downside to this mistake too: getting overwhelmed, and feeling stressed about a lack of control over your investment portfolio.

The Investment Company Institute says there are 95 million mutual fund shareholders in 54.2 million U.S. households. As of

May 2001, the latest for which figures were available, the average U.S. household had $119,700 in assets spread out among six mutual funds. What's appropriate or ideal?

Here are some ideas on this topic from money management pros. Be prepared, because their advice runs the gamut.

Rande Spiegelman, a CERTIFIED FINANCIAL PLANNER™ practitioner in San Francisco, says many investors are best served by owning just one index mutual fund, such as those that mimic the performance of the Wilshire 5000 Index. With this type of fund, Spiegelman reasons, you'll be getting broad stock-market exposure, including an array of small-, mid-, and large-cap companies.

By contrast, Alexandra Armstrong, a partner at the Washington, D.C. investment advisory firm Armstrong Welch & MacIntyre, says that 10 or 15 funds are entirely appropriate – for those with at least $1 million in assets.

These and other financial advisors say they've encountered some clients whose portfolios are completely out of control, with upwards of 30 or 40 funds. And sometimes the investors don't have the asset size to justify this extremely large number of accounts.

SOME SIMPLE SOLUTIONS

Having your investments spread out over too many accounts is, quite literally, spreading yourself to thin. Don't try to be a superhero and manage an overwhelmingly complex set of holdings.

- If you think the number of funds you own have gotten unwieldy, consolidate if necessary.
- If appropriate, consider index funds or build your own core portfolio of diversified mutual funds and/or individual stocks, bonds and funds so that there's no need for 10 or 20 miscellaneous accounts.
- You can also look into Spyders, Diamonds and QQQs. Don't let the names throw you. These are just the index-tracking stocks for the S&P 500, the Nasdaq, and the Dow Jones In-

dustrial Average, respectively. If you buy these investments, you'll be getting broad exposure to the market and again, you may not need to have a multitude of other funds.

A HIDDEN DANGER

Michael Kresh, of MD Kresh Financial Services, says he sees too many people who come into his office and "don't understand what they own." As a result, he warns that you shouldn't lose sight of a bigger problem caused by excessive funds: duplicating your investments. "The single biggest issue is portfolio overlap," Kresh says. "I'm more concerned about the amount of overlap than I am about how many funds you own."

$UMMARY $UCCESS $TRATEGY
TO CONQUER INVESTING MISTAKE #14:

Maintain a manageable number of mutual funds. There's no "right" number that's suitable for all investors. But if you spread your assets over too many accounts, you may pay excessive fees, get overwhelmed with statements, or duplicate your investments.

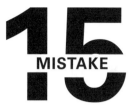

MISTAKE

FAILING TO REASSESS AND REBALANCE YOUR PORTFOLIO AS NEEDED

No one has to tell you to take your umbrella with you outdoors if you see threatening rain clouds. Not to do so just because you're in a rush to get out of the house would be short-sighted, right? By the same token, you have to check the weather, so to speak, with regard to your investment portfolio. When external forces shift, it's often prudent for you to reassess whether your portfolio also needs shifting.

Those investors who bypass such a review risk under-performing the market, taking on additional portfolio risk, hanging onto to inappropriate investments and possibly having improper asset allocation.

You should also be aware that sometimes one investment you own performs really well and begins to take up a larger percentage of your portfolio than intended. If this occurs, make sure you re-jigger that position so that the amount you own in any one stock or asset class is consistent with your intentions. You don't want even "good" investments to throw your asset allocation strategy out of whack.

According to Michael Kresh, of MD Kresh, "one of the reasons why investors have performed so much worse than expected is because a lot of funds allowed their stock positions to become very similar." With regards to the funds he picks, "We're very cautious about whether these fund managers really do have very different styles," Kresh notes, citing one fund that looks for broken down bonds and deep value, while another one seeks growth at a reasonable price.

 Ibbotson Investment Research has long shown the benefit of rebalancing. If nothing else will get you to rebalance your portfolio, perhaps this statistic will: During the past 25 years, rebalancing at least once a year on a portfolio with a target split of 60% stocks and 40% bonds cut the risk of the portfolio by nearly 20%.

Remember: You're starting with your investing plans as broadly laid out in your asset allocation strategy. When you get down to diversification, those plans are merely guidelines. They've got to have some wiggle room in them because circumstances invariably change.

TAKE A LOOK AT RISK

As you monitor your portfolio, one key factor you want to check is how much risk your investments possess. Surely you know about volatility, as triple-digit point swings on the Dow Jones Industrial Average seem to be commonplace now. But given the market's gyrations, you really need to get a handle on how risky your unique holdings are. One company that can help you determine this is RiskMetrics, a J.P. Morgan spin-off. The firm's web site, *www.riskgrades.com*, will "grade" the riskiness of any stock and most mutual funds.

FAVOR LOW BETA STOCKS

A stock's beta is simply a measure of its volatility, compared with a given benchmark. The most frequent benchmark investors use is the S&P 500 Index. If you have a stock with a beta of 1.0, that means it matches the volatility of the broader index. Any stock with a beta that is greater than 1.0 will experience more gyrations than the overall market, in both good and bad times. A stock with a beta of less than 1.0 will be less volatile than the general market.

So let's say you own a low-beta stock. It's a company with a beta of .75. When the market goes up or down, the stock will move in the same direction, but only 75% as much. Therefore, if the S&P 500 climbs 10% this same stock would go up by 7.5%. By the same token a 10% drop in the S&P 500 would produce only a 7.5% fall for this stock. What you need to take away from all this is that you should seek out low beta stocks if you want to minimize your worries about risk as you monitor your portfolio. You can visit S&P's Personal Wealth web site (*www.personalwealth.com*) (it's run in conjunction with BusinessWeek magazine), or Multex Investor (*www.multexinvestor.com*) to check the beta of any stock. Multex is a Reuters service that provides financial research and information.

Hugh Johnson, market strategist at First Albany, once told me that one smart way people can rebalance their investments wisely is to diminish risk in their portfolios. He suggested buying sectors of the market that are typically less volatile, such as health care, utility, and consumer-staples industries.

CHANGE WITH A PURPOSE

Don't make changes to your portfolio just for the sake of changing. And I'm certainly not advocating wholesale liquidating of your investments. However, you should certainly revisit your plan on a regular basis. Re-evaluate things. Think about it this way: If you buy a new car, it's great in the beginning. But after a while, the tires get a little worn. You have to change the oil, maybe put on a new pair of brakes. Your investment portfolio works the same way.

Companies change, markets change, and so do industries. What worked for you five years ago may not be as compelling today.

Make a point to re-examine your investments whenever broad economic conditions transform, industry conditions are altered, or major changes occur at the company in which you're investing. Some things to think about: Has the manager of that mutual fund you bought seven years ago left? Has a company's credit ratings been downgraded or have its financials began to deteriorate? Is the industry, in general, under pressure? These are some of the considerations worthy of your attention when you start to consider if it's time to rebalance your portfolio.

$UMMARY $UCCESS $TRATEGY

TO CONQUER INVESTING MISTAKE #15:

Rebalance your portfolio as needed. Your asset allocation can get out of whack if certain investments start to represent a larger portion of your overall portfolio than you intended.

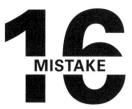

16
MISTAKE

FAILING TO ACT WHEN YOUR
PERSONAL SITUATION HAS CHANGED

The previous chapter talked about how and why you might need to tweak your investment portfolio if external factors change. This chapter is designed to get you thinking about smart ways you should be monitoring your portfolio if your personal situation changes.

If you remind yourself to consider your finances whenever you have a major event in your life – either personally or professionally – chances are you'll do a decent job of holding the proper investments.

> You should reassess your investments if you have a major personal or professional event. For instance: have you gotten married, had a child, or planned a new business venture? These are some reasons to reconsider your investment holdings and make sure they're right for the current time.

Investors who fail to re-evaluate their investment holdings when important changes have occurred in their lives may hold securities that are no longer appropriate for their needs. These investors also suffer from improper asset allocation.

If your review suggests that it's time to lighten up on a given investment, make preparations to do that. Discuss tax implications with your tax advisor. Consider what better-performing investment alternatives are available to you, and so forth. When you are successfully holding and monitoring your investments, you want to cull from your portfolio, not engage in wholesale selling.

Don't overdo it on either side – in terms of buying investments and keeping them forever, or selling them when you really should hang onto them.

Though some big-name investors have made a fortune by buying and holding, chances are you'll have to liquidate your holdings at some time. Warren Buffett is famous for saying he likes to "buy and hold forever." With his wealth, he certainly has that luxury. Most people don't.

Whatever you do, avoid the mistake that some investors make when they monitor their portfolios obsessively: these investors wind up going way overboard in switching in and out of stocks for all manner of reasons.

HOLDING PERIODS ON THE DECLINE

Just look at what happened during the Internet bubble.

According to research from Boston-based consulting firm Bain & Co., shareholders of many Internet companies typically hung onto their stocks for just a few days at a time. And that includes those Internet companies that are still around today like Yahoo!

Even larger, blue-chip companies had less loyal investors. Back in 1999, the average IBM shareholder owned Big Blue for just 9.2 months. Johnson and Johnson shareholders owned that company for 23.4 months before selling. And General Electric shareholders had an average holding period of 30.2 months.

The following data illustrate how investors are hanging onto stocks for less and less time.

Holding Period For Average Stock on NYSE

Year	Holding Period
1960	8.3 years
1970	5.3 years
1980	2.8 years
1990	2.2 years
2000	1.3 years

Source: Bain & Co.

To stay on top of when you might need to more actively monitor your portfolio, you might create a "life events" checklist or get one from a financial planner. This life events checklist is designed to get you to think about changes in your life that you have already experienced, or may experience in the future – changes that can have relevant financial and investment planning implications.

$UMMARY $UCCESS $TRATEGY

TO CONQUER INVESTING MISTAKE #16:

Change your investments when your personal situation or goals change substantially. If you experience a major life event, such as having a baby, getting married, or starting a business, assess whether your investments need updating.

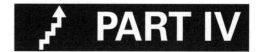

PART IV

SELLING SNAFUS

MISTAKE 17

NOT HAVING A SELL STRATEGY

There comes a time when every investor, from the novice to the sophisticated professional, must confront this question: Should I sell or should I hold?

For a lot of investors, this is one of the most agonizing decisions they make. It's so agonizing, in fact, that some don't make a decision at all – or they do so only by default. They *know* they should sell, or they *think* they should, but somehow they can't bring themselves to do so.

Indeed, the whole area of selling seems to be the greatest source of anxiety for investors. There's good news and bad news on this front. The bad news is that selling mistakes can cost you a fortune.

The good news is that you can conquer this problem. Over the course of the next few chapters, I'll tell you how. Before I do, though, a few observations.

Investors who lack a sell strategy are baffled about what investments to sell and why. Fear and other emotions guide their decisions. They often follow the herd and make poor decisions, such as dumping a stock prematurely or selling amid a market panic.

After considering your personal needs, investment philosophy and leanings, come up with a set of rules to guide why, when and under what circumstances you will sell a stock.

This creation of a selling strategy must be done at the outset – prior to buying a stock!

If more investors followed this simple rule, they would have a lot easier time down the road in determining when to hang on to investments and when to let them go.

For those stocks, bonds, currencies or other investments you already own, establish a sell strategy now to guide decision-making going forward.

And plan to give your selling strategy the proper time and attention it deserves.

> A study by Roper/Ameritrade survey found that consumers spend an average of 7.6 hours researching each investment they purchase. But precious little time and thought are given to the sell decision.

Some experts believe that almost any carefully thought out strategy can be workable. The key is to have some pre-established idea of what you will do, when you would do it, and why, under various circumstances. Of course, no one has a crystal ball. So your sell strategy isn't supposed to cover every possible scenario. But by and large, you should be able to assert what you would do given, say, a big run-up in your investments or big losses as well. When financial markets experience extreme volatility, as has been the case for the past decade, having a selling strategy becomes even more important. Otherwise, the topsy-turvy nature of the market may cause you to act impetuously.

Intellectually, most investors know that selling amid a market panic is a bad idea. Nevertheless, many people fall victim to this blunder. Often times, when broad based selling is occurring, it's because the individuals involved didn't have a plan. As a result, they are just following the herd.

But if you take a look at past stock-market trends, it's plain to see that dumping stock in a market sell-off typically has been a wrong move. The reason is because most investors don't know when to jump back into the markets. And those investors who pulled out of the financial markets after big market declines lost out in a big way.

> For example, if you stayed invested in the S&P 500 Index for the entire 2,528 trading days from 1980 through 1989, you would've racked up 17.5% average annual returns. But if you pulled out of just 10 of the best trading days during that decade, your average annual return got chopped down to 12.6%. People who missed the best 40 days during that 10-year span had a return of just 3.9%, according to Ibbotson Associates.

This is not to suggest that no matter what, you should always stay fully invested in equities – even when you are not comfortable doing so. On the contrary, your selling strategy should also fit nicely with your overall investing game plan. In other words, you should be able to sleep at night with whatever sell strategy you devise, as it pertains to your risk tolerance, time invested in the market, and so on.

Some smart selling strategies include employing 30-day moving averages, using stop-loss mechanisms, and relying on fundamental research, among others. When you use a stock's 30-day moving average as a guidepost for selling, you sell when it consistently falls below its trend, that 30-day average. Some investors also use 60 and 90-day moving averages to guide them.

A stop-loss mechanism helps to make selling automatic. And that's a big plus for many investors. A stop order puts a "floor" or a "ceiling" that defines when you will sell a security. So, if you buy a stock at $25 a share, you might put a floor at $17.50. What this means is that you're not willing to lose any more than 30% of your money. So if that $25 stock fell by $7.50 (or 30%) to $17.50, a sell order would automatically be triggered. On the upside, you could also put in a 30% ceiling. In this case, if the stock hits $32.50 a sell order would also be instantly triggered, letting you lock in your profits. Other people have less technical, though equally effective methods for investing successfully at the selling phase.

An example comes from trader Susan Kingsbury, who lives near Salt Lake City, Utah. In discussing her selling strategy, she once told me that she's able to sell her losing investments because she views them simply as "a cost of doing business." In that way, Kingsbury suggested she's able to take her lumps when need be without feeling so emotionally wracked over her decision to sell.

Here are three web sites that can help you calculate when it's time to sell a stock:

www.dynamictaxoptimizer.com

www.quicken.com

www.networthstrategies.com

Dynamic Tax Optimizer is a finance and accounting calculator engine that aids you in making selling decisions by showing you which decisions will result in the optimal after-tax returns. David Gottstein, head of Anchorage, Alaska-based Dynamic Capital Management, believes the tax-loss harvesting feature his firm offers makes it of particular value to investors who are deciding what to sell and when.

Another company, Smart Leaf (*www.smartleaf.com*) makes software that it sells to financial services professionals. That software helps your advisor recommend when a stock should be sold and when it should be kept. Smart Leaf CEO and founder Jerry Michael once explained to me that in making any educated sell decision, you really have to balance risk, taxes, your own estimate of future returns, as well as expenses.

$UMMARY $UCCESS $TRATEGY
TO CONQUER INVESTING MISTAKE# 17:

Create a selling strategy prior to actually purchasing any investment. Know in advance when you will sell a stock that rises, and when you will dump an investment that is tanking.

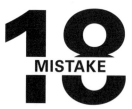

MISTAKE

18

FAILING TO STICK WITH YOUR
SELL STRATEGY

Frank Owen, the head of FR Owen & Associates in Charlotte, North Carolina, has been in business for nearly 25 years. He has 1,500 clients, most of them schoolteachers who work with kindergarten to 12th grade students. Like the bulk of the American public, these busy teachers "are not illiterate, but they are financially uninformed," says Owen.

Many of Owen's clients need help planning for retirement. For some, that means planning 30 years into the future. As a result, Owen tries to get his clients to think long-term.

For many investors who sell at the wrong time, Owen says it's because they're looking in the rear view mirror. "They need to focus on what's going to happen instead of what has happened," he says.

Owen also believes it's human nature to get scared about investing. Even for those people who do have a plan, "they tend to forget it when times get tough. That's partially the fault of the client, but also of the advisor who may not communicate regularly about the plan," Owen says.

"GUT INSTINCTS" ARE NO STRATEGY

It might be tempting to hang onto a losing investment because your "gut instincts" tells you to, or based on later research you've done that makes you think that a poor-performing stock will rebound. It may, in fact, come back. But don't wait around for it. Stick with your established game plan for consistency, investment discipline and, ultimately, the best overall investment performance. This way you won't have to say, "I coulda, woulda, shoulda" later on.

Investors who abandon their established sell strategy become undisciplined, suffer inconsistent or poor portfolio performance, and are more likely to sell at the wrong time for the wrong reasons.

That's what Owen has frequently witnessed. He says he's seen highly impressive looking action plans, all done up nicely with pretty graphics and printed on laser paper. It's a nice package, but it's little more than window dressing if the advice isn't followed. "You can get as fancy as you want to be. But if you don't implement the plan, it's just words on a piece of paper," Owen says.

To help you stick with your selling strategy, I recommend that you ask yourself the following three questions before you get rid of an investment:

1. Are my actions in keeping with my pre-established sell criteria?

2. Has this investment ceased to serve my investment needs?

3. Do I have a better, alternative investment in mind into which I can quickly place my money?

If the answers to all three questions are "YES," that's a good candidate to be sold from your portfolio.

Whatever happens, don't reverse course mid-way through your investing game plan and try to alter your selling game plan just to fit one individual stock that you don't want to sell. Neither should you get "trigger happy" just because the market falls unexpectedly. As long as your stop-loss limit hasn't been reached, or as long as the reason you bought a stock or a fund remains valid, you should probably hang onto that stock. Otherwise, you're defeating the whole purpose of having a written sell strategy. It's a guide that will improve your investing results with discipline and consistency.

$UMMARY $UCCESS $TRATEGY
TO CONQUER INVESTING MISTAKE #18:

Stick to your sell strategy. Don't abandon your game plan. Use stop-loss orders, and keep your strategy in black-and-white before you to remind you of your plans. Only sell, both winning and losing investments, according to your pre-set selling criteria.

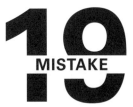

MISTAKE

LETTING YOUR EMOTIONS RULE
YOUR DECISION-MAKING PROCESS

One of the best things about the human body is that it works so marvelously – and when it doesn't, it gives us messages that something has gone afoul. When your body gets overworked, for example, you feel tired and a little achy – some signs that you need to take it easy. More serious aches and pains or chronic fatigue are your signals that perhaps you should go see a doctor. In short, when something is wrong with your body, you literally get a "bad feeling." Maybe that's why physicians use the word "disease" (translate: dis-ease) to describe the ailment or discomfort sick patients feel.

If only investing was that simple.

When investors get a pain in their gut – or any kind of "gut feeling" at all – more often than not heeding that feeling brings disaster, not relief. The reason? Acting on a "gut feeling" means you're letting your emotions guide your decision-making process. When this happens, you inevitably make poor choices, experts agree.

Want to know one of the most common "gut feelings" that emotion-wracked investors experience? It's the strong yet unfounded belief that a downtrodden stock will miraculously rebound and come back from some precipitous decline. But "most investors, I'm afraid, have a pretty slap-dash idea of what a stock's upside is," Harvard University finance professor Samuel Hayes once told me. He says part of the reason for investors' unrealistic expectations about a stock's future performance is that people get stuck thinking about the company's price history – something that has no bearing on how well the company will perform in the future.

If you're among those investors saying: "I'll sell when the stock comes back," just remember that any investment that has lost 50% of its value has to climb 100% to get back to break-even status. That's a tall order in any market condition.

Donn Sharer, a former vice president of financial services at MetLife, has an interesting hypothesis about what happens to people who buy stocks, and then watch their investments go down the tubes. In a nutshell, his theory is that people who lose money in the stock market go through stages not unlike individuals coming to grips with the death of a family member or loved one.

"It kind of mirrors the grieving process: there's denial, sadness, anger — all those emotions," Sharer theorizes. Sharer is no psychologist. But he may be on to something when it comes to the way investors behave when faced with a blow to their pocketbooks.

Experts long ago discovered that putting money at risk – and especially selling an investment – brings to the surface an array of emotional issues for investors. Ironically, you're just as likely to experience emotional bouts over selling winning investments as you are about selling losing ones. But those emotions must be overcome.

When emotions dictate your investing decisions, faulty judgment kicks in, impulsive behavior often emerges, and financial losses result. Being guided by emotions also leads to heightened anxiety about the investing process, sleepless nights, and obsessing over investments.

Greed and fear are two of the most dominant emotions you have to guard against. "There really is even a physiological issue surrounding fear, especially fear of loss. Fear is centered out of the brain stem, so it's very primal and much more intense," says Deanna Tillisch of Northwestern Mutual.

Feelings of loyalty, guilt and sentimentality are other common emotional barriers that get in the way of making smart selling decisions. Perhaps you inherited a stock from a parent or grandparent and feel obligated to keep it. Some investors hang onto losing stock because they don't want to hurt the feelings of their broker or their spouse who recommended it. Or maybe you work for a large company where everyone else buys company stock, so you fall in step – even though the investment doesn't suit your needs. Or maybe you *used* to work for the company and holding onto those shares makes you feel as if you're still "a part of the team" at your former employer.

No matter what, though, emotions have no role in your investment portfolio.

Needless to say, there's no magic wand, good luck charm or special pill you can take to get those emotions in check. (That's probably for the best, since such a thing would foster its own set of investment mistakes … as if we don't have enough issues to tackle!)

The best way to conquer your emotions while investing is to have a sell strategy, as described in Chapter 17. But there are some other things you can do to overcome the numerous and inevitable emotions that bubble up during the investing process.

DO YOU NEED PROFESSIONAL HELP?

One obvious solution is to hire a professional to take over the selling decisions for you. This may be absolutely necessary if you're one of those people who not only "falls in love with" an investment, but also "gets married" to it, blinded by it, and starts to believe the investment can do no wrong! If this scenario accurately describes you, divorce yourself from the process by retaining the services of a trustworthy, competent money manager. It may take some getting used to at first. But in the long run, you'll be glad you made the switch.

THE BUDDY SYSTEM

For those of you who bristle at the thought of paying a professional advisor and letting that person call the shots, another option is to enlist the help of a friend as an investment partner. That was an idea once suggested to me by Rishi Narang, then president and vice chairman of Tradeworx, a New York financial analytics firm. "When you have a trading partner, you tell each other what your plan is and the other guy's job is to hold you to it," said Narang, who uses this method with a pal he's known for a dozen years.

It's a good thing he adopted the buddy system, too, because Narang was married in July 2002. Before the "Big Day," he actively bought and sold stocks in a trading account he established to help pay for the wedding. But he always knew that his wife "would kill me if I lost too much money," Narang said jokingly. On a more serious note, any stock in that wedding-fund account that fell 5% immediately got sold because of a 5% stop-loss rule to which Narang adheres.

Occasionally, though, when a stock declines 5%, Narang doesn't want to cut bait. That's when his trading buddy steps in. "He tells me what I already know," Narang said, which is to unload the stock immediately, in accordance with his plan. Having a trading partner "makes a huge difference," according to Narang. "It's the same thing as having a spotter or a coach."

If you think you could benefit from a black-and-white reminder about your sell strategy — but not necessarily another person's involvement — an "investment policy statement" may be in order. "It's just a guiding document that articulates the specific goals of your investment plan, how much risk is acceptable, and the range of what you can invest in any asset class," explains Robert Wolfe, a CERTIFIED FINANCIAL PLANNER™ practitioner at Capital Planning Group in Fort Lauderdale, Fla.

In years past, only very wealthy individuals, families and pension plans used investment policy statements. Nowadays, smart investors in all income-brackets create their own investment policy statements. Wolfe uses them with all his clients because they "help take emotion out of the mix." As a financial advisor, "You have to be half technician and half psychologist these days," he believes.

A final strategy for dealing with the emotional roller coaster that investing throws us all on is to track your behavior in hopes of improving it.

Richard Geist is president of the Newton, Mass.-based Institute of Psychology and Investing, which researches the psychological aspects of financial decision-making.

Geist says that people "tend to make the same mistakes over and over."

"It may be helpful to write down what happened around the mistakes," counsels Geist, who is also a clinical instructor in the department of psychiatry at Harvard Medical School. "A few months later people often see a pattern," in their decision-making, he adds.

Geist figures that once people recognize how and why their faulty logic or poor judgment creeps in, they can begin to reverse those trends and become better investors.

Don't be guided by greed, fear of loss, sentimentality, guilt or any other emotion. The best antidote to these powerful emotions is having a sell strategy (See advice in Chapter 17). But you can also enlist the help of an investing buddy to help you stick to your investment game plan. Some people may have to hire a pro, and turn over to that person the responsibility of deciding when to sell various investments. This is advisable if you can't divorce yourself from the investing process because you find yourself "getting married" to a stock, bond or other investment.

It's also helpful to formulate an "investment policy statement," a black-and-white reminder of how you're supposed to be investing, what you're supposed to be investing in and under what circumstances you should sell.

Whatever you do, make a promise to yourself that from this day forward you will no longer base your sell decisions on impulses, hunches, or other emotional whims. Just remember that listening to your body is a great rule of thumb in medicine. But in investing, relying on that "gut feeling" can be hazardous to your wealth – a situation that just may cause you to really bust a gut.

$UMMARY $UCCESS $TRATEGY
TO CONQUER INVESTING MISTAKE #19:

Let your head, not your emotions, rule your decision-making process. Try to keep fear and greed in check. They can cause you to make irrational decisions.

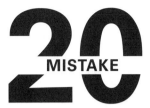

REFUSING TO ADMIT YOU MADE
A MISTAKE AND TO MOVE ON

Investors too stubborn to admit their mistakes often suffer the steepest losses of all. They hang onto losing investments for far too long, they stick with failing companies even as they fall into bankruptcy, and they throw off their asset allocation strategy. These investors may also adopt a demoralized, defeatist attitude about investing.

Does this sound like you?

If so, you've got to change your outlook.

Don't be stubborn. Cut your losses by using trigger points to sell declining securities. And forget about trying to "break even" on every single investment. Remember that savvy investors consider first their overall portfolio's performance. They focus on absolute returns. Then they worry about the individual stocks, bonds and other components. Finally, smart investors don't always make up their losses in the same place they got them. They "break even" by selling losing investments and replacing them with better-performing ones.

I remember one investor from Maryland I once interviewed. This retired gentleman refused to sell a stock, Plantronics, and had suffered big losses in the process. He bought the stock for around $50 a share in early 2000. A year later, it had fallen to $16. Headquartered in Santa Cruz, Calif., Plantronics makes earphone pieces and telephone headsets. As of June 2003, the stock changed hands for around $22. This investor thought his investment would be a sure winner. But he later came to think of it, in his words, as a "dog" in his portfolio. Still, he never sold the stock. He said he was waiting for the market to turn around and "validate" his belief in Plantronics.

I'm certainly not suggesting that Plantronics won't turn around. (This is, after all the company that made the headset that astronaut Neil Armstrong used to broadcast his famous "One small step for man" transmission from the moon in the 1969. And today, Plantronics is a leader in supplying hands-free devices for cell phones, something a growing number of states are requiring of drivers nationwide). What I am asserting though, is that this gentleman bought the stock with expectations of getting immediate double-digit growth. And three years later, that still hadn't happened.

"If you have cancer in an arm, you cut it out to save the rest of the body," reasons money manager and hedge fund expert Daniel Strachman. "The problem is, most investors don't want to do that."

Sometimes it can be tough to reverse course and change directions. Have you ever been in a car with a driver who was clearly lost, but he or she refused to stop and ask for directions? Just like that person could soon get back on the right road with a little proper guidance, so too could investors who make a u-turn when they realize they've gone the wrong way.

TAKE SOME SOLACE

If you are willing to sell your losers, at least you might take some solace in getting out of a losing position the right way. Nick Hodges, the CPA from Fullerton, CA, recommends carrying forward your loss for up to 15 years, as the law allows, or using it to offset capital gains.

Some people "also have real estate," he notes. "Offset those gains with stock losses," he advises.

You should also realize that it's O.K. to admit your investing mistakes – they will happen. The more important thing is: what are you doing to do about them? That's where your mettle as a serious and savvy investor gets tested.

"Everybody wants to talk about what they did right. You know, the cocktail party chatter where people claim to have made brilliant investments," says David Winters, chairman of the Mutual Series Funds. "But most people are never straight enough to say 'Hey, I did this wrong.'"

Not so for Winters, who makes a point to disclose to shareholders what went right – and wrong – in any given year.

Asked about investing mistakes he's made, Winters said: "We're cheapskates, and sometimes we've not been willing to pay up for stocks." As a result, he added, some good prospects "have gotten away from us."

But with the Mutual Series Funds' international funds posting three and five-year returns of 8-9%, most of the firm's shareholders are no doubt pleased with their overall results.

$UMMARY $UCCESS $TRATEGY
TO CONQUER INVESTING MISTAKE #20:

Admit your mistakes and move on. Don't waste time and money on investments that are clearly money-losing propositions. And don't justify hanging onto a sour investment by saying "I'll sell when it comes back." Some quick math: any stock that falls 50% must then rise 100% to break even.

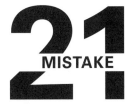

MISTAKE 21

MISSING OPPORTUNITIES
TO TAKE PROFITS

Investors who neglect to book their gains at the correct time rank among the most anguished of investors. In the bull market, many of these people owned stocks that generated tremendous profits. But these investors never saw one penny of those gains. It was sort of like they won the lottery jackpot, but wouldn't cash in their winning ticket. Worse still, some investors held out for even bigger gains only to watch their investments turn sour, resulting in financial losses.

Avoid the temptation to be greedy. Sell when you reach a pre-established target. For example, your investment has doubled or you've reached a required dollar amount for a specific goal such as saving for your kid's college education.

Realize that booking gains is part of adhering to a winning investment strategy. So don't fret too much over the prospect that you "might miss out" on future gains. Rather, look at selling opportunities where you've made a profit as indications that you are meeting your personal and financial objectives.

And remember the advice of financial expert Denis Walsh, of Money Concepts. Most of his clients are people in their 40s and 50s. They've often left a job or are between jobs. They're seeking help with their 401(k) because they've never had such a big chunk of money to invest for themselves.

The thing he sees happening is that some stocks perform almost "too well." By that, he explains: "It's almost automatic that if you have four or five types of investments, and one of them outperforms the market, (clients) will be resistant to taking some of those monies and moving it elsewhere."

In fact the investor's automatic reaction will be to put more money into the one fund that did well, according to Walsh. So he find himself fighting the client's urge to "go with something that's great."

At the same time, he has to explain to the client that the *more* a stock vastly outperforms the market or its industry, the *less* likely it is that such out-performance will continue in the future. So like many advisors, a big part of Walsh's job is educational. Money Concepts has 750 representatives around the country – – as well as affiliates in Ireland, Canada, New Zealand, and 40 regional offices. CPAs and tax professionals run about one-third of these offices. CERTIFIED FINANCIAL PLANNER™ professionals and other financial specialists head the rest.

TAKE THE MONEY AND RUN!

Even when investors sell for a sizeable profit, however, they sometimes second guess themselves. That was the case with Lara Oyetunde, who initially considered herself a "very conservative" investor.

For Oyetunde, that entailed being properly diversified, buying only mutual funds, and investing for the long-term. But amid the Internet craze of 1999, Oyetunde became intrigued by the possibility of making much bigger profits with individual stocks. So that summer, she dove into the equities market, buying shares of Intel for $57.25 apiece and Yahoo for $159 a share.

For several months thereafter, Yahoo traded all over the place, wreaking havoc on Oyetunde's nerves. "It was kind of fun, but definitely nerve-wracking," she said of the experience. She ultimately sold Yahoo for $184 a share. And by November 1999, she let her Intel shares go for $79.95 each. When Yahoo later shot up to about $205, Oyetunde regretted her decision. She said she was just getting comfortable with trusting her investing instincts but "panicked" and sold too early.

In hindsight, she likely made the right choice given the bear market that was to come beginning in early 2000.

$UMMARY $UCCESS $TRATEGY
TO CONQUER INVESTING MISTAKE #21:

Take your profits when the opportunity arises. Again, don't be greedy. Nor should you take money off the table prematurely. Use your sell strategy as a guide.

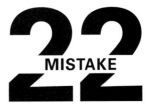

MISTAKE 22

EXCESSIVE TRADING

I know some people who visit the mall practically every other day – and then these shopaholics wonder why their credit card bills are so high. The same could be said for some investors. They engage in a form of shopping excess as well, in this case excessive trading of stocks, mutual funds, or other investments.

But trading too frequently leads to a number of problems: the generation of high commissions, short-term capital gains taxes, and portfolio under-performance.

To avoid this mistake, buy only well-researched securities. Buy only when you can truly afford it. Avoid getting a margin loan just because you're itching to get in on a "once in lifetime" deal. Buy only after you've carefully considered the risks involved; and buy only when you're positive the investment complements your existing portfolio and doesn't duplicate some holdings you already own. On the back end, sell only as per your pre-designed sell strategy. That's the best way to avoid excessive trading.

If you won't take my word for it, consider the story of a former day-trader I know who traded at the height of the Internet bubble. She had been a successful stockbroker at a major Wall Street brokerage before she took $50,000 of her money to begin full-time day-trading in 1998. She quickly learned how active trading resulted in stiff fees. By the time she stopped trading, she'd lost $18,630. Of that total, $15,040 was in commissions and execution expenses.

RESEARCH ON TRADING AND GENDER

University of California professor Terrance Odean also says over-trading affects the testosterone laden (that's you men out there!) more than the feminine sex. According to Odean's research, men trade 45% more actively than do women. Single men traded 67% more actively than single women. As a result, single women fared better performance wise – some 2.3 percentage points better per year over single men. Overall, women got better returns than men, 1.4 percentage points higher, according to Odean's research.

His findings were drawn from a study that Odean and another colleague did in which they examined 150,000 accounts from a discount broker and studied the trading patterns from 1991 through 1997. They found that on average, women achieve better returns than do men because women trade less often.

Odean also discovered that online trading has, predictably, led to people trading more frequently. In 1998, the number of online brokerage accounts stood at roughly 5 million. As of 2003, that figure quadrupled to an estimated 20.4 million online accounts, managing more than $3 trillion online, according to Forrester Research.

USE THE WEB THE RIGHT WAY

No one is suggesting that you stop any online trading in which you might engage. In fact, the web can be a tremendously valuable place to learn, educate yourself about investing, and cut costs too.

But since it's faster, easier and cheaper to trade online (and more thrilling as well, some investors say), just realize that you may be tempted to do a bit more armchair trading than is wise. For most people, the temptation to over-trade won't be too hard to resist because of their busy schedules and a million other matters to which they must attend. Perhaps that's why, according to Odean's research, it's the single crowd, especially unmarried males, that are most likely to spend excessive time at the computer screen trading.

Portfolio turnover rates are also very telling. Women tend to turnover their portfolio an average of 53% a year, while men did it at a rate of 77% a year. Part of Odean's research showed that people had been beating the market by about 2 percentage points a year before they moved online. And once they started online trading, they typically under-performed the market by more than 3 percentage points.

THE ONLINE TRADING BOOM

There are roughly 100 online brokerage firms in the U.S. with millions customer accounts, according to Gomez Advisors, a Concord, Mass., consulting firm. Professional day traders, however, number between 3,500 and 4,000 people nationwide, according to industry estimates. (Of course, this doesn't include traders who work for brokerage firms).

The head of a major day-trading group also once said that the vast majority of day traders lose money during their first four to six months. The losses typically range from $10,000 to $50,000.

In January 1999, Momentum Securities Management Co., one of the largest professional day trading firms in the U.S. released a survey about day-trading performance. The three month survey, which collected data from 107 traders in Momentum's six Texas offices, revealed that 58% of newcomers lost an average of $21,479. On a brighter note, nearly two-thirds of traders who got past a three-to-five month "learning curve" made an average of $28,426, the study said.

Critics of the survey argued that it didn't disclose how many traders actually made it through that initial three-month period. And some regulators say at least 80% of day traders lose money.

As a reminder, for most of you, adopt a long-term strategy to guide you through the investing process. Blow-by-blow trading in the markets should be reserved for only the most sophisticated of investors, people who trade for a living.

$UMMARY $UCCESS $TRATEGY
TO CONQUER INVESTING MISTAKE #22:

Trade less frequently. People who over-trade tend to make poor investment decisions and invest impulsively. Excessive trading can also frequently cause you to pay more commissions and more taxes to Uncle Sam.

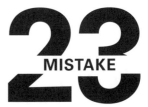

NOT TAKING TAXES INTO CONSIDERATION

The next chapter in this book will look at investors who place too much emphasis on taxes. At the other end of the spectrum are investors who give no thought whatsoever to taxes. This, too, is a mistake. Investors who don't take taxes into consideration wind up paying the government more taxes than necessary. They could have often saved a bundle with just a bit of planning or a little more patience.

Look at the pre- and post-tax ramifications of any investment decision: whether that decision is to buy, hold or sell. Recognize the benefits of paying long-term capital gains taxes, which currently top out at 20%. By contrast, depending on an investor's tax bracket, short-term gains can be taxed at a rate of nearly 40%, notes Lehman Brothers tax expert Robert Willens.

It may sound silly to say this, but one thing you should consider – especially if you plan to sell a large chunk of stock — is whether or not you'll actually have the money to pay any large tax bill. You don't want to get a big surprise from the government after April 15th.

CPA Nick Hodges can tick off a litany of tax mistakes he's seen investors make.

One of the biggies, according to Hodges, is not having any year-end planning with your financial intermediaries, in order to coordinate year-end stock sales and harvest the appropriate losses. It doesn't matter if you've not been diligent enough to do this in the past, or if your broker or planner hasn't been diligent enough in doing so, the fact remains: from now on, you're going to be responsible for making sure it gets done.

Hodges also sees some people who refuse to sell individual stock positions for fear of paying capital gains taxes. So what happens? The person rides the stock all the way down. They do avoid paying capital gains, but they also eliminated all the profits that could've helped pay those capital gains. For example, say you bought 500 shares of a stock at $35 a share, and one year later it rose to $56. With a proper sell strategy, after a 60% run-up you would probably be inclined to sell some of this stock and lock in your profits. But what if you didn't just because you didn't want to pay taxes? Well, now let's assume that your stock started to fall – and fall sharply. If it dropped back down to $35, you've lost a gross profit of $10,500 (500 shares X $21 a share price increase). If you paid a 20% capital gains tax on that $10,500, you'd give up $2,100 and keep $8,400. But by failing to sell, and watching the stock crash back to $35, you lose all your profit. Even worse, if the stock goes down to, say $22, you've incurred a loss.

Now which is better: to lose money, to "break even" or to net an $8,400 profit? Look at it this way: By taking your profits at the prudent time, you effectively use the gains you generate to pay the requisite taxes.

Another example of a tax-related investing mistake, as mentioned earlier in Chapter 7, is putting the right investments in the wrong accounts. Hodges knew of a fund in which there were over $300,000 worth of tax-exempt bonds inside of Individual Retirement Accounts. Again, the investors effectively took tax-free income and turned it into taxable income. Here's a brief example of a retirement-related investing mistake that occurred when the investor didn't properly consider tax consequences.

IN THEIR OWN WORDS:
INVESTORS SHARE LESSONS LEARNED

> My biggest investing error was converting my Individual Retirement Account to a Roth IRA at the very height of the market. That meant I paid taxes for four years on its highest-ever value, while it fell to half that amount in that time.
>
> John Voelcker

MUTUAL FUND RELATED TAX ERRORS

Have you ever erred in exchanging from one mutual fund to another fund within the same fund family? Unbeknownst to you, this exchange could create an unexpected capital gains tax when you think it's a tax-free exchange. So be careful here.

A final blunder: don't make the mistake of viewing your IRA as your short-term piggy bank. You probably know that you can get a tax deduction, subject to income limitations, on money you put into a regular IRA account. But what happens if you deposit money you can't really afford – just so you can save taxes? If you make a contribution you can't truly afford, you'll later likely tap the account, get hit with a 10% penalty, as well as have to pay ordinary income rates on the funds you withdrew.

$UMMARY $UCCESS $TRATEGY

TO CONQUER INVESTING MISTAKE #23:

Consider the tax implications of any selling decision. Ideally, you should hold a security more than 12 months to get favorable capital gains treatment. Any capital investment you own for less than 12 months is taxed at ordinary income rates, which are usually much higher.

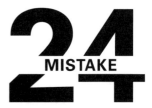

WORRYING TOO MUCH ABOUT TAXES

Is there any one out there who relishes paying taxes?

If so, I don't know him. The one blessing about paying taxes, of course, is the fact that since you owe them, that means there was some income on which to base those taxes. That's a plus. Besides that, however, I'm going to assume most of you are like me: you want to pay the least amount of taxes that is possible – and legal, of course!

If you are a high net worth individual, or if you own stock options, and you want more information about increasing your after-tax returns, a wonderful web site to use is *www.myStockOptions.com*. Run by Bruce Brumberg, a stock options expert who also has a background in securities law, myStockOptions.com offers you all the ins and outs of the tax ramifications of owning, holding or excercising incentive stock options and Non-qualified stock options.

One of the key messages consistently delivered by Brumberg, and the experts who write for his site, is that taxes should not drive your decisions. Ever.

To make the best buy, hold and selling decisions, you must first consider whether the investment makes solid financial sense – in terms of potential performance, risk to you, and so forth. Tax considerations, while very important, should nevertheless come second.

But this is one of those rules that no matter how many times you try to drive the message home to investors, many people simply won't listen. Please don't make that mistake.

Countless investors hang onto to stocks they should sell because of a fear of paying taxes. But this flawed thinking makes investors own the wrong investments for far too long. In many cases where a stock subsequently falls in value, investors would have been better off simply making whatever tax payments were due.

Don't let the tax tail wag the dog. First pick the most prudent investment strategy and individual investments. Then weigh the tax implications. In the long run, the returns you get from making good investment choices will outweigh any money you must fork over to Uncle Sam.

STRATEGIC IDEAS TO CUT TAXES

From a strategic standpoint, it's also a good idea to think about how to get the best after-tax returns from the investments you buy in the future.

Many experts think that the May 2003 tax cut passed by Congress on dividends will make dividend-paying stocks more attractive. Don't, however, expect the tax cut to juice up your near-term returns. Instead, the long-term (and more lasting) benefit to you will likely occur if publicly-traded companies start to increase their dividends. If that happens, those dividend-paying stocks will be highly sought after, especially since for years dividends have been getting slashed or eliminated altogether a few more ideas:

- You can get Standard & Poor's Earnings and Dividend Rankings on more than 3,400 U.S. companies through Standard & Poor's Stock Reports. S&P says the information is available through the 120,000 investment advisors and brokers that subscribe to Stock Reports, as well as through investor web sites sponsored by brokerage firms.

- Also, check out the American Association of Individual Investors' Guide to Dividend Reinvestment Plans. AAII members receive the guide free of charge each June. The publication explains how you can use the dividend reinvestment programs of hundreds of companies to buy additional stock at no commission. AAII is an independent, non-profit corporation formed in 1978. Its mission is to help individual investors learn to manage their own assets through education, research and information.

- Another strategy to consider is buying iShares, which have become tremendously popular. The reason investors like them is because they're good at reducing taxes and cutting costs. There are nearly 80 iShares funds segmented by sector, country, market cap, or investing style. For more information, call 800-iSHARES or log onto the web at *www.iShares.com*. iShares are offered through Barclays Global Investors.

- Add municipal bonds to your portfolio if you don't already own some. They are free from federal taxes, and in many parts of the country they are also exempt from state taxes. High net worth individuals, in particular, should have municipal bonds in their portfolios for tax-reduction purposes.

- A handful of companies now offer online services to help investors easily figure out the tax consequences of their investment choices. NetWorthStrategies.com of Bend, Oregon, which sells a product call StockOpter, is one such business. Dynamic Capital Management of Anchorage, Alaska is another. The latter company, owned by money manager David Gottstein, has a patented system called DynamicTaxOptimizer that helps investors figure out the best time to sell a stock or book losses for tax purposes.

One other tip: Some tax averse investors may be considering borrowing money from your broker (getting a margin loan) in order to exercise and hold onto stock options. Here's a word to the wise: Don't do it. In most cases you're better off using other funds.

$UMMARY $UCCESS $TRATEGY

TO CONQUER INVESTING MISTAKE #24:

Don't worry too much about taxes. Take taxes into account; but they shouldn't be the driving force behind your decisions. Any investment you buy or sell should make economic and rational investment sense first. Tax considerations are secondary.

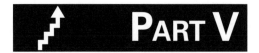

PART V

FINANCIAL ADVISOR FOUL-UPS

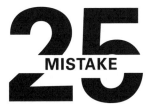

OMITTING INDEPENDENT RESEARCH

We all know someone who loves to have designer clothing or brand name goods. Some people are lured by advertising come-ons. Other consumers have a desire to "keep up with the Joneses." For whatever reason, many of these individuals wouldn't dream of shopping at retail outlets where they can't purchase items that don't have a recognized label of some sort.

Interestingly, this "bigger is better" kind of thinking seems to extend from Main Street to Wall Street. Many investors who are looking for financial research, information and advice also automatically flock to the biggest, most well-known investment firms and brokerages. In most cases, these institutions have been around for many decades and are household names.

As a rule of thumb, it certainly is good practice to consider doing business with established institutions from any industry. After all, you have to figure that if a company has been around 50 years or more, it's probably been doing something right. But the problem with this logic in the financial services world is that all too often many investors have an automatic tendency to seek counsel, products and services *only* from the major Wall Street players. In particular, some investors rely solely on Wall Street research, while completely disregarding (often to their detriment) independent financial services firms that also have a lot to offer.

> Think about your own situation for a minute. Whom do you rely on for investment research? For many of you, the answer will be that you are using a big Wall Street outfit, a company known in the industry as a "bulge bracket" firm.

If this describes you, I want you to think about other options available to you. My goal here is not to make you yank all your money from the investment firm where you accounts are now held or to not buy research from that firm. Rather, I simply want to you to be aware of the dangers of relying on any single source of information. Moreover, I want you to discover the tremendous benefits of using independent research. And finally, I want you to realize that while many independent research shops may be "off brand" names, and not familiar to you, this doesn't make then second-rate in terms of quality. In fact, many of them regularly produce research that rivals their larger peers.

I believe that depending too heavily on Wall Street analysts, even well-known ones, can sometimes cause the average investor to buy an investment – and especially to sell it – at the wrong time. It can also lead to an individual purchasing inappropriate securities that don't meet their needs. Investors who rely unduly on Wall Street pros are often simply following the pack, and jumping in too late on supposedly "good" investments.

To avoid these mistakes, here are some key points to keep in mind.

- **Be discriminating in how you view research.**

    In general, look critically at Wall Street research when the firm has an investment banking relationship with the company it is covering. In an ideal world, there is supposed to be a "Chinese Wall" that separates the invest-ment banking side of a brokerage firm's operations from its research division. In reality, however, this is sometimes not the case. And critics say some brokerages may not be as critical of companies they cover, when the brokerage firm wants to underwrite initial public offerings (IPOs) or do mergers and acquisition work, and other advisory services for that corporation. A 2002 BusinessWeek cover story, dubbed "The Investor Betrayed," cited research conflicts of interest and several Wall Street scandals as reasons why investors no longer trusted many brokerages. Indeed, as of June 2003, investors had won a proposed $1 billion settlement from 309 companies that issued IPOs in the late 1990s. These companies, mainly telecommunica-tions companies and Internet businesses, were widely touted by Wall Street analysts.

• **Know how to really interpret Wall Street research**

Only 1% of all analyst recommendations are sell ratings, according to First Call, which tracks corporate earnings. Logic alone tells you that of all the thousands of publicly-traded companies that are rated by analysts, way more than 1% of them should be considered "sell" candidates. So understand that many Wall Street ratings are inflated, according to Chuck Hill, research chief at First Call. Thus, "strong buy" means buy the stock, "buy" means "hold," and "hold" really means "sell," says Hill.

• **If you have the time and desire, do much of your own due diligence.**

Otherwise, pay a trusted broker, financial planner or ad-visor. Develop a relationship with that person - and hold him or her accountable for investing recommendations. (For more information on how to do that, see Chapter 27).

Also, if you do start to seriously do your own research, keep in mind the following list of "red flags" in company announcements, quarterly corporate earnings reports, or any SEC filings:

- a "going concern" notation from an auditor
- big drops in revenues or profits
- lawsuits that could potentially be very costly
- wholesale management shake-ups

ANALYSTS REMAIN OPTIMISTIC

A *Wall Street Journal* article from February 2003 noted that most Wall Street analysts remained unshaken in their unbridled optimism about stocks. In short, most of the analysts rating stocks offered the belief that those companies would post above-average, double-digit growth over the next several years. These predictions fly in the face of the fact that corporate earnings historically grow at about the same rate as the overall economy over time. And 10%-plus growth is nowhere on the radar screen for the U.S. economy in the near future. Still, analysts expected 345 companies in the S&P 500 Index to boost their earnings by more than 10% a year during the next three to five years. Another 123 companies were seen growing their earnings by more than 15%.

It would be great if these forecasts came true. But it seems like a long-shot that this will happen for many of these companies. Again, I'm not suggesting that analysts have no clue in their forecasts. As a note, for instance, soon after the *Wall Street Journal* article, stock prices surged tremendously. After hitting it's low on March 11, 2003 the market staged a three-month rally, with the Dow Jones Industrial Average rising 21%, the S&P 500 adding 23%, and the technology-heavy Nasdaq gaining 28%. It remains to be seen though, if corporate earnings will follow suit.

EXISTING INDEPENDENT SOURCES

If you want independent research today, it's actually plentiful to find. One major player that is widely respected is Standard & Poor's. Most investors think of S&P in the fixed-income arena. You probably know that S&P rates bonds, assigning some as investment grade securities, others as "junk" bonds, and so forth. But did you also know that S&P is an extremely established and trusted source of stock-research information for institutional investors? Pension funds and mutual fund managers in particular often turn to S&P and its sizeable equity research division.

S&P's stock pickers have done very well in making market calls – even in down markets. For instance, in 2001 S&P's stock picks posted gains of 22%. Meanwhile, the Dow lost 7%, the S&P 500 Index fell 11%, and the Nasdaq dropped 13%. You can use S&P's stock rating system, called STARS, which is found on the company's web site. During an interview, S&P equity research chief Ken Shea once told me: "We really pride ourselves on our independence, and the fact that S&P has been around for over 100 years. This is no fly by night operation."

Value Line is another trusted source of quality financial research. It too fiercely guards its status as an independent venue from which investors can get unbiased information. Once, when I was doing a story on this subject, Value Line research chief Stephen Sanborn said: "We don't have any investment banking relationships. We don't do corporate business. And we don't even let our analysts buy or sell stocks that they follow." Maybe that's why no less than billionaire Warren Buffett and Peter Lynch, of Fidelity fame, have both espoused the value of Value Line's research.

Weiss Ratings Inc. is a third solid source of independent research. The firm offers what it calls "financial safety ratings" on insurance companies, HMOs, banks and mutual funds.

RATING INDEPENDENT RESEARCH

By now, some of you may be saying: Oh, sure there's independent research out there, but how good is it? Excellent question. The answer is: much of it is very good – if you know where to turn. Like anything else, of course, you have independent firms with outstanding track records, such as Argus Research, and other ones with mediocre results. But according to one source, Investars, four of the five top research firms are independent companies.

Here are the three other ways to get information about independent research – and to compare it to research from traditional Wall Street firms.

- Go to *www.investars.com.*

    Investars is run by Kei Kianpoor, who's told me during several interviews in recent times that the value his firm offers is that it tells you how your portfolio would've performed if you followed a given firm's recommendations. Investars assesses both Wall Street and independent research firms' results.

    Regarding independent research entities, Investars has given high marks to Best Independent Research LLC. Best, founded in December 2002, is a consortium of five independent equities research firms. BIR member firms are Callard Research, LLC (Chicago, IL), Channel Trend (Dallas, TX), Columbine Capital Services (Colorado Springs, CO), Ford Equity Research (San Diego, CA), Global Capital Institute (managing partner - Chicago, IL), and Market Profile Theorems (Seattle, WA). As of 2003, these firms were among the top of Investars' one-year, two-year and three-year rankings by stock, industry and total portfolio.

    If you contact some of these firms to get their research, be prepared for sticker shock: many of them have very pricey research.

- Use *www.bnyjaywalk.com*. Jaywalk is a division of the Bank of New York that also offers good independent research and information. It's primarily geared toward institutional investors, so you can probably most readily access it through a broker or financial advisor that receives BNY Jaywalk's research.

- Subscribe to the Hulbert Financial Digest (*www.hulbertdigest.com*) for the most comprehensive information anywhere about investment newsletters that offer independent research. The publication, now a service of CBS MarketWatch, is run by Mark Hulbert. Hulbert follows 160 investment newsletters and the 500+ portfolios they recommend.

THE FUTURE OF INDEPENDENT RESEARCH

Here's another reason you should start to take independent research much more seriously: chances are you're going to be getting it one way or another. According to John Meserve, the president of BNY Jaywalk, his company has well over 1,000 clients and business grew 20% in 2002.

Wall Street firms are also recognizing that investors want independent research.

In March 2003, CSFB – a unit of Credit Suisse Group – was reportedly exploring launching an independent stock-research company under the name DLJ Research. DLJ stands for Donaldson, Lufkin & Jenrette, a company that Credit Suisse First Boston bought in the year 2000.

But in June 2003, CSFB squashed plans to launch that independent research operation. Still, according to the $1.4 billion Wall Street settlement involving 10 major investment dealers and banks, the firms are required to contract with at least three independent research providers and make available to clients that research, as well as their own research for five years.

$UMMARY $UCCESS $TRATEGY

TO CONQUER INVESTING MISTAKE #25:

Don't rely solely on Wall Street analysts. Independent research is often of very high quality. And getting differing opinions can frequently give you valuable insights into potential investments.

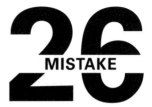

MISTAKE 26

NEGLECTING TO CHECK YOUR BROKER OR FINANCIAL PLANNER'S HISTORY

The three-year downturn in the stock market that began in 2000 convinced a lot of investors that it was time for help. As a result, many former do-it-yourselfers turned to stockbrokers, financial planners and others for investment advice. But even if you pulled off a miracle, and didn't get badly hurt during that period, having a financial advisor, or perhaps several advisors, can help you immensely. Conversely, if you have an unqualified advisor, that can hurt you tremendously, as you'll later see from reading one investor's troubles in this chapter.

Some data from the Investment Company Institute, the mutual fund industry trade group, reveals the extent to which investors these days rely on financial intermediaries.

According to the ICI's 2003 Fact Book, only 13% of the money in stock and bond funds has come directly from an individual retail investor. The remaining 87% of the money has passed through an intermediary, such as a CERTIFIED FINANCIAL PLANNER™ practitioner or stockbroker. (401(k) plans are also included in this total).

Other ICI data also reveal the extent to which people go to their financial advisors. According to the 2001 Profile of Mutual Fund

Shareholders, 69% of mutual fund owners either strongly agreed, or somewhat agreed, with the following statement:

"I tend to rely on the advice of a professional advisor when making fund purchase and sales decisions."

Summing up how investors probably feel, ICI spokesman John Collins puts it this way: "I'm fairly confident that I could make a decent vegetarian Indian meal. But I'm also inclined to go to a restaurant where it's already made, or where there are experts who cook that type of cuisine."

In his *Finish Rich Workbook,* best-selling author David Bach offers this insight:

"Enlisting the help of a financial advisor is not a sign of laziness or weakness or ignorance. To the contrary, it's a the smart thing to do." He goes on to write: "Think about it. Rich people almost always work with financial professionals. In fact, they usually have teams of attorneys, accountants, and financial planners who help them make sure their money is working hard for them. According to one recent study, nine out of ten people with more than $100,000 to invest prefer to work with a financial advisor. This is something to keep in mind if you are not yet as rich as you want to be."

If you do turn your finances over to a professional, or simply want to get some input and perspective before you make your own investing decisions, it's crucial that you pick the right kind of financial advisor – and that you check out that person's credentials.

So many investors carelessly enlist the "help" of ill-qualified or unscrupulous financial advisors – advisors who later turn out to "help themselves" to the investors money, or who make decisions that are not in the best interest of their clients.

To avoid this scenario, and for other practical reasons that will be discussed in this chapter, it is crucial that you do your homework and investigate the background of any potential financial advisor.

By "investigate" I don't mean you're going to do a full-scale background check on the individual, trying to figure out if the person's ever got a speeding ticket or what his neighbors think of him. I simply mean you should assess the person's professional track record, education, work experience, and whether or not he or she is skilled in the area or areas in which you need help.

If you don't check out your financial advisor, that's like jumping into the shower before putting your hand in there to test the water temperature. You might get burned.

Sometimes, careful diligent research still won't unearth a con artist who is determined to scam you and other investors. After all, it's possible that a no-good advisor has yet to be busted for his or her wrongdoing, so there's no record of that fact. But at least you can have a weeding out process to eliminate potential advisors who do have major blemishes on their record, and are therefore clearly undesirable.

Investors who neglect to check out their advisor's history subject themselves to people who may be inexperienced, unprofessional, or unqualified. That was the case for one New Jersey investor who says she wound up with an incompetent advisor.

IN THEIR OWN WORDS: INVESTORS SHARE LESSONS LEARNED

LESSONS LEARNED

> I listened to my daughter's advice to get a planner to help me invest about $10,000 wisely. The planner was a Wall Street advisor with hardly any experience and apparently not enough clients to keep his job. After I turned over my $10,000 to him, he lost his job

> and had never completed some paperwork properly to have my money transferred from one fund to an account at his firm. Apparently, he was trying to transfer money from an IRA to a money market account and the system wouldn't allow it. To make the story short, it took 11 months to correct the problem. The money sat idle without gaining any interest. The matter has finally been resolved, but I had to pay fees to both firms during the entire period although my money was held up. The major lesson learned is to not go with just any planner referred to you. Many of them are clueless as to simple procedures of transferring funds.
>
> Ida Spruell
>
> Paterson, New Jersey

In extreme cases, an investor may hire someone with regulatory blotches on their record – a big red flag because the advisor may have mistreated other investors. Individuals who are ignorant about their broker or financial planner's background also sometimes lack confidence or trust in that advisor.

When you are in the market for a financial intermediary, here are some guidelines to follow:

- **Interview at least three prospects.** Ask for recommendations, then call those clients and ask what kind of service and advice they've received and whether or not they've been happy with the individual in question.

- **Ask for Parts 1 and 2 of the person's ADV form**, which discloses his or her professional regulatory history. Boston Globe personal finance columnist Charles Jaffe, the author of *The Right Way To Hire Financial Help,* has been quoted as saying the ADV form "is a complete deal breaker for me."

He said that if you ask a broker for the complete form, and he only sends Part 1, "I don't even need to check" Part 2.

- **Also consult the National Association of Securities** **Dealers** to learn a stockbroker's professional, educational and regulatory history, including whether the individual has been fined or sanctioned for wrongdoing. In addition to having a very good web site, *www.NASD.com*, the NASD maintains a Public Disclosure Information Center that you can call at 800-289-9999.

- If the person claims to be a CERTIFIED FINANCIAL PLANNER™ practitioner or a Chartered Financial Analyst, **call to the appropriate professional organizations** (the Certified Financial Planner Board of Standards and the Association for Investment Management and Research, respectively) to verify those credentials and make sure the person is in good standing.

- **Finally, you can contact your state securities agencies** via the North American Securities Administrators Association *(www.NASAA.org)* to get more information about individual brokers or brokerage firms with whom you might consider doing business.

In general, you want to hire someone who is skillful, sensitive to your needs, experienced, and communicative in a way that you like. For instance, if you strongly prefer to do business in person or by telephone, but the advisor indicates that he mainly deals with clients via e-mail, the two of you likely won't have the best chemistry and rapport. It's also enlightening to ask potential advisors about their "typical clients" and about how many clients they have whose situations are similar to yours. If you're a 33-year old single parent with a $35,000 a year income, it's probably not wise to hire an advisor who works almost exclusively with retired couples, or with business owners earning $250,000 annually.

COMMISSIONS VS. FLAT FEES

Whenever you hire a financial advisor, you also want to know how that individual will be paid. Most often, it will be on a commission basis, a flat-fee arrangement, or some combination thereof.

Frank Owen, the CFP® practitioner from F.R. Owen & Associates, says he tells his clients up front that he works on commission. At the same time, he says it's a misconception that "if someone is getting a commission they're just pushing a product and taking you to the cleaners." His advice on picking an advisor: "check their pedigree and make sure they have your interest at heart."

HIGH-TOUCH SERVICE

Let me offer you a case in point of such a financial advisor, an individual who is really earning his keep. The person is Kevin Albritton, the head of AFS, a financial services firm founded in January 1996. Not only is Albritton very-well credentialed – with MCRS, CLU, ChFC, and CFP® designations – but he makes a point to be involved in professional industry associations and to constantly challenge himself to learn and keep up with changing practices and ideas.

Best of all, however, is his approach to dealing with clients. It's something he calls the "Financial consulting process." It starts with a discovery/introductory meeting where he spends an hour with clients learning about their situation, telling them about his own background and expertise, and, if necessary, offering some introductory financial education. A two-hour meeting follows. In this next confab, the client brings financial data and other documents and they continue to discuss issues of concern. At a third meeting, Albritton presents an action plan identifying challenges, telling his clients how to eliminate dangers and solve problems, answering questions and generally trying to help the client make smarter decisions. A fourth meeting follows, if necessary, to review the financial action plan, answer questions and make suggestions to implement the best strategies. Another meeting occurs 45 days later, to make sure the client is on track and executing the agreed-upon strategies. Finally, quarterly meetings take place. I outline this process in detail because it's unique. It's a high-touch approach that many investors want, but unfortunately, don't get.

$UMMARY $UCCESS $TRATEGY

TO CONQUER INVESTING MISTAKE# 26:

Check out your broker or financial planner's background. Get references, call NASD's Public Disclosure Information Center at 800-289-9999, and ask potential advisors for Parts 1 and 2 of their ADV Forms, which disclose their professional and regulatory history.

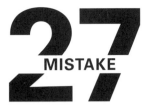

FIRING A BROKER OR PLANNER WITHOUT GOOD CAUSE – OR NOT FIRING ONE WHEN NECESSARY

I sympathize with stockbrokers these days.

They're having a tough time, with the slide in the capital markets, layoffs happening industry-wide, and corporate mergers among financial services firms resulting in even more pink slips.

To top it all off, investors are getting more than a little testy with their brokers. In fact, many people with beaten down portfolios are second-guessing their stockbrokers and financial advisors.

More to the point, an increasing number of individual investors are sending their brokers packing because, in the customers' minds, they're getting inefficient service, a lack of value or substandard performance. Mind you, most investors aren't becoming pure do-it-yourselfers. Many investors used to think they could hold down a full-time job, look after the kids, visit the in-laws, handle the grocery shopping, attend the town council meeting, read the Sunday paper – *and* manage their investments alone. Those days are long gone. These days, even as investors are giving their brokers the ax, they're seeking out smarter, better advisors. Even if this means they have to pay more to get them.

If you are unsatisfied with your broker or financial planner, you may have entertained thoughts of canning him or her. But is that really necessary? If you're upset because your portfolio has gone done recently, that's hardly justification to send your advisor packing. Even if you focus on absolute returns, it's probably not realistic to demand portfolio gains every single year. It's also unreasonable to fire someone just because one or two recommendations they made didn't pan out.

TAKE A CUE FROM THE RICH

It's particularly noteworthy that well-to-do investors don't make a practice of hopping from one advisor to the next. In fact, many well-heeled investors typically stick with their advisors for long periods of time. A survey by Matthew Greenwald & Associates, the New York polling firm, found that nearly 90% of affluent individuals stay with their first financial advisor. Greenwald & Associates surveyed 805 people under the age of 60, with more than $150,000 in annual household income.

The Greenwald & Associates survey also asked what investors were seeking in a financial advisor. And even wealthy, presumably more sophisticated investors still want good old-fashioned financial education. The poll said 73% of those surveyed were looking for someone to teach them about financial planning.

TO FIRE OR NOT? – THAT IS THE QUESTION

With this information in mind, here are six reasons that you might go ahead and fire your broker or financial planner – along with some tips about when you shouldn't.

By the way, this information isn't just helpful for anyone who uses a financial intermediary to invest. It's also practical guidance for brokers, money managers and financial advisors who want to know how to retain clients – in up and down markets.

1) I Inherited My Broker

There's a saying that, in life, we can't choose our parents and family members. That's true. But it's certainly not the case for our brokers. Yet, hoards of investors remain locked in the uncomfortable position of having "inherited" a broker. In many cases, these investors feel no connection or have little, if any, rapport with their advisors.

Think about whether you "inherited" your broker. If so, it probably happened when you inherited some money from a family member or loved one. In the process, you inherited the broker who was managing those funds. Many adults also often default to using the brokers their parents used.

Others get assigned a "new" broker after their original broker quits to join another firm, leaves the industry, retires, or loses his job in a merger. Whatever the reason, it can make you a little squeamish to have to deal with a new or unfamiliar broker or financial planner. Does this mean you should let the person go?

Not necessarily. The key is to judge how well the broker attempts to address your needs. (Don't fall for someone just because he says: "Your grandfather was always very happy here.") Smart brokers know that the getting-to-know-you period can be an uneasy time. So it's wise for them to give these clients extra attention during this transition.

2) I lost HOW MUCH money?!?

Is there anything worse for an investor? You get your quarterly statement or a phone call from your broker telling you that a stock you were heavily invested in has crashed, leaving you with huge financial losses.

Do you scream at the broker? (Why not, you figure: it was

her recommendation in the first place). Well, you could throw a tantrum. But it probably wouldn't do you much good. Taking a beating in the stock market – or in any market for that matter – is always a painful thing. Nevertheless, it doesn't make sense to summarily dismiss your broker just because one or two investments didn't work out. Firing a broker or planner under these circumstances is especially foolish if you've enjoyed an otherwise satisfactory, long-term relationship.

Instead, view the "bad" recommendation in the context of all the other suggestions the advisor has made. On balance, have the "good" recommendations far outweighed the bad? If so, stay put.

But woe to the broker who is consistently giving his or her customers bad advice and touting stocks that only head south. "If you aren't making money and the broker is, that's the best reason to fire him or her," Judith Berkey once told me. She's an investor and part-time computer consultant who lives in the suburbs of Washington D.C.

Think about it this way: why would you *pay* someone money to *lose* more of your money? That's like continuing to shop at a department store that you know always stocks inferior merchandise and has lousy customer service.

One caveat, though, to investors: if you know you lack the time, skills or inclination to manage your own brokerage account, seek out a competent professional. Besides, "it's folly to think that individual investors, as a group can outperform professionals, as a group," says Leonard Weiss, head of Weiss Wealth Management in Birmingham, Mich. Weiss, an industry veteran of 25 years, says he spends 50 hours a week studying the market. Yet he doesn't hold himself out as an all-knowing stock-market guru.

When it comes to stock-picking, "I don't know if my next decision is going to be my best one or my worst one," admits Weiss. "But if you let me make 10 or 20 decisions, I don't think I'll fail you because the process is what makes me good, not me."

3) Buy, buy, buy – now!

Nothing irritates investors more than when stockbrokers and financial advisors only seem interested in pushing a product. That's what happened to Tukufu Zuberi, a sociology professor at the University of Pennsylvania in Philadelphia. He finally had to fire his broker after he realized "the only time she called was to pitch a stock and it was just overbearing."

In this day and age, brokers should be doing more than just trying to generate commissions. They must offer value-added service because "among banks, brokerages and insurance firms, everyone is competing for the same assets," says Frank Bianchi, head of American Management Systems, a Fairfax, Va. consulting firm that provides CRM, or customer relationship management, software and other services to the financial services industry.

4) That's simply not right

Any stockbroker, financial planner or advisor who does things that are not in the client's best interest should be fired. What are some examples? Making unauthorized trades, "churning" a customer's account by buying and selling securities just to get commissions, and so forth. Investors don't take these things lightly – and they shouldn't. A record number of people are accusing their brokers of improper dealings. Just look at arbitration claims being filed with the NASD, which handles 90% of all investment disputes between customers and brokers. Through June 2003, NASD new arbitration filings hit 4,654 cases, up 25% from the comparable period in 2002.

Many times, arbitration disputes involve complaints from investors who lost money, and now have a case of "sour grapes." Of course, there are plenty of instances where an investor does have a legitimate gripe, like when a broker puts the client's money into investments that are clearly unsuitable for the client, given his or her goals, risk tolerance, age, etc.

DON'T TOLERATE CROOKS

It almost goes without saying, but any financial advisor who does something illegal is courting the wrath of his or her clients — and possibly worse consequences. What's illegal? Stealing comes to mind. "Borrowing" money from one client's account temporarily to put those funds someplace else is another example of illegal activity.

When a dispute moves beyond a point of a misunderstanding – say you told your broker to sell $10,000 worth of shares, but he thought you said to sell 10,000 shares – and involves downright intentional dishonesty, you have a duty to take action.

Investors who let corrupt brokers off the hook are allowing themselves to get taken advantage of and, in some instances, ripped off. Unfortunately, investors who don't do anything about unscrupulous brokers feed into what is often a pattern of abuse. Because a broker gets away with misconduct, he repeats bad behavior with future customers. Consequently, an unknown number of unsuspecting investors get scammed.

Think about it this way: if your car was stolen, you'd certainly report it to the police, wouldn't you? By the same token, don't take any illegal shenanigans from a broker. Report a broker's illegal activity immediately to a branch manager. Inform regulators or consumer groups about misconduct by independent investment advisors. Document everything. Put your complaints in writing. You may need written support if you have to go to arbitration, Wall Street's dispute-resolution process.

I remember writing back in the 1990s about a woman name Janie Thomas. She was a high-powered stockbroker in Merrill Lynch's Las Vegas branch. Thomas billed herself as the "broker to the stars" and boasted that she had numerous celebrity clients – including actress/singer Barbra Streisand and singer Paul Anka. But authorities say Thomas was the real performer. She allegedly created phony offshore accounts and lied to people about how well their investments were doing. The 32-year-old Thomas eventually skipped town (with her husband in tow) and has never been found. But her clients didn't take their plight lying down. They complained – and got compensated by Merrill Lynch — to the tune of an estimated $16.5 million. To Merrill's credit, it made all the investors whole.

5) Same Advice, Different Client

Brokers who offer only boilerplate advice or give cookie-cutter suggestions aren't doing their jobs. Period. "People can get generic financial planning and asset allocation recommendations free off the Internet. So good financial advisors really need to offer people customized solutions," says Robert Wolfe, a CERTIFIED FINANCIAL PLANNER™ practitioner with Capital Planning Group in Fort Lauderdale, Fla. "To the extent that a broker or advisor isn't doing that, he or she should be replaced," Wolfe adds.

Getting personalized service and value-added products and information is a top concern for Gregory Beckstrom, an investor from Minneapolis. In early 2001, he decided that he "needed more expert assistance." So he closed his account with a discount brokerage and turned his sizeable portfolio over to a broker at full-service firm.

"A lot of us got our fingers burned" in 2000, says Beckstrom, a geologist at an engineering firm. He used to obsess over his investment holdings. But "now I sleep better at night," Beckstrom says, adding that his current asset allocation mix is tailor-made for his needs.

6) Promises, Promises

Another investor turnoff: brokers who raise clients' hopes of achieving unrealistic returns. What's unrealistic? Anytime an advisor tells you that a certain investment is "guaranteed" to appreciate, or that you can expect 25% annual returns in the stock market — even though historically stocks have risen by about 10% a year. Even if you have an advisor who talks about more reasonable returns, you should make a point of remembering those conversations — and later hold the broker accountable.

Tukufu Zuberi, the Philadelphia investor, practices this strategy. "Brokers usually try to promise you 10% to 15% annual returns," he said. "So now, when I meet with my advisors I bring the past year's (performance) report and I ask them why the target was or wasn't achieved."

In some cases, you may need to have your advisors lower those expected return figures — or show you how they'll make up a shortfall, a difficult task in today's market.

And don't be pacified by brokers who simply try to convince you that everything is fine because they're "monitoring" the situation. "Monitoring is good," Zuberi notes. "But that's not enough."

PARTING COMPANY

Remember: Individuals who stick with brokers that should be fired experience dissatisfaction with their mix of investments or the specific securities chosen. They get frustrated about the investing process. They obtain little, if any, value-added service. And they often feel that they've received bad counsel because they are saddled with lackluster or poor-performing investments.

Breaking up is always hard to do, but sometimes it's necessary to give your broker or planner the ax. If you do so, just make sure you have good cause. Also, if you do part company with your financial advisor, be sure to get all your financial documents. Before you make the split, ask for current statements from the banks and brokerage firms with which you're doing business.

$UMMARY $UCCESS $TRATEGY
TO CONQUER INVESTING MISTAKE# 27:

Keep a financial advisor who is working in your best interest – and fire one that isn't. Good advisors don't just push products. They try to understand your overall financial situation and your personal needs. They also actively work to help you reach your goals.

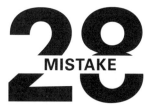

MISTAKE 28

BEING DISHONEST OR GIVING YOUR ADVISORS INCOMPLETE INFORMATION

When you go to the doctor for an annual physical exam, or complaining of a backache, what's the first thing you'll probably be asked to do? Chances are a nurse will say, to put it bluntly: "Strip."

In order for the doctor to properly evaluate you, you'll probably have to bare yourself a bit.

The same principle holds true when you deal with financial advisors. Yet, too many investors – especially high net worth clients – refuse to disrobe, so to speak, in from of their stockbrokers or financial planners. These investors keep their cards "close to the vest" and decline to reveal all kind of personal, yet very pertinent, information. In some cases, wealthy investors "forget" to tell one broker about another large account that is held at another brokerage firm. At other times, investors omit personal information, such as the fact that they've been laid off – and have been out of work for the past six months.

Without an accurate picture of an investor's financial situation, an advisor is likely to offer an inaccurate diagnosis of what steps or strategies can benefit the investor. This means the investor's holdings may fare worse than the overall market and carry more risk.

To avoid this pitfall, it's vital that you are truthful and thorough in giving your financial advisor information. And don't worry about them trying to make a buck off of you. Just because you tell them about other assets you own, doesn't mean they'll bother you about those accounts. Yes, it is possible that they may tell you about the benefits of "consolidating" those accounts – no doubt with their firm. But chances are, they won't make an issue of it. And remember, the truth of the matter is there is value in having fewer funds, because you have less paperwork to track and you may be able to pay lower fees with higher account balances.

But a primary reason that you need to be upfront with your advisors is because they are often making recommendations based largely on the information you give them. They might recommend certain stocks, bonds or other assets, not knowing that you already have those securities. Then you would suffer from "portfolio over-lap" or a duplication of your investments. This situation could also very easily cause your asset allocation to be thrown off balance. The end result would be that your overall portfolio may not per-form as well as expected.

ACCOUNT AGGREGATION

Some firms will also be able to offer you one of the most popular new services being offered by financial services firms: account aggregation. This is an online feature that allows you to have a snapshot view of all your money matters: assets, liabilities, credit card debts, investments, and even frequent flyer miles. Though consumer advocates say account aggregation raises privacy and security concerns, this service may be helpful for those with com-plicated, dynamic lives.

ENCOURAGE DIALOGUE AMONG YOUR ADVISORS

Bruce Schwenger, the CEO of Harris*direct*, an online brokerage, told me that his company is well aware that it typically has only about

20% of a client's assets. No matter, though. Schwenger's firm encourages a "team approach." Its financial specialists employ a collaborative strategy in working with an investor's other advisors, including insurance specialists, accountants, attorneys or other financial pros.

Some people mistakenly think that their CPA – who might only do their taxes right now – really has no need to know their other financial business. Nothing could be further from the truth. And besides, your CPA may just become your financial advisor in the future. According to American Institute of Certified Public Accountants (AICPA), about 66,000 CPAs are now, or are in the process of becoming, registered investment advisors. CPAs are getting away from their traditional roles in part because clients need assistance in several areas of financial planning. This is good news for you, because your CPA's background in taxes and accounting may well enhance his or her ability to service your financial needs.

HONESTY REALLY IS THE BEST POLICY

Didn't your mother (or someone with good sense) always say: "Honesty is the best policy?" That truism is valuable to you as an investor too. So be truthful. Disclose all assets you own, even if you don't intend to marshal those assets under one roof. Also, let advisors know about life-changing events, such as divorce, because this will impact your finances.

A big challenge for financial advisors is keeping up with changes in their clients' lives. If you don't tell your advisor that you've had a death in the family, lost your job, got a fabulous new position paying twice your previous salary, have gotten remarried, or had a child, etc., how would they know? (Well, OK. If you're a woman, and you came strolling into their office 8 months pregnant, hopefully they'd have a clue.). But you get my point. Most investors want their advisors to be conscientious and communicative. But you've got to do your fair share of communicating as well. The telephone rings both ways.

$UMMARY $UCCESS $TRATEGY

TO CONQUER INVESTING MISTAKE# 28:

Give your financial advisors honest and complete information. An advisor can't fully help you or give you the best possible recommendations if he or she is only privy to part of your overall financial picture.

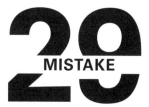

TAKING AN ADVISOR'S RECOMMENDATIONS ON BLIND FAITH

Investors who accept their advisors' every word without question may end up buying investments not in keeping with their comfort level for risk. Because they fear offending or second-guessing their broker, these investors keep quiet about decisions made by the advisor with which they don't agree. The result: the investor suffers the financial repercussions of poor decisions, and they sometimes sell investments at the wrong time. Furthermore, by taking a "hands off" approach with their advisors, these investors aren't truly learning about or developing a real appreciation for the investing process.

> On June 4, 2003, the yield on the 10-year Treasury note fell to 3.29%, hitting its lowest level in 45 years. That same day the Dow topped 9,000 for the first time since August 2002. And technology stocks were on fire, with Motorola rising 5.5% in a single day, Sun Microsystems soaring 6.6%, and Applied Materials gaining 5.2%. Depending on if you were a stock or a bond investor, you might have gotten a call from your broker advising you to buy or sell some of

these securities. Would you have been comfortable with any of them? What would you have done?

If your advisor makes a buy or sell recommendation that is inconsistent with your investment strategy, question the merit of that recommendation. Ask the advisor why deviating from your pre-set strategy is prudent, necessary or justifiable. Get comfortable asking your advisors to explain the rationale behind their suggestions.

Healthcare patients often get a "second opinion" when their doctors diagnose illnesses or make medical recommendations. Sometimes you may also need to get a "second opinion."

The idea here isn't to arbitrarily second-guess everything your broker or financial planner recommends. On the contrary, the more you trust your advisor, and feel secure in the knowledge that he or she is working in your best interest, the less you'll feel compelled to doubt or question that person's advice.

What I'm suggesting for all investors, though, is that you not shy away from talking to your advisors about why they recommend certain investments. It's particularly important for you to have these discussions if you feel the investment is a little too risky for your taste, or if you don't understand the investment and why it would complement or bolster your investing objectives.

$UMMARY $UCCESS $TRATEGY
TO CONQUER INVESTING MISTAKE# 29:

Listen to your advisor's recommendations – but don't take every suggestion on blind faith. Remember: you are ultimately responsible for ensuring your financial well-being. If you don't understand why a suggestion is being made, ask questions.

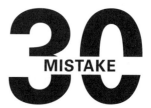

MISTAKE

BEING AN ABSENTEE OR DIFFICULT CLIENT

Based on my decade of experience as a financial journalist, and having listened to literally more than 1,000 financial planners, stockbrokers and others tell me about the investors with whom they deal, I can safely say that there are generally three types of clients:

1) The "absentee" client

2) The "difficult" client – also known as the "pain in the butt" client; and

3) The "ideal" client

My goal in this chapter is to help you get into category number three. In this final chapter, I'll tell you about serious mistakes you may be making in dealing with your financial intermediary that can cost you in more ways than just money. I'll also tell you how to make sure that you're one of your advisor's favorite customers, the ones they also call "dream" clients.

WHAT YOUR ADVISOR WON'T TELL YOU

This is information that your stockbroker or financial advisor would probably never dream of telling you. (Well, actually they might *dream* about it, but they wouldn't dare actually *say* it). And can you really blame them for not wanting to offend you? On the other hand, I can candidly tell you this information because I'm a third party. So trust me when I clue you in on this stuff, and believe me when I say that if you take the following do's and don'ts to heart, you'll have much better, much more effective relationships with your financial advisors. That, in turn, will make you happier about your finances, more knowledgeable about investing, and it probably will improve your portfolio performance as well.

Let's start with a brief overview of the typical investors: the "absentee," "difficult" and "ideal" clients. Then I'll give you the do's and don'ts you should follow.

THE ABSENTEE CLIENT

As the name suggests, an "absentee" client is largely away from or out of contact with his or her advisors. If you're an "absentee" client you may think that you're doing your broker or financial planner a favor. After all, you don't place demands on your advisor's time. You don't call them on the phone to fret over the fact that the Dow fell 200 points or that another Enron-type scandal has been unearthed. You don't insist on many in-person meetings. In fact, you really don't insist on much service, attention, or hand-holding at all. You're so out of touch with your advisor, though, that you're pretty much off his or her radar screen. And that is a definite mistake.

Absentee clients may suffer from a lack of information or knowledge about where their finances really stand. Because they only deal with their advisor's once a year – if that often – they probably don't have their portfolios assessed or rebalanced as frequently as might be necessary. These individuals also don't get much value-added insights from their advisors – simply because the broker or planner never connects with them to lend their expertise.

THE DIFFICULT CLIENT

We've all encountered difficult people before. Depending on the situation, they can be rude, offensive, unreasonable to talk to, and sometimes out of control. Now imagine that personality type – and picture that the person has just lost $10,000 or $20,000. Their overbearing personality is likely to *really* kick into overdrive.

But some other investors who are difficult clients aren't nasty people to deal with. It's just that they're sometimes ultra-whiny or they make completely unreasonable demands on their advisors' time. This is the investor who calls his or her broker practically every day – sometimes two or three times a day. This same individual has probably had half a dozen one-hour meetings in his or her advisor's office, and then turned those meetings into three-hour marathons.

Still another type of difficult client second-guesses almost every single thing his or her advisor says or does. It's one thing to question advice or recommendations that you don't understand, as I suggest you do. But it's another thing to contradict your broker because of some gossip you heard on an Internet investing chat room. This type of client gives his advisors big-time headaches. They sometimes cringe when they take your phone calls. They often dread talking to you, or meeting in person, simply because they know your patterns and unrealistic expectations. To top it all off, the difficult client who monopolizes an advisor's time will get haughty – or downright upset – if the advisor dares to try to bill the investor for that excessive time.

THE IDEAL CLIENT

Unlike the absentee client, and the difficult client, the ideal client knows how to strike the proper tone, balance and philosophy in dealing with his or her advisors. This individual is fully engaged in the process of investing and communicates clearly, concisely and regularly with financial advisors. To the advisor, an ideal client is neither incognito, nor ever-present. This person is, nonetheless, consistently on the advisor's mind. When you are an "ideal" or "dream" client, your advisor will think of you when reading an article or something of interest and send it to you. The advisor will call you up to see how you're doing and if you feel comfortable and on track with your financial goals.

The ideal client knows how to get his or her questions answered, stay in touch on a reasonable basis with financial advisors, and maintain a pleasant attitude during the process. As a result, the ideal clients' advisors *want* to work with them. Advisors want to further educate ideal clients financially. They take special pleasure in seeing those clients' money grow. And advisors especially enjoy witnessing an "ideal" client reach his or her goals.

In some cases, advisors may relish it when "difficult" clients meet their goals too. But in these instances, it's more likely that the advisor is feeling a sense of relief: "Whew!" he's thinking. "Now this person won't bug me as much!"

What I'm telling you here is not rocket science. And it's not that financial advisors don't want to talk to, interact with and help *all* their clients. Believe me, they do. But it's human nature to *especially* want to help those people you *like*.

I have had many, many advisors tell me, flat out, that when they are initially being interviewed by prospective clients, the "interview process" is really going both ways. Advisors are sizing you up, just as much as you are evaluating them. Advisors try not to take on investors that they personally don't like. Don't you do the same thing when you're seeking out business relationships?

So as an individual client, what can and should you do to get "most favored investor" status with your financial advisors?

Here are a few don'ts:

- **Don't call your advisor only to whine about one portfolio statement.** Focus on absolute returns. If you did, you wouldn't want to bite off your planner or broker's head if that one fund he recommended dropped by 7% but your overall portfolio is up 11%.

- **Don't focus on the negative.** When you call and say "did you hear that the Nasdaq is off 100 points?" you make your advisor think that you've not learned what proper investing is about. You're focusing on short-term, negative events and in all likelihood your planner is trying to get you to think about your long-term strategy. As a minor aside, the question, "Did you hear about the Nasdaq?" is also somewhat irritating and insulting. Of course they know! They follow the markets just as well as you do, if not better.

- **Don't second-guess your advisor unnecessarily.** Please try not to run to your financial planner asking: "Why don't I own XYZ stock?" just because you heard some Wall Street guru talking about it on television or radio. Whatever that person was recommending probably doesn't fit your personal situation.

- **Don't make unreasonable demands on your advisor's time.** Limit phone calls to what's necessary. Don't call too frequently or stay on the phone for an inordinate amount of time. Book face-to-face appointments when you think you need them, and resist the urge to "pop by" their office unexpectedly or unannounced. That's highly inconsiderate. Like you, your advisor has a million things to do. He or she could also be occupied with other clients in the office.

- **Don't let yourself be forgotten.** If your advisor has numerous clients, it's all too easy to slip into the ranks of being an "absentee" client. Stay in touch with periodic phone calls, and update your advisor if there are any big changes in your life that could affect your financial goals and needs.

Here are some do's you'd be wise to practice:

- **Do say "thank you."** You'd be surprised how far a simple verbal expression of gratitude, or even better a handwritten thank you note, can go. Your advisor will remember your thoughtfulness and you will stand out in his or her mind, because so few clients take the time to show their appreciation.

- **Do follow through on your advisor's recommendations.** It's frustrating for advisors when you sit in their office, nod your head in agreement with a plan of action they suggest, then fail to take any action.

- **Do come prepared for meetings.** If you've been asked to bring documents, come with a list of financial goals or whatever, keep your end of the bargain. Don't waste your advisor's time with meetings you're not ready to have.

- **Do be willing to pay for what you get.** Many investors want stop-everything-now service from their advisors, outstanding research, tailor-made investment products, and so forth. But they're not willing to pay for these things. That's not reasonable.

- **Do become a client who is liked and whose calls are enjoyed.** Remember, you're dealing with another human being. And chances are you'd get a lot better everything – better advice, better quality of information, more hand-holding if necessary, etc. – simply by being nice. A tip: send a holiday or birthday card. If you've got good advisors, let them know that they are valued and appreciated.

And just because there are plenty of financial planners out there – at last count more than 250,000 people identified themselves as financial planners – don't think you can treat your financial advisors as if they're a dime a dozen. Listen to the following advice from an investor who's found out how crucial it is to have the right financial advisor.

IN THEIR OWN WORDS: INVESTORS SHARE LESSONS LEARNED

My entire investing career has been one mistake after another. This is a result of not working with a good advisor. In the past 15 years, I have worked with seven investment counselors. I didn't realize how important it was to work with someone who understood and took the time to communicate. There were years when I did not speak to my advisor. I was a small potato and not very active, and I accepted that there was no reason for me to have a conversation with my agent.

In October of 1987, like most Americans, I lost money. I was scared and because I did not have a good relationship with my agent, I locked in my loss of $7,000. I stayed away from the market for years. I thought my next two advisors would be good because I knew them personally though my work in the community and my church. Another mistake. This did not guarantee that they had my best interest in mind. The fellow from my church, after he got my money locked into a plan which once again lost money, wouldn't even answer a question when I saw him in church.

I think what helped me turn the corner was finding a great accountant. After working with this gentleman for a couple of years, I went to him for advice about a new agent. He recommended a wonderful man who treats me like I'm important no matter how much money I have. He works well with both me and my husband. I even recommended him to an older friend of mine. She is now able to sleep at night without fear. I will probably be with my current advisor until death do us part. I feel confident and on track for the first time ever.

Getting the right person should not be taken lightly. Not only must they know their stuff, but they must have a great amount of emotional intelligence, sensitivity and communication skills.

Veronica Holcomb

Owner, VJ Holcomb & Associates

Like in all industries, it takes time and perseverance to find someone who is skilled and expert in the subject matters in which you need help – whether it's taxes, insurance, investment planning or whatever. Furthermore, there's no guarantee that the most qualified or knowledgeable person you find will click with you, or will want your business. It may not be anything personal, but that person could already be swamped with new clients or existing ones for that matter. One point of information, though, is that an abundance of fresh talent is constantly entering the field. The Bureau of Labor Statistics forecasts 40% growth in the financial planning profession between 1998 and the year 2008.

$UMMARY $UCCESS $TRATEGY
TO CONQUER INVESTING MISTAKE# 30:

Strive to become an "ideal" client who is engaged in the process of investing, but not over-bearing. Don't be a pesky "difficult" client who is a nuisance to financial advisors. But neither should you be an "absentee" investor who is readily forgotten.

I hope the information in this and all the other chapters proved valuable and eye-opening to you. I'm confident that if you conquer these 30 costly investing mistakes, you will definitely multiply your wealth!

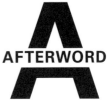

Mistakes are a natural part of life. We all make mistakes: from goofs on the job to saying or doing the wrong things concerning our family members and friends. So it's unreasonable to assume that investing will be any different. Investing mistakes will inevitably occur. Nevertheless, I've often seen how difficult it is for people to talk about and admit their investing mishaps. Indeed, some people would sooner reveal very personal flaws or moral errors in judgment, rather than admit than their lack of investing prowess. It is my aim to help reduce the shame, guilt and embarrassment that many people feel about having made investing mistakes. Furthermore, I hope that by reading this book you will be informed, empowered and inspired to act.

I would love to hear about your investing successes or how you were able to correct any investing mistakes.

If you have a story you'd like to share, write to me personally at lynnette@InvestingSuccess.net.

I'm also collecting tales from investors who are courageous enough to admit their past shortcomings, and explain what they learned from those mistakes. Look at the front of this book for future titles planned in the *Investing Success*™ series. Then write and let me know if you happen to fit into any of those groups.

If you'd like to be included in an upcoming
***Investing Success*™ book, send your tale to**
mystory@InvestingSuccess.net.

Your knowledge and experience could help other investors avoid the pitfalls you've encountered. And if your story is selected to be included in an upcoming *Investing Success*™ title, you'll get a free, autographed copy of the book.

I look forward to hearing from you.

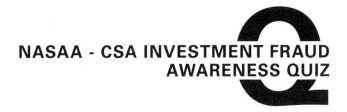

NASAA - CSA INVESTMENT FRAUD AWARENESS QUIZ

The North American Securities Administrators Association (NASAA) is a membership organization of the 66 state, provincial and territorial securities administrators in the 50 states, the District of Columbia, Canada, Mexico, and Puerto Rico. In the United States, NASAA is the voice of the 50 state securities agencies responsible for grass-roots investor protection and efficient capital formation. The Canadian Securities Administrators (CSA) is the umbrella organization representing the 13 provincial and territorial securities commissions.

1. Which of the following phrases should raise your concern about an investment?

a. High rate of return

b. Risk-free

c. Your investment is guaranteed against loss

d. You must invest now

e. All of the above

2. Securities laws protect investors by requiring companies to:

a. Show profits before they can sell stock

b. Provide investors with specific information about the company

c. Pay dividends

d. Repay investors who have lost money

3. In which situation are you taking the least amount of risk?

a. Buying a Certificate of Deposit (CD), in United States, or a Guaranteed Investment Certificate (GIC), in Canada, from a bank

b. Investing with someone you know through your church or community association

c. Investing offshore

d. Investing with someone who contacted you by phone

4. A fellow book club member tells you about an investment opportunity that has earned returns of 20% during the past year. Your investments have been performing poorly and you're interested in earning higher returns. This person is your friend and you trust them. What should you do?

a. Ask your friend for more information about the investment so that you can understand the risks before you make a decision

b. Invest only a small amount to see how things go before making a larger investment

c. Call your securities regulator to see if the investment has been registered or is properly exempted for sale

d. a and c

5. Which of the following should you rely upon when making an investment decision?

a. Testimonials of other investors

b. Advertisements and news stories in the media or on the Internet

c. Technical data that you don't really understand

d. Information filed with your securities regulator

6. Ways to protect yourself from investment fraud include:

a. Read all disclosure documents about an investment

b. Seek advice from an independent and objective source

c. Be skeptical and ask questions

d. Never write the check/cheque for an investment in the name of your salesperson

e. All of the above

7. When dealing with a securities salesperson who is considered reputable, you should do all the following except:

a. Request copies of opening account documentation to verify that your investment goals and objectives are stated correctly

b. Open and review all correspondence and account statements when you receive them

c. Verify your written account statements with information you can obtain online

d. Allow the salesperson to manage your assets as they see fit because they are the expert

e. Evaluate your salesperson's recommendations by doing your own independent research

8. Which of the following are frequently used to defraud the public?

a. Short-term promissory notes

b. Prime bank investments

c. Offshore investments to avoid taxes

d. Nigerian advance fee letters

e. All of the above

9. The role of government securities regulators is to:

a. Sell shares to investors

b. Act as an association for securities dealers and advisers

c. Regulate securities markets, the investment industry and protect investors

d. All of the above

10. You have been working closely with your securities salesperson for years. Recently your salesperson asked you to invest in a product that he/she is really excited about, however, the recommendation seems very different from financial products you have invested in previously. Which of the following should you do?

a. Agree to make the investment because you have done business with your salesperson for years and trust them implicitly

b. Check with your securities regulator to see if they have any information on the investment product

c. Check with your securities regulator to see if the securities salesperson is authorized to sell the product in question

d. Rely upon the written material the salesperson gives you

e. a & d only

f. b & c only

11. An investment is likely to be legitimate if:

a. The promotional materials and company website look professional

b. The company has a prestigious office location

c. Other investors are receiving quick up-front returns

d. The company has an official-sounding name

e. None of the above

12. Who insures you against investment losses?

a. No one; this is the risk you take when you invest

b. My securities regulator

c. The company selling the investment

d. The Securities Investor Protection Corporation (SIPC) in United States or the Canadian Investor Protection Fund (CIPF) in Canada

Answers

1. Answer: e
Unusually high rates of return should be viewed as a cause for concern about an investment and would indicate a high-risk investment. Investigate all risk-free promises. Guarantees should also raise concern. Legitimate investments are not guaranteed against loss. Suggesting that you must invest "now" is generally

a high-pressure tactic used by swindlers to get the money before investors can change their minds or obtain more information.

2. Answer: b
Securities regulation is based on a disclosure system - laws requiring companies to provide investors with specific information. This ensures that investors have access to the information they need in order to make sound investment decisions. Companies do not have to show profits nor pay dividends in order to sell stock to investors. Also, companies are not required to repay investors who have lost money by investing in their shares.

3. Answer: a
Buying a CD or GIC is low risk, but you should investigate insurance levels in the event of the bank's failure. You should also consider inflation risk when dealing with low return investments. If you are going to invest with someone you know through your church or community association, you should ensure that both the person and the investment are properly registered/licensed with your securities regulator. You should thoroughly investigate **before** investing your hard-earned money. Investing offshore is not a guarantee of tax benefits. In addition, when you invest offshore, you are giving up some of the protections provided by your securities regulator. Investing with someone who calls you with an investment opportunity is also very risky. You should always be skeptical of telephone pitches.

4. Answer: d
You should never make an investment based simply on word-of-mouth, even if the recommendation comes from a family member, friend or acquaintance. Fraudulent schemes are frequently perpetuated this way. The promise of quick, high returns should also alert you to a possible scam. As a general rule, risk and return are proportional; the higher the return, the higher the risk. Even if a company looks and sounds legitimate, you should always check it out. Therefore, ask for more information about the investment and call your securities regulator to see if the investment has been registered or exempted for sale.

5. Answer: d

Information filed on an investment with your securities regulator can include disclosure documents, such as a prospectus or offering memorandum, and is meant to provide you with valuable information in order for you to make a wise investment decision. This is your best source of information about the history of the company and the risks associated with the investment. When shopping for investments, you should base your decisions on your own financial situation. If you don't understand an investment or if it feels too risky, don't invest in it.

News stories may be factual, but may not provide investors with enough information on which to base an investment decision. Ads are not necessarily factual. Be aware that con artists use advertisements, technical language, fake testimonials, and news stories to make their schemes appear legitimate.

6. Answer: e

Before making an investment, do your research and ensure that you understand what you are buying, the risks involved and if it is suitable for your personal financial situation. You can obtain written materials from your salesperson, go to the library, use the Internet, and/or get an opinion from another professional. Contact your securities regulator to ask about the salesperson's background and to verify proper licensing or registration of the investment and salesperson. Never transfer money in the name of a salesperson. Your check/cheque or fund transfer should always be directed to the company in which you are investing or to your brokerage/investment firm to settle your account.

7. Answer: d

Registered/licensed securities salespeople and their administrative staff can and do make errors. These errors and mistakes can be costly and need to be caught and corrected as soon as possible. More importantly, there have been instances where salespeople have intentionally abused their clients' trust through excessive trading in their accounts, selling them inappropriate financial products and outright fraud. Generally speaking, your salesperson should never buy or sell a security without first getting your approval.

8. Answer: e

With the presence of con artists and the ever-increasing complexity of financial products and markets, today's investors need to be well informed. The abovementioned items are all "scams" but represent only a small number of fraudulent investments that are currently being sold to unwitting investors. NASAA provides a current list of these scams that you can review at *www.nasaa.org.* Consumers need to maintain a heightened sense of caution when investing. Additionally, if the investment is something you are not familiar with, be sure to gather information and understand the product **prior to investing.** Consult with your securities regulator and review its website for additional investor education materials and information on scams.

9. Answer: c

Securities regulators administer the laws in their jurisdiction. One of their key mandates is to protect investors by ensuring that the rules and regulations are followed. Securities regulators do not sell shares directly to the public, but oversee the companies that do. They do not represent the industry, but provide protection to investors through rules, regulations and educational programs.

10. Answer: f

It is important to ask for and obtain written details of the investment recommendations you receive **before you make any decisions.** This could include a prospectus, an offering memorandum, research reports and other information. You should also contact your securities regulators for information relating to the registration or exemption status of the securities product in addition to checking to see if your salesperson is registered/licensed to sell the investment product. You should **always** assess your investment objectives before making an investment in this, or any other product, to determine the risks involved, even if the recommendation comes from someone that you have done business with for many years.

11. Answer: e

You should not judge the legitimacy of an investment by the following: the look of the written promotional materials you receive; where the company's office is located; its website whether other investors received quick up-front returns; or the name of the company. All of these things may be done to lure investors into a scheme. Do your homework. Obtain information about the company from reputable sources such as the SEDAR website for Canadian publicly traded companies (*www.sedar.com*) or the EDGAR website for U.S. public securities filings (*www.sec.gov/ edgar.html*) and call your securities regulator **before** you invest.

12. Answer: a

Any investment involves some degree of risk. You should know what degree of risk you are willing to take in order to meet your financial goals and objectives. Securities regulators protect investors by ensuring that securities laws and rules are abided by, but they do not insure investments. Be aware that there have been many problems with companies that falsely inform investors that their investments are guaranteed or insured. SIPC (*www.sipc.com*) in United States, and CIPF (*www.cipf.ca*) in Canada, do not insure investments or cover declines in investment value or fraudulent sales. SIPC and CIPF provide coverage in limited circumstances and with set dollar limits in the event of insolvency of a member brokerage firm. Investigate **before** you invest since you alone are bearing the risk involved with your investments.

Author's Note: Investment Fraud Awareness Quiz reprinted with permission from NASAA

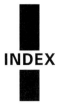

INDEX

NOTES

NOTES

NOTES

NOTES

**Advantage
World Press**

Investing Success™ Order Form

Online orders: www.InvestingSuccess.net

Fax orders: (914) 835-0398

Phone orders: (800) 431-1579

Mail orders: Book Clearing House
46 Purdy Street
Harrison, NY 10528

Name:_____

Address: _____

City: _____ State: _____Zip: _____

Country: _____

Telephone: (   )_____

Email address: _____

Investing Success™ **$24.95 ea.** qty_____

No. of Books_____

Subtotal $_____

Tax $_____

Add $1.50 sales tax for each item shipped to New Jersey

Shipping and handling: Shipping $_____
$3.50 for standard shipping;
$5.50 for Priority Mail

Total Order Amount (in U.S. dollars)$_____

Payment:
❐ Check   ❐ Credit Card
❐ Visa   ❐ MasterCard   ❐ AMEX   ❐ Discover

Name on card: _____

Card Number: _____

Exp. Date _____ / _____

Signature _____

Bulk Purchase Discount Available